wclt   withdrawn

B. SAUNDERS COMPANY
Division of Elsevier Inc.

00 John F. Kennedy Boulevard, Suite 1800 • Philadelphia, PA 19103-2899

ttp://www.theclinics.com

**SURGICAL ONCOLOGY CLINICS
OF NORTH AMERICA**
October 2007
Editor: Catherine Bewick

Volume 16, Number 4
ISSN 1055-3207
ISBN-13: 978-1-4160-5129-9
ISBN-10: 1-4160-5129-5

The ideas and opinions expressed in the *Surgical Oncology Clinics of North America* do not necessarily reflect those of the Publisher. The Publisher does not assume any responsibility for any injury and/or damage to persons or property arising out of or related to any use of the material contained in this periodical. The reader is advised to check the appropriate medical literature and the product information currently provided by the manufacturer of each drug to be administered to verify the dosage, the method and duration of administration, or contra-indications. It is the responsibility of the treating physician or other health care professional, relying on independent experience and knowledge of the patient, to determine drug dosages and the best treatment for the patient. Mention of any product in this issue should not be construed as endorsement by the contributors, editors, or the Publisher of the product or manufacturers' claims.

Surgical Oncology Clinics of North America (ISSN 1055-3207) is published quarterly by Elsevier Inc., 360 Park Avenue South, New York, NY 10010-1710. Months of publication are January, April, July, and October. Business and editorial offices: 1600 John F. Kennedy Boulevard, Suite 1800, Philadelphia, PA 19103-2899. Customer service office: 6277 Sea Harbor Drive, Orlando, FL 32887–4800. Periodicals postage paid at New York, NY, and additional mailing offices. Subscription prices are $202.00 per year (US individuals), $308.00 (US institutions) $102.00 (US student/resident), $232.00 (Canadian individuals), $375.00 (Canadian institutions), $137.00 (Canadian student/resident), $272.00 (foreign individuals), $375.00 (foreign institutions), and $137.00 (foreign student/resident). Foreign air speed delivery is included in all *Clinics* subscription prices. All prices are subject to change without notice. POST-MASTER: Send address changes to *Surgical Oncology Clinics of North America*, Elsevier Periodicals Customer Service, 6277 Sea Harbor Drive, Orlando, FL 32887–4800. **Customer Service: 1-800-654-2452 (US). From outside the United States, call 1-407-345-4000. E-mail: hhspcs@wbsaunders.com.**

Reprints. For copies of 100 or more, of articles in this publication, please contact the Commercial Reprints Department, Elsevier Inc., 360 Park Avenue South, New York, New York 10010-1710. Tel. (212) 633-3813 Fax: (212) 462-1935 email: reprints@elsevier.com.

Surgical Oncology Clinics of North America is covered in *Index Medicus* and *EMBASE/Excerpta Medica, Current Contents/Clinical Medicine,* and *ISI/BIOMED.*

Printed in the United States of America.

theclin

SURGIC
ONCOLOGY CLINIC
OF NORTH AMERIC

Tumor Immunolog
for the Practicing Surgeor

GUEST EDITOR
Robert P. Sticca, MD

CONSULTING EDITOR
Nicholas J. Petrelli, MD

October 2007 • Volume 16 • Number 4

SAUNDERS

An Imprint of Elsevier, Inc.
PHILADELPHIA   LONDON   TORONTO   MONTREAL   SYDNEY   TOKYO

CONSULTING EDITOR

NICHOLAS J. PETRELLI, MD, Bank of America Endowed Medical Director, Helen F. Graham Cancer Center at Christiana Care Health System, Newark, Delaware; and Professor of Surgery, Thomas Jefferson University, Philadelphia, Pennsylvania

GUEST EDITOR

ROBERT P. STICCA, MD, FACS, Department of Surgery, University of North Dakota School of Medicine and Health Sciences, Grand Forks, North Dakota

CONTRIBUTORS

NICOLE M. AGOSTINO, DO, Department of Internal Medicine, Lehigh Valley Hospital and Health Network, Allentown, Pennsylvania

ARJUMAND ALI, MD, Department of Surgery, Lehigh Valley Hospital and Health Network, Allentown, Pennsylvania

ROBERT J. AMATO, DO, Director, Genitourinary Oncology Program, The Methodist Hospital Research Institute, Houston, Texas

WILLIAM E. CARSON III, MD, Professor of Surgery, Division of Surgical Oncology, The Ohio State University School of Medicine; and Associate Director for Clinical Research, The Ohio State University Comprehensive Cancer Center, Columbus, Ohio

TIMOTHY CLAY, PhD, Associate Professor, Duke University Medical Center, Durham, North Carolina

CHARLES G. DRAKE, MD, PhD, Assistant Professor of Oncology, Immunology, and Urology, Johns Hopkins Sidney Kimmel Comprehensive Cancer Center, Baltimore, Maryland

SOLDANO FERRONE, MD, PhD, Professor of Surgery and Associate Director for Faculty Career Development and Advancement, Hillman Cancer Center, University of Pittsburgh Cancer Institute, Pittsburgh, Pennsylvania

BERNARD A. FOX, PhD, Laboratory of Molecular and Tumor Immunology, Robert W. Franz Cancer Research Center, Earle A. Chiles Research Institute, Providence Portland Medical Center; Department of Environmental and Biomolecular Systems; Department of Molecular Microbiology and Immunology; and OHSU Cancer Institute, Oregon Health and Science University, Portland, Oregon

JOSEPH F. GROSSO, PhD, Johns Hopkins Sidney Kimmel Comprehensive Cancer Center, Baltimore, Maryland

RUDOLF A. HATZ, MD, PhD, Department of Surgery, Laboratory of Clinical and Experimental Tumor Immunology, Grosshadern Medical Center, Ludwig-Maximilians-University Munich, Munich, Germany

DAVID M. HEIMANN, MD, Department of Surgical Oncology, Fox Chase Cancer Center, Philadelphia, Pennsylvania

AMY HOBEIKA, PhD, Assistant Professor, Department of Surgery, Duke University Medical Center, Durham, North Carolina

KARL-WALTER JAUCH, MD, PhD, Department of Surgery, Laboratory of Clinical and Experimental Tumor Immunology, Grosshadern Medical Center, Ludwig-Maximilians-University Munich, Munich, Germany

HOWARD L. KAUFMAN, MD, Associate Professor of Surgery, The Tumor Immunology Laboratory, and Chief, Division of Surgical Oncology, Columbia University, New York, New York

SEUNGHEE KIM-SCHULZE, PhD, Assistant Professor of Surgical Science, The Tumor Immunology Laboratory, Division of Surgical Oncology, Columbia University, New York, New York

MEDINA C. KUSHEN, MD, Neurosurgery Resident, Section of Neurosurgery, The University of Chicago Hospital, Chicago, Illinois

LEE LANGER, BS, Department of Surgery, Duke University Medical Center, Durham, North Carolina

MACIEJ S. LESNIAK, MD, Director, Neurosurgical Oncology and the University of Chicago Brain Tumor Center, Section of Neurosurgery, The University of Chicago Hospital, Chicago, Illinois

MARGARET I. LIANG, BS, The Ohio State University School of Medicine, Columbus, Ohio

H. KIM LYERLY, MD, Professor, Department of Surgery, Duke University Medical Center; and Director, Comprehensive Cancer Center, Durham, North Carolina

FRANCESCO M. MARINCOLA, MD, Chief, Infectious Disease and Immunogenetics Section, Department of Transfusion Medicine, Clinical Center, National Institutes of Health, Bethesda, Maryland

ROGER W. MELVOLD, PhD, Professor and Chairman, Department of Microbiology and Immunology, University of North Dakota School of Medicine and Health Sciences, Grand Forks, North Dakota

LILAH F. MORRIS, MD, Department of Surgery, UCLA Medical Center, Los Angeles, California

MICHAEL MORSE, MD, Associate Professor, Department of Medicine, Duke University Medical Center, Durham, North Carolina

PAUL J. MOSCA, MD, PhD, Chief, Section of Surgical Oncology, andn Vice-Chair for Research, Department of Surgery, Lehigh Valley Hospital and Health Network, Allentown, Pennsylvania

SURESH G. NAIR, MD, Fellowship Director, Hematology-Oncology, Department of Internal Medicine, Lehigh Valley Hospital and Health Network, Allentown, Pennsylvania

JANET M.D. PLATE, PhD, Professor, Division of Oncology and Hematology, Department of Immunology/Microbiology, Rush University Medical Center, Chicago, Illinois

ANTONI RIBAS, MD, Department of Surgery, UCLA Medical Center, Department of Medicine; and Jonsson Comprehensive Cancer Center, University of California at Los Angeles, Los Angeles, California

CRISTIANO RUMIO, PhD, Associate Professor, Universita'degli Studi di Milano, Department of Human Morphology, Milan, Italy

DOMINIK RÜTTINGER, MD, Department of Surgery, Laboratory of Clinical and Experimental Tumor Immunology, Grosshadern Medical Center, Ludwig-Maximilians-University Munich, Munich, Germany

MARIANNA SABATINO, MD, Visiting Fellow, Infectious Disease and Immunogenetics Section, Department of Transfusion Medicine, Clinical Center, National Institutes of Health, Bethesda, Maryland

SILVIA SELLERI, PhD, Visiting Fellow, Infectious Disease and Immunogenetics Section, Department of Transfusion Medicine, Clinical Center, National Institutes of Health, Bethesda, Maryland; Universita'degli Studi di Milano, Department of Human Morphology, Milan, Italy

ADAM M. SONABEND, MD, Research Associate, Section of Neurosurgery, The University of Chicago Hospital, Chicago, Illinois

ALEXANDER STARODUB, MD, Department of Medicine, Duke University Medical Center, Durham, North Carolina

JONATHAN A. STICCA, BA, Department of Pathology and Laboratory Medicine, Medical University of South Carolina, Charleston, South Carolina

ROBERT P. STICCA, MD, FACS, Department of Surgery, University of North Dakota School of Medicine and Health Sciences, Grand Forks, North Dakota

BRET TABACK, MD, Assistant Professor of Surgery, The Tumor Immunology Laboratory, Division of Surgical Oncology, Columbia University, New York, New York

ENA WANG, MD, Staff Scientist, Infectious Disease and Immunogenetics Section, Department of Transfusion Medicine, Clinical Center, National Institutes of Health, Bethesda, Maryland

LOUIS M. WEINER, MD, Vice President, Translational Research; and Chairman, Department of Medical Oncology, Fox Chase Cancer Center, Philadelphia, Pennsylvania

THERESA L. WHITESIDE, PhD, Professor of Pathology, Immunology, and Otolaryngology, and Director, Immunologic Monitoring and Cellular Products Laboratory, Hillman Cancer Center, University of Pittsburgh Cancer Institute, Pittsburgh, Pennsylvania

CONTENTS

The immune system is one of the most important means by which more complex animals protect themselves from external threats. There are two immune systems: the innate and the adaptive. The innate is the most basic and has existed for the longest time; the adaptive immune system is a more recent evolutionary development. The immune system plays a critical role in surveillance and prevention of malignancy. It is only when malignant cells develop mechanisms to escape the immune system that they become clinically significant tumors. Our knowledge of the immune system has grown enormously. We have begun to understand not only the mechanisms by which it protects us but also the ways in which it can inflict injury on the body. We are also learning about how it communicates with the environment and how its various components interact within the body. With this information, we are learning how to manipulate it to our greater benefit.

Without clinical information, accurate follow-up, high-quality sample collection, and preservation, scientific conclusions are only based on theoretical assumptions that are unlikely to lead to clinical breakthroughs. In this article we discuss our understanding of the relationship between cancer cells and the host immune response. We emphasize the critical role that future clinical investigations, led by surgical oncologists, may have for the assessment of the validity of the disparate hypotheses so far formulated at the bench side.

Current Immunotherapeutic Strategies in Pancreatic Cancer 919
Janet M.D. Plate

The immune systems of patients with newly diagnosed pancreatic cancers are functional, with T-cell responses capable of responding to tumor antigen presentation. Pancreatic tumors have been demonstrated to express tumor antigens as mutated, altered, underglycosylated and/or inappropriately overexpressed proteins. Considering these two facts, it should be possible for patients' bodies to recognize their tumors as foreign and to reject them. A number of clinical trials have been initiated to exploit this immune activation to eradicate or stabilize tumor growth. Immunotherapeutic trials include the specific testing of a variety of tumor vaccines, of cytokines as adjuvants or directed cytotoxicity, and of monoclonal antibodies to target specific molecules. This article reviews evidence for immune-cell activation and function in patients with pancreatic cancer, and evidence that pancreatic tumor cells express tumor antigens, or mutated (or altered) proteins. Nevertheless, tumors survive immune attacks by producing products that help them to circumvent effector T cells. The article thus examines complications of immune evasion by cancer cells, as well as the challenges of trying to exploit the immune system in solid tumors where tumor cell products can turn off invading immune T cells set to kill them. Finally, the article discusses the choices of a variety of clinical trials using immune modulation for patients with pancreatic cancer.

Current Immunotherapeutic Strategies in Malignant Melanoma 945
Nicole M. Agostino, Arjumand Ali, Suresh G. Nair, and Paul J. Mosca

The basis of immunotherapy for melanoma is the existence of melanoma-associated antigens that can be targeted by the immune system. Identification of many of these antigens has enabled investigators to develop a wide array of immunotherapy strategies for the treatment of melanoma. Although several of these strategies have been shown to induce antitumor immune responses in some patients, robust clinical responses have been observed less frequently. With exciting recent advancements in this field, however, there is promise of generating potent immunologic responses and translating them more consistently into durable clinical responses. This article reviews several current approaches to immunotherapy for melanoma and describes the key role that surgeons play in advancing this area of oncology.

Current Immunotherapeutic Strategies in Renal Cell Carcinoma 975
Robert J. Amato

Advanced renal cell carcinoma remains resistant to drug-, hormone-, and cytokine-based therapies. Promising new immunotherapeutic approaches include monoclonal antibodies, kinase inhibitors, mammalian target of rapamycin inhibition, dendritic cell, and tumor antigen vaccines. Most of these approaches have yet to produce clinical responses significantly superior to those of previous standard therapies, although most are well tolerated and elicit relatively high rates of stable disease. Two recently approved agents, a kinase inhibitor and a mTOR inhibitor, are recommended for use as first-line therapies against renal cell carcinoma. An additional approved tyrosine kinase inhibitor, sorafenib, is recommended as second-line therapy. More clinical research on these agents and their use in combination, especially sequentially, is warranted.

Immunotherapy has emerged as a promising tool in the management of malignant central nervous system tumors. Despite improvement in patient survival, traditional approaches, which consist mostly of surgery, radiotherapy, and chemotherapy, have been largely unsuccessful in permanently controlling these aggressive tumors. Immunotherapeutic strategies offer not only a novel approach but also an advantage in a way other modalities have been failing. Specifically, the capabilities of the immune system to recognize altered cells while leaving normal cells intact offer tremendous advantage over the conventional therapeutic approaches. This article summarizes our current understanding of immunotherapeutic treatment modalities used in clinical trials for management of malignant central nervous system tumors.

FORTHCOMING ISSUES

RECENT ISSUES

THE CLINICS ARE NOW ONLINE!

Access your subscription at:
http://www.theclinics.com

ELSEVIER
SAUNDERS

Surg Oncol Clin N Am
16 (2007) xv–xvi

SURGICAL
ONCOLOGY CLINICS
OF NORTH AMERICA

Foreword

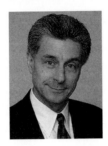

Nicholas J. Petrelli, MD
Consulting Editor

This edition of the *Surgical Oncology Clinics of North America* is devoted to tumor immunology. The guest editor is Robert P. Sticca, MD. Dr. Sticca is Chair of Surgery and Program Director for the General Surgery Residency at the University of North Dakota. Dr. Sticca received his general surgery training from Boston University, and this was followed by a surgical oncology fellowship at the Roswell Park Cancer Institute. His basic science and research has centered around dendritic cell vaccines for melanoma and renal cell cancer, and thymidylate synthase variation in human colorectal tumors.

Dr. Sticca has put together an expert group of investigators with several discussions centered around the current immunotherapeutic strategies in solid tumors. The role of cancer vaccines in both therapy and prevention is also discussed. Cancer is felt to be the result of several sequential events, including transformation by viruses or environmental carcinogens, such as radiation and chemicals, genetic predisposition, and tumor promoters. The theory of immune surveillance states that the immune system constantly recognizes and eliminates tumor cells. If a tumor escapes immune surveillance and grows too large for the immune system to kill, the result is cancer. Immune surveillance is likely to be successful against virus-induced tumors that express foreign peptides. Tumors vary greatly in their immunogenicity and even tumors who have antigens which can be recognized by the host immune system can evade immune elimination. Several immunotherapies have been tested in human trials, including melanoma vaccines. Melanoma vaccines have induced tumor remission in some patients, and whole protein, peptide, and recombinant vaccines are also being developed. Heat shock proteins from tumor cells are also being tested as possible vaccines. Lastly, tumor antigen pulsed autologous dendritic cells are being tested for their ability to stimulate a tumor specific immune response.

All of the issues above are described in detail by experts in the field of tumor immunology. Dr. Sticca has emphasized to the authors to develop articles in tumor immunology that would be applicable and educational for the practicing surgeon. I believe Dr. Sticca and his authors have been successful in achieving this goal.

Nicholas J. Petrelli, MD
Helen F. Graham Cancer Center
Christiana Care Health Services
4701 Ogletown-Stanton Road
Suite 1213
Newark, DE 19713, USA

Thomas Jefferson University
College Building
1025 Walnut Street
Philadelphia, PA 19107, USA

E-mail address: npetrelli@christianacare.org

ELSEVIER
SAUNDERS

Surg Oncol Clin N Am
16 (2007) xvii–xviii

SURGICAL
ONCOLOGY CLINICS
OF NORTH AMERICA

Preface

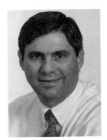

Robert P. Sticca, MD, FACS
Guest Editor

The importance of the immune system in cancer has been recognized for over 100 years, but it has only been in the past two decades that the knowledge of the immune system's interaction (or lack thereof) with malignant cells has been characterized enough to allow for meaningful therapeutic interventions. The discipline of tumor immunology has expanded greatly over the past 20 years. A great deal of time, effort, and resources has been spent on the research of the relationship between the host immune system and altered cells of malignancy in the hopes of developing new and effective treatment options for cancer. The results of these expenditures are now coming to fruition as new immunotherapeutic treatments have been developed and, in some cases, implemented, improving disease free and overall survival for patients who have solid tumors. In addition to advances in molecular immunology, an understanding of the genetic basis of immune recognition and response to malignancy has allowed both basic scientists and clinicians to use the immune system in the diagnosis and management of cancer. Although the interactions between the immune system and tumor cell are complex and have not been completely elucidated to date, these interactions have been better characterized in many malignancies, allowing effective therapies to be developed.

This issue of *Surgical Oncology Clinics of North America* is organized as both a review for practicing surgeons as well as a current update for individuals who are well versed in immunotherapy. The first seven articles are written as a review of the basic concepts in tumor immunology. Much knowledge has been added to the domain of basic immunology over the past

doi:10.1016/j.soc.2007.08.001

two decades; therefore, the first section of the first article is included as a brief review of basic immunology for surgeons who have not had any recent exposure to the latest in basic immunologic principles. The last eight articles are written as an update of current information and immunotherapy for many of the most common disease sites of cancer. I am indebted to several of the world's leading tumor immunology authors from some of the most prominent immunotherapy centers, who have contributed to this issue to bring the reader the most current state of the art information in tumor immunology.

Though many of the steps in immune recognition and reaction to malignant cells are now better understood, there remains much to be discovered. The potential for manipulation of the immune system to better recognize and eradicate transformed cells offers much promise for an effective, long-lasting treatment option in many solid tumors. Although immunotherapy may not be appropriate for all clinical situations, better understanding of the conditions which are appropriate for an effective immune response will allow clinicians to use this valuable treatment modality in addition to current treatment options. The use of immunotherapeutic treatments, such as monoclonal antibodies, has now become a standard part of treatment regimens for some malignancies, and it is only a matter of time before other forms of immunotherapy such as vaccination become part of the standard treatment options for solid tumors. The attraction of a nontoxic, nondebilitating form of therapy, such as immunotherapy, is great.

The use of immunotherapy cannot occur without appropriate and timely clinical trials to delineate the activity and benefits of immunotherapeutic regimens in the treatment of malignancies. The surgeon's role in the investigation and implementation of immunotherapy is critical, for in many cases only surgeons can identify appropriate patients and obtain the necessary tissue specimens for the development of tumor specific immunotherapy. It is my hope that the surgical community will continue to accept and maintain the vital role that it plays in the development of this valuable weapon in the fight against malignancy.

Robert P. Sticca, MD, FACS
Department of Surgery
University of North Dakota
School of Medicine and Health Sciences
501 North Columbia Road, Room 5108
Grand Forks, ND 58203, USA

E-mail address: rsticca@medicine.nodak.edu

ELSEVIER
SAUNDERS

Surg Oncol Clin N Am
16 (2007) 711–735

SURGICAL
ONCOLOGY CLINICS
OF NORTH AMERICA

Basic and Tumor Immunology: A Review

Roger W. Melvold, PhD[a],
Robert P. Sticca, MD, FACS[b],*

[a]Department of Microbiology and Immunology, University of North Dakota
School of Medicine and Health Sciences, 501 North Columbia Road,
Grand Forks, ND 58202-9037, USA
[b]Department of Surgery, University of North Dakota School of Medicine and Health Sciences,
501 North Columbia Road, Grand Forks, ND 58202-9037, USA

Review of basic immunology

Overview

Every organism in nature, from the simplest microbe to the most complex forms of plants and animals, seeks to protect itself against the threats presented by other organisms. The immune system is one of the most important means by which more complex animals protect themselves from being invaded—and perhaps ingested—by microbes and parasites. There are, in fact, two immune systems: the innate and the adaptive. The innate is the most basic and has existed for the longest time, although its importance and mechanisms only recently have received the attention they deserve. The adaptive immune system is a more recent evolutionary development, probably arising in the jawless fishes and restricted to their descendants.

Many of the features of the immune system have been long recognized and exploited by humans, even in an absence of any understanding of its nature. For example, the ancient peoples of Mesopotamia and Egypt and China recognized that for many diseases, individuals who survived the disease were protected against future recurrences and that this protection could be transferred to others by means that amounted to primitive forms of vaccination. In the modern era, our knowledge of the immune system has grown enormously. We have begun to understand not only the mechanisms by which it protects us but also the ways in which it can inflict injury on the

* Corresponding author.
E-mail address: rsticca@medicine.nodak.edu (R.P. Sticca).

1055-3207/07/$ - see front matter © 2007 Elsevier Inc. All rights reserved.
doi:10.1016/j.soc.2007.08.003
surgonc.theclinics.com

body. We are also learning about how it communicates with the environment and how its various components interact within the body. With this information, we are learning how to manipulate it to our greater benefit.

Recognition: self and non-self

Recognition of invasion of infection requires the ability to distinguish self from non-self; what cells and molecules should be present within an individual's body and which should not. Where the presence of non-self is detected, subsequent decisions must be made with respect to the level of the threat imposed by non-self and what to do about it. If judged harmless, it may be ignored. If deemed harmful, it may be isolated and contained or eliminated altogether. Non-self may include cells and molecules, such as microbes, parasites, and toxins, that enter the body. It also may include new proteins or molecules that arise within the body, such as the malignant transformation of normal cells into cancerous ones expressing mutated or inappropriately expressed gene products that act as "non-self."

The distinctions between self and non-self are made by two types of receptors. One type is used by the innate system and consists of receptors that have been "hard wired" into our genomes and are, in most cases, able to recognize and bind molecules produced by infectious organisms (eg, bacteria) but not by host (eg, human) cells. In some cases, these receptors do not recognize microbes/microbial products directly but detect their presence indirectly through the recognition and binding of "stress signals"—molecules produced by cells that have become infected. The receptors of the innate immune system are identical, or nearly so, among the members of a given species.

The second type of receptor is used by the adaptive immune system and consists of a vast number of receptors that are formed by lymphocytes through the random rearrangement of DNA encoding a relatively small number of genes. These are the immunoglobulins (antibodies) produced by B lymphocytes and the T-cell receptors (TCRs) generated by T lymphocytes. Because these receptors are generated by a random process during lymphocyte development within each individual, each individual has a unique "repertoire" of such receptors, although there is considerable overlap among individuals. Because the receptors of the adaptive immune system are randomly generated, some are useful, some are not, and some are potentially dangerous. Developing lymphocytes undergo selective processes within the thymus to promote expansion of those most able to function within the body and eliminate those capable of reacting against self molecules/tissues.

The innate immune response

Some form of innate immune response can be found in practically all multicellular animals and even in plants. The innate system can be divided into two general parts. The first is a set of barriers.

1. Mechanical barriers (eg, the skin and mucous membranes)
2. Chemical barriers (eg, the high acidity of the stomach, the salts and mild acidity of the skin, secretion of various enzymes and other microcidal molecules produced by many different types of cells)
3. Biologic barriers (eg, commensal microbes that occupy various parts of the body)

The second part of the innate immune system is based on the activity of a set of cells and molecules that can detect the presence of microbes and act against them once detected. One of the primary features of the innate immune response is that it is based on pre-existing molecules and cell types that can act immediately upon contact with infectious agents or other threats. This feature is distinct from the adaptive response, in which 1 to 2 weeks or more may be required to generate and activate the necessary cells and molecules. The innate system is generally composed of cells and molecules that bear receptors (or, in the case of molecules, binding sites) that can recognize molecular structures (pathogen-associated molecular patterns) present on numerous types of microbes but not on host cells. The receptors and binding sites that recognize the pathogen-associated molecular patterns are called pattern recognition receptors (PRRs). PRRs are found on a wide variety of host cells, phagocytes in particular. Among the noncellular PRRs are some complement components, such as C3b and MBL (mannan-binding lectin). PRRs are "hard wired" into host genomes as a result of their long evolutionary separation from microbes and are expressed without any additional chromosomal rearrangement, as occurs in the generation of antibodies and TCRs. As a result, the genetic variation seen within a population for a given PRR is limited, and these receptors are consistent among individuals within that population. In humans, one of the prominent types of PRRs are Toll-like receptors (TLRs) expressed on numerous cell types, especially by phagocytes and other leukocytes and by epithelial cells. Eleven TLRs (eg, TLR1, TLR2) have been identified in humans. TLR2, for example, recognizes and binds peptidoglycan and many other bacterial molecules, whereas TLR4 binds bacterial lipopolysaccharide, and TLR3 binds viral dsRNA. Not all TLRs bind solely to structures on microbes. TLR4, for example, also can bind to various "stress molecules" that appear on the surfaces of infected host cells, which allows those infected cells to be identified and destroyed.

Binding of TLRs and other PRRs expressed on phagocytic cells by microbe-associated molecules (pathogen-associated molecular patterns) triggers the activation of those phagocytes. Activated phagocytes become enlarged, increase their production of antimicrobial products, and begin to ingest and degrade microbes. Once activated, they may increase their motility and begin to actively "hunt" additional microbes. The innate system becomes active immediately upon contact with invasive microbes and is responsible for "holding the fort" while the adaptive immune response is generated, whereupon the innate and adaptive systems may interact cooperatively in performing some immune responses. The initial activation of adaptive immune responses depends on ongoing innate immune responses. The ingestion and degradation of microbial cells and molecules allow certain of these phagocytes, the so-called "antigen-presenting cells" (APCs), to redisplay fragments of those ingested and degraded molecules on their surfaces to initiate the activation of T lymphocytes and the development of subsequent adaptive immune responses. The soluble PRRs of the complement system operate in innate and the adaptive immune responses and are described in more detail later in the article.

Natural killer cells

Natural killer (NK) cells are part of the lymphoid lineage but are distinct from T and B lymphocytes because they do not express the specialized receptors associated with the adaptive immune response. Instead they have two other types of receptors that determine their ability to identify and kill targeted host cells: killer activation receptors and killer inhibition receptors. NK cells are important elements in innate defenses against virally infected and cancerous host cells. Host cells that are stressed as a result of viral infection or transformation into tumor cells may express surface molecules termed "stress signals." Two of the primary stress signals in human cells are called MICA and MICB. By way of their killer activation receptors, NK cells are able to identify and bind to such stressed cells. Binding of MICA or MICB by killer activation receptors triggers the NK cells to kill the cells to which they are bound. Before proceeding to kill, however, the NK cells use their killer inhibition receptors to scan the attached cell to determine the level of major histocompatibility complex (MHC) class I molecules expressed on its surface. MHC class I molecules are expressed on all nucleated cells of the body and serve as a way of alerting T lymphocytes to the presence of infectious or abnormal proteins within the cell. The expression of these molecules is often reduced in infected or transformed cells as a mechanism of evading the immune response. If the NK cell determines that the targeted cell has reduced MHC class I expression, it proceeds to kill the cell. If the MHC class I expression is normal or elevated, however, it cancels its killing program and releases the targeted cell.

The adaptive immune response

The adaptive immune system can be viewed as a group of mechanisms that permit the immune system to generate immune responses that are far more focused and intensified than those of the innate immune system. The adaptive immune system also allows the development of immunologic memory, whereby the immune system can "remember" stimuli that it has previously encountered and respond to subsequent encounters with greater speed and intensity. In contrast, the innate immune system views each such encounter as if it were the first and is unable to "mold" its response against infectious agents to which it is repeatedly exposed. The adaptive immune system is an "add on" to the more ancient innate system, appearing in the vertebrate lineage.

Adaptive immune responses are based on the activities of T lymphocytes (also called T cells) and B lymphocytes (B cells). B cells develop from stem cells in the bone marrow, as do T cells. Cells destined to become T cells migrate from the bone marrow at an early stage and move to the thymus, where they complete their differentiation. The key to the adaptive immune system is the presence of the extremely variable antigen-specific receptors of the T lymphocytes (called TCRs) and B lymphocytes (called B-cell receptors [BCRs], immunoglobulins, or antibodies, depending on the context). Unlike the genomically stable receptors of the innate immune system, the receptors of the adaptive immune system are generated anew in the somatic lymphocytes of each individual by the random shuffling and uniting of the DNA encoding a relatively small number of genes to produce an array of millions of receptors that can be further modified somatically through the introduction of small mutations and other irregularities. As a result, although receptors of the innate immune system are finite (perhaps a hundred different types, each of which is highly consistent among individuals within a species), each individual hypothetically could express adaptive immune receptors that range into billions or trillions of different varieties. Because they are generated by a random process, the range of available adaptive receptors of a given individual (the "immunologic repertoire" of that individual) also differs somewhat from other members of the same species.

Because of physical and physiologic constraints on the immune system, the hypothetical maximum number of receptors is never actually achieved in any given individual; however, it is estimated that the pool of TCRs and BCRs in an average adult is capable of recognizing and selectively binding to at least 10 million different molecular structures. Each individual lymphocyte develops such that all of its receptors have the same specificity, and when it proliferates, its clonal descendants maintain the same specificity. As a result, the ability of an individual to distinguish among at least 10 million different structures means that the individual contains at least 10 million different clones of lymphocytes, each capable of recognizing a different structure.

When the antigen-specific receptor of a T or B lymphocyte binds to the appropriate target structure (antigen), the stage is set for lymphocyte activation. Because these cells have destructive capabilities, however, their activation and activity are closely regulated and require not only binding of the TCR or BCR but also the simultaneous receipt of multiple additional signals.

Structure of B-cell and T-cell antigen receptors

TCRs and BCRs (immunoglobulins or antibodies) have some similarity of structure (Fig. 1). TCRs are always membrane bound. Immunoglobulins are membrane bound on B cells until the B cells enter a stage of terminal differentiation and become plasma cells. Plasma cells cease formation of membrane immunoglobulin and switch to synthesis and secretion of a soluble form of the immunoglobulin (having the same antigenic specificity). Membrane-bound BCRs consist of four chains (two identical heavy chains and two identical light chains), whereas TCRs consist of two heterodimers. There are two types of BCR light chains (κ and λ) and five types of heavy chains (A, D, E, G, M). Four types of chains comprise TCRs—α, β, γ, and δ—and TCR heterodimers expressed by any given T cell are either α-β or γ-δ combinations. All of the chains, whether for BCRs or TCRs, are glycoproteins and can be divided into a constant region and a variable region. Constant regions display a limited amount of variability among B cells or T cells within an individual's body (or among different individuals), whereas the variable regions display an enormous amount of variability within and among individuals.

Antigen presentation and T-cell activation

Most adaptive immune responses begin with the activation of T lymphocytes (T cells) after interaction with a group of cells known as APCs, including dendritic cells, macrophages, and B lymphocytes. Activation of naïve T cells is primarily mediated by dendritic cells and usually occurs in lymph nodes. Reactivation of previously activated T cells can be done by any of the APCs and can occur in the body tissues and lymphoid aggregations (eg, lymph nodes, spleen, Peyer's patches, tonsils). This interaction is

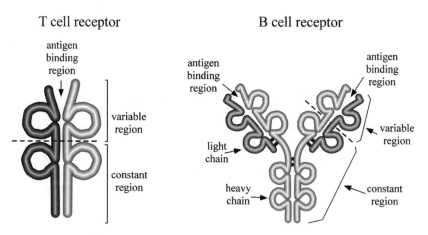

Fig. 1. Structure of T-cell and B-cell antigen receptors.

necessary, in part, because of the special requirements of the TCR but also because APCs can provide additional signals to the T cells that regulate their activation. APCs present antigens to T cells in two different ways (Fig. 2). T cells respond primarily to protein/peptide antigens.

1. APCs are capable of ingesting and degrading material derived from infectious organisms and the debris of dead cells and most other materials. Phagosomes that contain the ingested materials fuse with lysosomes that contain degradative enzymes to form phagolysosomes. Phagolysosomes then can fuse with other organelles that contain newly synthesized MHC class II molecules. Peptides that result from degradation of ingested proteins are loaded onto the MHC class II molecules and are transported to the surface, where (still associated with the MHC class II molecules) they are exposed to T cells that may make contact with the APC.

2. APCs also can degrade and present proteins/peptides that are synthesized within their own cytoplasm, including proteins encoded by infectious organisms within the cytoplasm (eg, viruses) and normal cellular proteins that are worn out, malformed, or in excessive amounts. These various peptides are then loaded within the endoplasmic reticulum onto

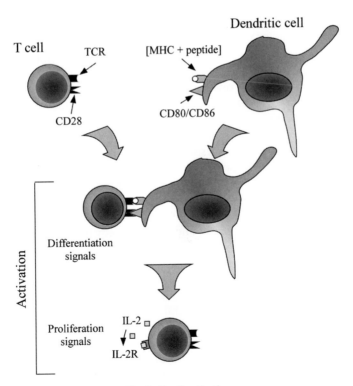

Fig. 2. T-cell activation.

newly formed MHC class I molecules. The MHC class I molecules, bearing their peptides, move to the cell surface, where the peptides (still associated with the MHC class I molecules) are exposed to T cells that may make contact with the APC.

With respect to interactions with APCs, T cells are divided into two categories; CD4+ and CD8+. Cells that express CD4 molecules concentrate on peptides presented by MHC class II molecules. They "sample" the many different (peptide + MHC class II) combinations on the APC surface, and if one of them fits the TCR tightly, a signal is transmitted to the T-cell nucleus that provides part of the stimulus for activation. Subsequent binding of CD80 and CD86 (also called B7.1 and B7.2) molecules on the APCs with CD28 molecules on the T cell initiate differentiation of the T cell into an activated state. Part of this differentiation involves synthesis by the T cells of a soluble cytokine (interleukin-2 [IL-2]), which serves as a proliferation signal, and a high affinity receptor (IL-2R) for the cytokine. After differentiation and proliferation, the newly activated CD4+ T cells leave the lymph nodes to recirculate throughout the body. CD8+ T cells concentrate on peptides presented by MHC class I molecules. They "sample" the numerous (peptide + MHC class I) combinations on the APC surface, and if one of them binds the TCR tightly, an activation signal to the T-cell nucleus provides part of the stimulus for activation. Like CD4+ T cells, binding of CD80 and CD86 to CD28 molecules on the T cell initiates differentiation, including production of IL-2 and IL-R. CD8+ T cells that undergo activation often depend on IL-2 from neighboring CD4+ T cells to help their initial proliferation until their own IL-2 production is sufficient. Like CD4+ T cells, newly activated CD8+ T cells leave the lymph nodes to recirculate throughout the body.

MHC class I molecules are expressed on all nucleated cells of the body, whereas MHC class II molecules are expressed only by APCs. Because of the costimulatory signals provided by APCs, naïve (unactivated) CD4+ and CD8+ T cells must interact with [peptide + MHC] on those APCs to become activated, and this occurs primarily in lymph nodes. Once activated, however, T cells recirculate throughout the body, looking for the same [peptide + MHC] combination that bound their receptor to initiate their activation. In the case of CD4+ T cells, they remain restricted to interaction with APCs because those are the only cells that express MHC class II. Because all nucleated cells express MHC class I molecules, however, activated CD8+ T cells can interact with APCs and non-APCs within the body tissues.

CD4+ T cells undergo a further differentiation during or shortly after their activation and enter into one of two general pathways of differentiation: T helper 1 (Th1) or T helper 2 (Th2). Which pathway is taken is the result of numerous factors, including local cytokine environments, the types of APCs with which they interact, the intensity with which their TCRs bind to the [peptide + MHC II], and perhaps even the nature of the particular infectious organism that provides the antigenic stimulus. Th1 CD4+ T cells are primarily (but not exclusively) involved in cell-mediated responses, whereas Th2 CD4+ T cells are primarily involved in regulation of the activation and antibody secretion by B cells.

T-cell–mediated cellular immune responses

This category of responses does not involve antibodies and includes two types of responses: delayed-type hypersensitivity and cytotoxic T lymphocytes (CTLs) (Fig. 3). Delayed-type hypersensitivity responses are mediated by activated CD4+ Th1 (or simply Th1) cells. These Th1 cells may encounter APCs in the tissues that are presenting the appropriate [peptide + MHC II] and bind to them. This action triggers reactivation of the Th1 cells, which then secrete cytokines to attract and activate phagocytic macrophages. Activation of the macrophages by Th1 cells occurs through the binding of surface molecules on the two cells and secretion of interferon-γ (IFN-γ) by the Th1 cells to provide a potent activation signal for the macrophages. The activated macrophages then attack the antigenic stimulus, but because they have no intrinsic antigenic specificity, "innocent bystander" cells and tissues often can be damaged. Th1 cells provide specificity to delayed-type hypersensitivity responses but do not themselves act directly against the antigenic stimulus (eg, infectious organism). Instead, they recruit and focus the activity of the nonspecific macrophages against the stimulus.

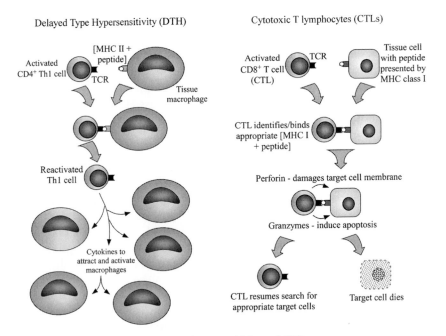

Fig. 3. Delayed-type hypersensitivity and CTL responses.

CTL responses are mediated by activated CD8+ T cells. Unlike CD4+ T cells, CTLs act directly against their targets (usually infected host cells) by direct action that involves cell-to-cell contact. Activated CD8+ cells recirculate throughout the body looking for the [peptide + MHC I] combinations that fit their TCRs. They may find these on either APCs or non-APC cells. (Recall that all nucleated cells express MHC class I molecules.) Upon encountering and binding to cells that express the appropriate [peptide + MHC I], CTLs damage the targeted cells by secreting molecules that damage their membranes and induce the targeted cells to undergo apoptotic cellular suicide. The CTLs are not damaged in the process and seek other target cells. The damage induced by CTLs is highly selective and involves only those appropriately targeted cells to which they bind; there is no innocent bystander damage, as seen in delayed-type hypersensitivity responses.

The role of genetic variability in immune responsiveness

The MHC I and II molecules that are responsible for presentation of peptide fragments are highly polymorphic molecules. There are literally hundreds of allelic forms of these molecules among the individuals of a given species, and they are inherited as autosomal codominant mendelian genes. Each individual is able to express only a limited subset of the allelic variants present in the population, however. Within the human MHC, the human leukocyte antigen (HLA) complex on chromosome 6, humans have three genetic loci encoding MHC class I molecules (HLA-A, HLA-B, HLA-C). Because of the large number of alleles in the population, most individuals inherit different alleles at each locus from their two parents and can express as many as six different allelic forms of MHC class I molecules. A total of seven to eight loci encode the two separate heterodimer chains that form three MHC class II molecules: DP, DQ, and DR. Like HLA-A, -B and -C, most individuals are heterozygous at the MHC class II loci. Because of the various ways in which these heterodimeric molecules can be assembled, the APCs of most individuals can express approximately 12 different MHC class II heterodimers.

As a result of this diversity, most individuals who are not closely related express different limited subsets of the MHC molecules present in the population. The allelic variation produces MHC class I and II molecules with slight structural differences that dictate what peptide fragments bind most efficiently to them for presentation. Each individual, expressing a particular subset of MHC molecules on his or her cells, presents certain peptide fragments to T cells more or less effectively than would another individual who has different HLA alleles. The result is that the subset of available T cells likely to be activated would differ between the two individuals, although there would be considerable overlap, and those individuals might show differences in their responsiveness to particular antigens. Many HLA class I and II alleles are associated with the ability to respond well or poorly to particular infectious agents and the risk for autoimmunity triggered by particular self-molecules. The human immune response is not monolithic and displays variations in the spectrum of antigens to which any individual's immune system responds.

B-cell activation

Initial activation of B cells, like that of T cells, occurs primarily in lymph nodes. Newly developed naïve B cells migrate from the bone marrow to the lymph nodes. Upon arrival in the lymph nodes, naïve B cells express only the IgM isotype on their surfaces but quickly begin to coexpress IgD having the same antigenic specificity as their IgM. In the lymph nodes, they can mingle with activated T cells and antigenic debris carried into the lymph nodes by certain types of dendritic cells. (It should be noted that dendritic cells do not ingest all of the material with which they come into contact but also carry some of it attached to their surfaces.) Within the lymph nodes, naïve B cells may find antigen that binds to their surface and provides a partial signal for activation. The other signals required for activation come from activated Th2 cells that provide signals mediated by soluble cytokines (particularly IL-4) and the interaction of membrane molecules on the two cells. Upon receipt of the full array of activation signals, the B cells become activated and begin to proliferate. Then they leave the lymph nodes. Unlike activated T cells that constantly recirculate through the body, activated B cells remain largely resident in the bone marrow and spleen, with minimal recirculation that is restricted to other lymphoid tissues.

Upon activation, B cells undergo differentiation (Fig. 4). They cease expression of IgD and express only IgM on their surfaces. They then enter one of two differentiation pathways to become either plasma cells or memory B cells. B cells that differentiate into plasma cells enlarge and cease surface IgM expression. Instead, they secrete large amounts of soluble IgM until they "burn out" and die within days to weeks. Memory B cells retain their smaller size and surface expression of IgM, lying quiescently in the bone marrow and spleen. Occasionally, some of them migrate back into the lymph nodes (or other lymphoid aggregations, such as the Peyer's patches or tonsils), where they have a new opportunity to interact with antigen and Th2 cells. Should their surface BCRs again bind to appropriate antigen, although they also receive appropriate signals from Th2 cells, they become reactivated and begin a new round of differentiation and proliferation.

During the proliferation of reactivated memory B cells, two independent types of changes can occur in some of them with respect to the antibody molecules they express. One of these changes is somatic hypermutation, by which small mutations may occur in the DNA that encodes the antigen-binding regions. If these changes increase the intensity of binding to their specific antigen, the memory cells proliferate even more rapidly when

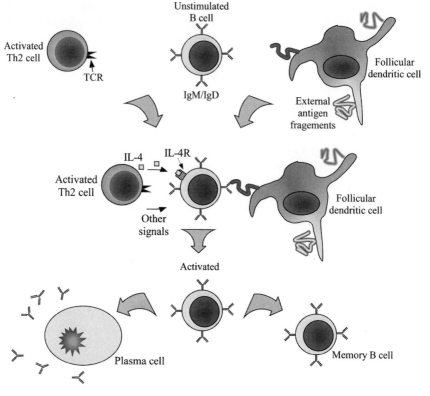

Fig. 4. B-cell activation.

they bind to that antigen. As a result, repeated exposure to an antigenic stimulus can result in a fine tuning that leads to the production of antibodies that bind with increasing intensity and efficiency—a phenomenon termed "affinity maturation." The other change that occurs in some proliferating memory B cells is the isotype switch. In this process, deletions of intervening DNA segments allow the memory B cells to change from production of IgM to production of IgG, IgA, or IgE while retaining the same antigenic specificity. Essentially, the heavy chain constant regions are altered while the remainder of the immunoglobulin structure remains unchanged. Whether the switch is to IgG, IgA, or IgE is determined by the cytokine signals received from the Th2 cells involved in the reactivation. Because the different immunoglobulin isotypes have differing capacities for participating in various immune responses, having multiple isotypes directed against the same antigenic stimulus broadens the spectrum of immune responses that can be generated effectively against that stimulus. After reactivation, memory B cells again enter either the plasma cell or memory B cell pathway and migrate back to the bone marrow and spleen. Cells that become plasma cells secrete soluble antibodies until they die, whereas memory cells remain quiescent again until they recirculate back to the lymphoid tissues. Memory B cells can undergo repeated rounds of reactivation, somatic hypermutation, and isotype switching.

Functional specialization of antibody isotypes

The five isotypes—IgM, IgD, IgG, IgA, and IgE—differ in their ability to engage in immune responses.

IgM. When expressed on the B-cell surface, IgM is a single Y-shaped monomeric unit (see Fig. 1). Its secreted form is a pentamer that combines fine monomeric units having ten antigen-binding sites, however. IgM is effective in the activation of serum complement, and its ten binding sites make it efficient at agglutination, which is the aggregation of multiple antigens. It is the first isotype produced after encounter with a particular antigenic stimulus.

IgD. This isotype is expressed as a monomeric unit on the surface of naïve B cells between the time they enter lymph nodes and undergo their initial activation. Its role and function are unknown.

IgG. IgG is expressed as a monomeric unit whether on the B-cell surface or in secreted form. It is the most common isotype in normal serum (75%–85%). It is highly effective in activating serum complement, stimulating opsonization (increased phagocytic activity), neutralizing the ability of infectious organisms to bind to host cells, and mediating antibody-dependent cellular cytotoxicity (the ability of NK cells and eosinophils to bind and destroy infectious organisms that have been "tagged" by antibodies). The four subtypes of IgG (IgG1, IgG2, IgG3, IgG4) have different functional specialties.

IgA. IgA is expressed as a monomer on B-cell surfaces but can be secreted as either a monomeric or dimeric form. The dimeric form has four binding sites and can be picked up by certain specialized epithelial cells and transported from the body to the external surfaces, where it is incorporated into fluids such as tears, intestinal and respiratory mucous surfaces, breast secretions, and urogenital membrane secretions. Approximately 10% to 15% of serum immunoglobulin is composed of monomeric and dimeric IgA.

IgE. IgE is monomeric whether on the B-cell surface or secreted. Secreted IgE is found at extremely low levels (<1%) in the serum because it is rapidly adsorbed onto the surface of mast cells, whose surfaces express high levels of receptors that bind to the Fc end of free IgE molecules (IgE molecules whose antigen-binding regions are still unbound and available). Mast cells are coated with IgE antibodies that can bind to specific antigens that may come into their vicinity. Binding of IgE triggers release of cytoplamic mast cell granules, which are involved in allergic and asthmatic responses.

The role of complement in innate and adaptive immune responses

Complement is the collective term for a set of serum proteins (components) that become activated via three different pathways. Two of these pathways—the alternative pathway and the mannan-binding lectin pathway—occur in the absence of antibody and are considered part of the innate immune system. The third pathway—the classic pathway—is initiated by IgG and IgM antibodies that already have bound to their specific antigens. All three pathways of activation result in three types of responses: (1) production of a membrane attack complex, which can disrupt the membranes of infectious microbes and cause their lytic death, (2) attachment of fragments of complement components to microbial surfaces, which renders them more susceptible to ingestion and degradation by phagocytes, and (3) chemotaxis and activation of leukocytes to the sites of infection to generate inflammatory responses. These responses are summarized in Fig. 5.

Primary and secondary immune responses in the adaptive immune system

Primary immune responses occur upon the initial encounter with a particular antigenic stimulus. In general, 1 to 2 weeks are required for these responses to develop to a level at which they are sufficient to begin effective action against infectious organisms. Repeated exposure (or continuous

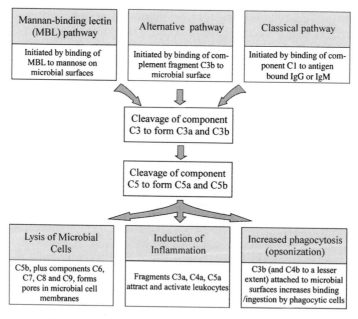

Fig. 5. Activation pathways and functions of complement.

exposure) to the antigenic stimulus, however, produces secondary responses that are characterized by more rapid development (several days instead of 1 or 2 weeks), elevated levels of activity, and longer persistence. This is the basis for immunologic memory, a phenomenon not seen in the innate immune system. This change is caused by the fact that the activation and proliferation of lymphocytes during primary responses provide a larger pool of available lymphocytes with the appropriate specificity that already has undergone some degree of activation. Although IgM is the predominant antibody produced in primary responses, the IgG isotype is also predominant in secondary response because of the isotype switching that occurs in reactivated memory B cells.

Regulation

The immune system is a double-edged sword. It has the ability to destroy infectious agents, and infected host cells carry the possibility of attacking normal body molecules, cells, and tissues unless carefully regulated. This regulation occurs at several levels.

1. *Elimination of potentially self-reactive T cells in the thymus.* As T cells undergo development within the thymus, they undergo a process called negative selection, which causes most self-reactive T cells to undergo apoptosis before they have an opportunity to leave the thymus and disperse to the rest of the body.
2. *The role of APCs in activating T cells.* Activation of naïve T cells in lymph nodes requires the intervention of APCs. Naïve T cells that encounter appropriate [peptide + MHC] on non-APC cells that are unable to provide the additional necessary signals cause these naïve T cells to enter a permanent state in inactivation or anergy. The random, uncontrolled activation of naïve T cells in the body tissues is prevented.
3. *Inactivation signals.* Activated lymphocytes are useful only as long as they are needed. If allowed to persist beyond that point, they become potential agents for self-injury. After activation, T cells begin to express a surface molecule called CD152 (or CTLA-4). CD152 competes with CD28 for binding to CD80/CD86. When bound, it provides an internal signal that inactivates the T cell. Activated T cells carry with them a mechanism for inactivating themselves and preventing excessive accumulation.
4. *Regulatory T cells.* Various T cells have been found to regulate and reduce the activity of other lymphocytes. The mechanisms by which these regulatory cells exert their effects are not yet well understood. The best known of these is a CD4+ T population called T regulatory cells, which inhibit the activity of other T cells directed against self-antigens and infectious agents. Although it may seem odd to reduce activity against infectious agents, it should be noted that some types of responses produce unacceptable inflammatory injury to certain tissues (eg, the eye and the

central nervous system). In these cases, regulatory T cells are among several mechanisms used to promote noninflammatory responses.

5. *Mutual inhibition of Th1 and Th2 cells.* Most responses to antigenic stimuli involve a mix of Th1 and Th2 responses. This balance is maintained by the mutual inhibition exerted by Th1 T cells against Th2 cells and vice versa. IL-4 and -10 and T-cell growth factor-β produced by Th2 cells inhibits the activity of Th1 cells, whereas IFN-γ produced by Th1 cells inhibits the activity of Th2 cells.

6. *T-cell regulation of B-cell activation.* More than 99% of B-cell activations require participation and regulation by T cells. This action helps prevent the random and uncontrolled production of potentially self-reactive antibodies.

Review of tumor immunology

Overview

The importance of the immune system in surveillance and prevention of malignancy has been hypothesized since the early twentieth century. The past three or four decades have seen an explosion of knowledge in molecular immunology that has led to an understanding of immune functions that are vitally important in each individual's response to malignant transformation. Although from an evolutionary standpoint the immune system's primary function has been to defend the host against infectious invaders, the immune system's role in eliminating autologous transformed cells may be equally important in higher vertebrates. Several lines of evidence indicate the immune system's importance in preventing proliferation of malignant cells. The basic roles of the immune system in the major aspects of tumor immunology are summarized in Table 1.

Immune surveillance

Macfarlane Burnet proposed the concept of immune surveillance in the 1950s. This concept refers to the continual surveillance for—and destruction of—abnormal or mutated cells by the immune system. Although this concept has been debated since its original proposal, the role of the immune system in surveillance for malignant cells is supported by several lines of evidence. The frequency and complexity of cell replication predisposes to the development of many malignant or potentially malignant cells throughout each individual's lifetime, yet only a small proportion of mammals develop malignancy during their existence. In humans, most malignancies develop in the later years of life as the mathematical probability (based on the error rate in chromosome replication and the sheer number of cell divisions that occur) of malignant cells gaining the appropriate mutations to escape the immune system increases. With aging of the immune system there also

Table 1
Roles of the immune system in tumor immunology

Roll of immune system	Evidence		Clinical examples
	Clinical	Experimental	
Immune surveillance	Increased rate of malignancy in immunodeficient patients Mononuclear cell infiltrates around tumors	Gene-targeted (knockout) and lymphocyte subset– depleted immunodeficient mouse models	Patients who have AIDS Transplant patients
Immunoediting	Increased rate of cancer in elderly persons	Higher immunogenicity of tumors from immunodeficient mice	Cancer transmitted from organ donors
Tumor destruction	Spontaneous regression of malignances	Tumor-infiltrating lymphocytes found in tumors that recognize tumor antigens	Melanoma
	Response to immunotherapy	Numerous animal models with immunotherapy-based tumor regression	Sarcoma
	Mononuclear cell infiltrates around tumors		Colorectal cancer
Tumor promotion	Increased rate of malignancy in chronic inflammation and infection	Tumor necrosis factor knockout mice do not develop tumors	*H pylori* gastric cancer
		Tumor-associated macrophages promote tumors	Hepatitis B hepatocellular cancer

may be decreased ability to recognize and eradicate abnormal cells. The low rate of actual malignancy, especially in the earlier years of life, indicates that some protective mechanism continually surveys and eradicates abnormal cells generated in the normal process of cell division and replication, namely immune surveillance.

Other clinical and experimental observations support the role of the immune system in surveillance of malignancy. Clinically there have been several reports of spontaneous regression of documented malignancies, primarily melanomas, which are most likely mediated by the immune system. Immunodeficiency, either clinically induced (eg, transplant patients) or occurring naturally (eg, patients who have AIDS) is well known to increase susceptibility to certain types of malignancies. In the past two decades, molecularly defined murine models that tested specific aspects of immunodeficiency have supported strongly the concept of immune surveillance in cancer. Pathologically it is common to see intense immune cell infiltrates around established tumors (eg, melanoma and colon cancer), which indicates an attempted response to the tumor by the host immune system.

Despite increasing evidence that supports the concept of immune surveillance, individuals with normally functioning immune systems still develop malignancy. The explanation for this clinical fact is related to the failure of the immune system to eradicate all malignant cells at the outset, leading to clinically aggressive tumors that already have escaped the host's defense mechanism.

Tumor antigens

The primary means for the host immune system to differentiate tumor cells as foreign is through the recognition of different types of abnormal molecules (tumor antigens) produced by the tumor cell that are identified as non-self by the host's immune system. Tumor antigens are generated by the tumor cell in various ways, including mutation of normal self-proteins, overexpression or aberrant expression of normal self-proteins, glycoproteins or glycolipids, and foreign protein products of oncogenes or oncogenic viruses. Without the expression of tumor antigens, it would be difficult—if not impossible—for the host to identify and react against malignant cells. A wide variety of molecules can serve as tumor antigens, although their ability to invoke an immune response depends on several factors, including immunogenicity, degree of expression, and accessibility to the cells of the immune system. There are several major categories of tumor antigens, which are classified by molecular structure and source (Table 2).

Mutated self-gene products

Mutations that lead to abnormal protein products can develop in genes in which the mutation is necessary for the development of malignancy (proto-oncogenes and tumor-suppressor genes) or random genes in the genome whose products are not necessary for malignancy. In either case, when these mutated gene products are expressed, they can be processed by the MHC class I or class II antigen-processing pathway and recognized as foreign by the immune system. In some cases this can serve as the basis for a subsequent host immune reaction against the tumor cells that bear these antigens.

Normal cell proteins abnormally or aberrantly expressed

Normal cell proteins that are absent or expressed in low levels in normal cells can serve as tumor antigens in malignant cells. Although these proteins are normal in structure and function, in the conventional state they are

Table 2
Categories of tumor antigens

Tumor antigen category	Cause of antigenicity	Example
Mutated self gene products (proto-oncogenes, tumor suppressor genes or random genes)	Abnormal molecular structure caused by mutation	Proto-oncogene: *Ras* Tumor suppressor gene: *p53* Random gene: *p91*
Normal cell proteins, which are not expressed or expressed in low levels in normal cells	Aberrant or abnormal expression (overexpression or expression in dedifferentiated cells)	Overexpression: tyrosinase, MART, gp100, *Her-2/neu* Dedifferentiated: CEA, AFP Aberrant: Cancer testis antigens
Glycolipids or glycoproteins	Overexpression or abnormal structure	Mucins: Muc-1, CA19-9, CA 125 Gangliosides: GM_2, GD_2 Blood group antigens
Oncogenic virus products	Foreign proteins	*DNA virus* Cervical cancer: HPV E6 and E7 proteins Lymphoma: EBV EBNA-1 protein *RNA virus* T-cell leukemia/lymphoma: HTLV-1

Abbreviations: AFP, alpha-fetoprotein; CEA, carcinoembryonic antigen; EBNA, Epstein-Barr nuclear antigen; EBV, Epstein-Barr virus; HTLV, human T-cell lymphotrophic virus; HPV, human papillomavirus; MART, melanoma antigen recognized by T cells.

believed to induce tolerance in the immune system because of their low level expression. When overexpressed in transformed cells they can stimulate an antitumor immune response. These tumor antigens have been studied most extensively in melanoma (eg, tyrosinase, melanoma antigen recognized by T cells) and have been used for several immunotherapeutic clinical trials.

Some proteins are normally expressed during differentiation but are not expressed in normal tissues. These proteins (eg, carcinoembryonic antigen in colon cancer) may be aberrantly expressed in dedifferentiated malignant cells and can serve as tumor antigens. Other proteins normally expressed on certain cell lines, such as germ cells, can be aberrantly expressed on malignant somatic cells leading to recognition as tumor antigens. This type of tumor antigen includes the cancer testis antigens, which can be expressed in a wide variety of tumors.

Abnormal glycolipids or glycoproteins

Many tumors overexpress normal or express abnormal cell surface glycolipids or glycoproteins, which can serve as tumor antigens with appropriate immune recognition. Included in this category of tumor antigens are mucins

(CA-125, CA-19-9, MUC-1), gangliosides (GM_2, GD_2), and blood group antigens. These antigens can be used for diagnostic or therapeutic purposes and may contribute to the malignant behavior of the tumor through characteristics such as tissue invasion and metastases.

Oncogenic virus products

DNA and RNA viruses have been shown to induce tumors in humans. The protein products of viral replication can be processed internally and expressed on the tumor cell surface in combination with MHC class I. These peptides are highly immunogenic, and the immune system plays an important role in preventing tumors induced by these viruses through immune surveillance. Examples of human DNA virus induced tumors include Epstein-Barr virus, which can lead to B-cell lymphomas, and human papillomavirus, which can lead to cervical cancer. Adult T-cell leukemia and lymphoma is caused by a RNA retrovirus, human T-cell lymphotrophic virus 1.

Immune response to tumors

The innate and adaptive immune responses have been shown to be active in destruction of tumor cells. Although there is some crossover between components of the innate and adaptive immune responses in tumor immunity, we discuss the principal components of the effector mechanisms of these responses in relation to malignant cells.

Innate immune response to tumor cells

NK cells can kill target cells without the need for prior activation. This phenomenon is primarily effective in virally infected and stressed cells but also plays a role in malignant cells (which may be regarded as stressed cells). NK cells kill tumor cells in which MHC class I molecules (which at normal levels inhibit NK cells) are absent or underexpressed. Many tumors lose expression of MHC class I molecules during malignant transformation while they continue to express ligands that activate NK cells, which makes them particularly susceptible to NK cell killing. Virally induced tumors, such as Epstein-Barr virus lymphomas, exhibit viral antigens that are recognized by NK cells, which makes them susceptible to NK cell killing.

Macrophages may recognize some tumor antigens leading to tumoricidal activity. Increased effectiveness in killing tumor cells has been observed in vitro and probably occurs in vivo in conjunction with cytokine activation, such as IFN-γ. The mechanisms of tumor cell killing by macrophages is the same as with infectious microorganisms, namely the intra- or extracellular release of lysosomal enzymes, reactive oxygen intermediates, and nitric oxide. Macrophages also can secrete tumor necrosis factor, which can lead to tumor cell death.

Cytokines are active in innate and adaptive immunity, mediating and regulating the less specific immune reactions of the innate immune system and the highly specific reactions of the adaptive immune system. They can play a role in tumor immunology through several effector mechanisms. Although many cytokines play a role in tumor immunology, the principal cytokines in the innate response to tumor cells are as follows. Tumor necrosis factor activates endothelial cells and can cause coagulation, leading to tumor necrosis and directly stimulating apoptosis. IL-12, IL-15, and the type I interferons (IFN-α, IFN-β) stimulate NK cells, which leads to proliferation and increased cytotoxic activity.

Adaptive immune response to tumor cells

CTLs are the primary mechanism of tumor cell killing of the adaptive immune response. CD8+ T cells (CTLs) specific for tumor antigens have been demonstrated in many different types of solid tumors in vivo and have been shown to cause tumor cell destruction in vitro. Inflammatory infiltrates derived from some solid tumors contain CTLs that are capable of killing the tumors from which they are isolated (termed "tumor infiltrating lymphocytes"). In many cases, generation of tumoricidal CTLs requires the participation of APCs (or dendritic cells) to present the relevant tumor antigen to the CTLs in the appropriate conditions for an antigen-specific immune response. MHC class I and class II molecules must be present to stimulate the production of CTLs because the APCs express both classes of MHC molecules, whereas tumor cells often do not express MHC class II molecules (costimulatory molecules). T-helper cells (CD4+ cells) play a role in the antitumor immune reaction by providing cytokines that stimulate CTL development and secrete IFN-γ, which can activate the cytotoxic activity of macrophages. Finally, CTLs are probably the effector mechanism for immune surveillance through eradication of mutated cells, destroying these malignant or premalignant cells before their ability to replicate and metastasize.

The host immune system can generate specific antibodies against tumor antigens, which can lead to cytotoxic reactions against the antigen-bearing tumor cells. Antibodies can bind to a wide variety of tumor antigens, including polysaccharides, lipids, and proteins, which broadens the number of tumor antigens that can be exploited by the host immune system for cytotoxic reactions. This is in contrast to T-cell antigen receptors, which recognize only protein-derived antigens. The mechanisms of cell killing mediated by antibodies include antibody-dependent cell-mediated cytotoxicity and complement-mediated cytotoxicity.

Tumor escape from immune response

Malignant tumors have developed various mechanisms to evade the host immune response. When a tumor possesses the right combination of mechanisms to evade the immune response along with the appropriate growth characteristics and environment, the result is a clinically apparent tumor.

Tumor characteristics

The growth rate of some aggressive tumors can overwhelm immune responses before the development of an adequate immune response can occur. In many cases, tumor antigens are only weakly immunogenic, which limits the development of a cytotoxic immune response against the tumor cells. The immune system often eradicates strongly immunogenic cells, which allows growth of the weakly immunogenic cell clones within the tumor and subsequent evasion of the immune response, a process called tumor editing.

Tumor cells may not express the necessary costimulatory molecules to stimulate an immune response. Tumor cells also may selectively lose expression of immunogenic antigens because of their genetic instability and high mitotic rates. Loss of these antigens can confer a growth advantage as long as the antigenic molecule is not required for cell growth. Tumor antigens also may induce immunologic tolerance in the immune system, which has been shown to increase tumor growth in experimental models. Immunogenic antigens may be shielded from immune recognition by other molecules, such as mucopolysaccharides, a process called antigen masking. Tumor cells can secrete or express factors that suppress or block the immune response, including transforming growth factor-β, which inhibits lymphocytes and macrophages, and Fas ligand, which can lead to lymphocyte cell death.

Tumor environment

The environment in which the tumor generates and grows may inhibit the immune response against it. The tumor microenvironment has been shown to be acidic or with a lower O_2 tension in some cases inhibiting or destroying the cells of the immune system. In these cases the tumor can adapt to the altered local environment, whereas the cells of the immune system cannot. Regulatory T cells in the tumor may inhibit the functions of the immune system cells through the production of inhibitory cytokines. This action has been demonstrated in animal models, in which increased numbers of regulatory T cells have been found in some tumors. When depleted of regulatory T cells by experimental techniques, improved antitumor immunity has been demonstrated in animal models.

Therapeutic interventions

Many different types of immunotherapeutic interventions are currently in use or under investigation for cancer therapy. They are discussed in detail in many of the articles in this issue. We briefly list and define the principal methods of therapeutic interventions in tumor immunology, referring the reader to the other articles for a more in-depth discussion of the rationale and justification for these treatment methods.

Active immunotherapy

Active stimulation of the host's own immune system holds the most promise for a durable response to malignant transformation of cells.

Currently, this is an area of intense research because the appeal of a long-lasting, nontoxic, nondebilitating method of treatment for malignancy is obvious.

Vaccination. A wide variety of vaccination techniques have been used in an attempt to stimulate host immunity against malignant cells, including vaccination with tumor antigens either purified or derived from whole tumor cells or tumor lysates, dendritic cell vaccines that express tumor cell antigens introduced through various techniques (eg, tumor antigen gene transfection, direct tumor antigen pulsation, or dendritic-tumor cell fusion), DNA vaccines that use DNA encoding for tumor antigens, and viral vector vaccines that use viral vectors that encode for tumor antigens and stimulatory cytokines. The development of functional cancer vaccines is much more complex than vaccines against infectious organisms because of cancer cells' adaptability to different conditions that the immune system displays and the various ways in which tumor cells circumvent the immune system.

Host immunity enhancement through tumor cell modification. The host immune system can be enhanced by genetically engineering tumor cells to produce absent factors that, when missing, aid the tumor cells in immune escape. Tumor cells often do not express costimulatory molecules, which impedes the immune reaction. Tumor cells can be removed and costimulatory genes can be transfected into them. When reinjected, these tumor cells can stimulate immune reactions and generate CTLs that subsequently react against all viable tumor cells present in the host. Antitumor immunity also can be enhanced by transfecting tumor cells with cytokine genes. When secreted by the tumor cells in vivo, these genes also can stimulate adaptive immune responses (CTLs) against the transfected tumor cells, which also cross-react with the nontransfected tumor cells, leading to tumor destruction.

Impede inhibitory pathways. Tumors can exploit normal inhibitory pathways of the immune system to hinder their recognition and destruction. These pathways function to control the immune reaction from developing autoimmune reactions (self-tolerance) and regulate the immune response to the appropriate conditions and location. By blocking these normal inhibitory pathways, tumor immunity can be enhanced. A concern is the development of autoimmune reactions, which has been the limiting factor in this type of therapy.

Nonspecific stimulation. Stimulation of the immune system can occur in a nonspecific manner with substances that enhance or activate certain aspects of the immune system. This represents the oldest form of immunotherapy for cancers, dating back to Coley's attempts in the 1890s to stimulate the immune system with bacterial toxins ("Coley's toxins") after he observed that some patients experienced tumor regression after bacterial infections. Bacillus Calmette-Guerin, a mycobacterial extract that causes an inflammatory response and activates macrophages, has been injected directly into various tumors and had some reported responses. Antibodies used in a nonspecific fashion to stimulate or suppress functions of the immune system are currently under investigation. Cytokines that enhance the immune response also represent a nonspecific immune enhancement technique.

Passive immunotherapy. The transfer of effector agents, such as antibodies and T cells for the treatment of malignancy, is termed passive immunotherapy. Although these methods of immunotherapy are not as specific or long-lasting as adaptive immunotherapy techniques, they are quicker and more commercially adaptable to larger populations of oncology patients.

Antitumor antibodies. Several different antitumor monoclonal antibodies have been developed over the past decade for tumor-specific immunotherapy. Currently more than 100 different monoclonal antibodies are in use or under evaluation for use as therapeutic agents in various malignancies. Monoclonal antibodies have been shown to improve survival in several solid tumors, including breast, lung, and colon. The mechanism of action of monoclonal antibodies is partly determined by the antigenic target of the antibody. These mechanisms include the accepted mechanisms for antibody-mediated defense against foreign antigens, such as complement activation, opsonization, phagocytosis, and specific mechanisms, such as activation of intrinsic apoptosis pathways, inhibition of vascular growth factors (bevacizumab), and inhibition of growth signaling pathways (trastuzumab, cetuzimab, panitumumab). Monoclonal antibodies have been coupled with cytotoxic agents (eg, ricin, diphtheria toxin, radioisotopes) to improve efficacy.

Adoptive cellular therapy. The use of cultured immune cells with antitumor activity transferred into a tumor-bearing host is adoptive cellular immunity. Encouraging results using autologous tumor-infiltrating lymphocytes expanded in culture with IL-2 stimulation have been demonstrated in melanoma and renal cell carcinoma. Isolation of lymphocytes from the peripheral blood, derived from NK cells (LAK cells), has demonstrated antitumor activity in some murine and human trials.

Graft-versus-leukemia effect. In patients who have leukemia, administration of T cells combined with stem cell transplant can induce a graft-mediated immune reaction against the leukemia cells. Graft-versus-host disease can occur.

Although there is ample evidence that the immune system plays a vital role in maintenance and prevention of malignant transformation, clinically apparent tumors develop when the tumor escapes immune system recognition. The field of tumor immunology attempts to manipulate the immune system to recognize and eradicate the offending malignancy. Recent evidence indicates that the potential to use the immune system for successful therapeutic interventions in fighting established malignancy is great, with several immunotherapeutic methods currently in use and many more under investigation.

ELSEVIER
SAUNDERS

Surg Oncol Clin N Am
16 (2007) 737–753

SURGICAL
ONCOLOGY CLINICS
OF NORTH AMERICA

Tumor Microenvironment and the Immune Response

Silvia Selleri, PhD[a,b], Cristiano Rumio, PhD[b],
Marianna Sabatino, MD[a],
Francesco M. Marincola, MD[a], Ena Wang, MD[a,*]

[a]Infectious Disease and Immunogenetics Section, Department of Transfusion Medicine,
Clinical Center, National Institutes of Health, Bethesda, MD 20892, USA
[b]Universita' degli Studi di Milano, Department of Human Morphology,
via Mangiagalli 31, 20133 Milan, Italy

"A few observations and much reasoning lead to error; many observations and a little reasoning to truth." Alexis Carrel (The Nobel Prize in Physiology or Medicine, 1912)

Accurate observation is the fundamental preliminary step that opens the door to scientific investigation. Within the community interested in biomedical research, nobody more than surgeons has the opportunity to observe human pathology as it evolves in natural conditions or in response to treatment and relate the findings to the bench scientists. Comprehensive observation may be particularly important when complex biologic phenomena are studied that cannot be explained readily by monothematic explanations provided by experimental models. Human cancer, in particular, is a fastidious scientific challenge that aggravates the innate complexity of human biology by adding capricious permutations to natural homeostatic mechanisms caused by the intrinsic genetic instability of cancer cells [1]. Because genetic changes accumulate randomly in time, each patient's cancer progresses into a private pathologic entity that cannot be represented accurately by the minimization of experimental variance applied to the testing of hypotheses in in vivo animal models or in in vitro experimental systems using conventional cancer cell lines [2]. Despite the enormous progress that basic biomedical sciences achieved in the last decades in the

Silvia Selleri is partially supported by FIRC (Federazione Italiana per la Ricerca sul Cancro).
* Corresponding author.
E-mail address: ewang@cc.nih.gov (E. Wang).

1055-3207/07/$ - see front matter. Published by Elsevier Inc.
doi:10.1016/j.soc.2007.07.002
surgonc.theclinics.com

understanding of specific biologic processes, cancer mortality has minimally changed, which reflects our limited ability to translate such knowledge into practical benefit for the patient [3]. It is our contention that this is partly caused by the unfortunate shift in priorities by the scientific establishment favoring theoretical investigations over direct clinical observation [4]. In this context, surgeons suffered a diminished role despite their privileged place at the bedside and should regain control while modern technology is providing the unprecedented opportunity to study human disease at the whole genome level.

The study of the tumor microenvironment in which the dialog between cancer cells and the host primarily occurs exemplifies the opportunity to study human cancers directly with the purpose of sifting through direct observation among the broad range of theories developed through experimental observation those relevant to human disease. For example, in animal models, interleukin(IL)-23 can either promote or hamper cancer growth [5–10]; however, information about its bioavailability in human cancers, modality of expression, and biologic effects—information that can potentially provide insight into the interpretation of such models—is limited.

Without clinical information, accurate follow-up, high-quality sample collection, and preservation, scientific conclusions are only based on theoretical assumptions that are unlikely to lead to clinical breakthroughs. In this article we discuss our understanding of the relationship between cancer cells and the host immune response. We emphasize the critical role that future clinical investigations, led by surgical oncologists, may have for the assessment of the validity of the disparate hypotheses so far formulated at the bench side.

Evidence of immune surveillance in cancer

Cancer is a systemic disease caused by cells that have lost the ability to control their growth and maintain their programmed organ tropism. Although random mutations occur incessantly during cancer progression, in the primary stages and for a long time during the metastatization process, human cancers retain characteristics typical of their tissue of origin and, most importantly, retain a phenotype closely related to that of normal autologous cells of the same lineage from which they derived [11,12]. Although some animal cancer models express mutated proteins that are recognized by immune cells as "non-self" antigens [13], most human tumors express nonmutated normal proteins that are part of the normal function of the cell lineage from which they originated. For instance, the expression of classic melanoma differentiation antigens is shared by melanoma cells and normal melanocytes as part of the differentiation process responsible for the production of pigment [14,15]. Most cancer cells behave immunologically like normal cells and are not spontaneously capable of inducing strong immune responses similar to those induced by transplanted heterologous organs, which bear heterologous human leukocyte antigen molecules on their surface.

Although human cancers most likely represent "self" tissues, numerous lines of evidence support the notion that the immune system is cognitive of autologous tumor and produces antibodies [16,17] and T cells that recognize specific cancer cells [18,19]. The reason for this recognition is better explained by the pathophysiology of autoimmune reactions than by that of allotransplant rejection. Although cancer cells are similar to the rest of the host cells, they revert to an embryonic stage and produce pro-factors that alter the environment around them most often to their own benefit. This production results in a chronic inflammatory process that characterizes the biology of most cancers compared with normal healthy tissues and assimilates them to tissues that suffer chronic or acute insults, which are at the basis of autoimmune phenomena [20].

In the early stages of cancer development, it is likely that the innate part of the immune system, a term that describes our inborn defenses that sense potential threats independent of previous exposure, recognizes cancer cells as abnormal. Because some of the factors produced by cancer cells may provide signals that alarm the host immune system, effector immune mechanisms are stimulated to destroy them, which results in a reduced incidence of cancer development. This phenomenon is generally termed "immune surveillance." It has been described extensively in animal models [21–23] and is supported in humans by the observation that congenital or acquired immunodeficiency is associated with increased prevalence of various types of cancer [24–28]. Immune surveillance plays an important role in the early stages of oncogenesis and generally leads to the elimination of cancer cells or their restraint in situ [29].

In time, under selective pressure by the immune system, tumor cells that survived this first line of defense undergo a process referred to as immunoediting. Probably at that stage they refine the production of factors that may promote their survival by eliminating factors with immune stimulatory properties and retaining factors that foster angiogenesis, tissue regeneration, and growth or can reduce the ability of immune effector cells to perform their function. For example, inhibitory cytokines, such as IL-4, IL-6, and IL-10, are often expressed by tumors and may have complex but overall immune suppressive effects on the infiltrating immune cells in natural conditions [30–32]. In response to cytokines produced by tumor cells, mononuclear phagocytes express specialized and polarized functional properties [33,34], which in turn promote tumor cell proliferation and modulate adaptive immunity (a term that refers to the arm of the immune response that requires previous exposure to an antigen to acquire specific recognition) by controlling the activation of T, B, natural killer, and natural killer T cells [35]. The dominant phenotype of macrophages that infiltrate tumors is that of weakly immunoreactive cells involved in tissue remodeling and down-modulation of destructive inflammatory processes (referred to as M2 macrophages because they participate in polarized T helper cell 2 reactions). As a net result, M2 macrophages promote tumor progression, tissue repair, and remodeling [36] and have immunoregulatory functions [34].

Chemokines, colony stimulating factor-1, and vascular endothelial growth factor-A produced by tumor cells and infiltrating M2 macrophages further recruit tumor-associated macrophages and sustain their survival in tumors [20]. Activated macrophage and tumor cells produce growth factors such as insulin-like growth factor, nerve growth factor, and epithelium growth factor. As tumor cells adapt to this first line of defense of the organism, they acquire properties that not only allow avoidance of effector mechanisms but also foster their growth through the recruitment of immune cells that produce soluble factors, such as cytokines, chemokines, growth, and angiogenic factors that help the development of an environment that favors tumor growth [20,37–39]. It is this chronic inflammatory process that subsequently fosters the growth of cancer and establishes the premise for a possible immune reaction that, when properly activated, leads to tumor rejection if conditions are met that equate to the biologic process that activates flares of autoimmunity [20].

In humans, the immune response is clearly involved in the dialog of the host with tumor cells. In particular, the adaptive arm of the immune response, which includes antigen-specific T cells and antibody-producing B cells, has been shown in several tumor models to be capable of specifically recognizing tumor-associated antigens. In melanoma, tumor-infiltrating lymphocytes (TIL) can be expanded readily from metastases in the presence of the IL-2. TIL can recognize autologous tumor cells and melanoma cells from other patients that share the same human leukocyte antigen phenotype of the person from whom they were generated. TILs do not recognize autologous or foreign normal cells, however. This observation represents the best evidence in humans that the immune system can naturally mount T-cell–mediated immune responses that are specifically directed against cancer cells [40]. The presence of TIL at the tumor site is associated with increased ability of circulating lymphocytes from patients with cancer to recognize tumor cells, which suggests that the tumor-bearing status induces the activation of systemic immune response in a kind of self-immunization process similar to those reactivities observed in patients who have with chronic autoimmune disease [41].

Research has shown that patients who have cancer display strong T-cell reactivities against proteins that are expressed only by cancer cells and not by normal cells—with the exception of testes—and are referred to as cancer testes antigens [18,42]. Because the testes are an immunoprivileged organ and their cells do not express the human leukocyte antigen molecules necessary to present antigen to immune cells, it can be concluded that also the T-cell–mediated immune responses directed against cancer testes antigens are directed specifically against cancer cells in natural conditions. Research has shown that patients who have cancer bear in their circulation high titers of antibodies that recognize most often cancer testes antigens [16], which suggests that B cells are naturally involved in the recognition of cancer cells.

The observation that T-cell and antibody responses can be detected in the blood and within cancerous lesions of tumor-bearing patients questions the role that the adaptive immune response may play in the control of cancer growth [31,43,44]. To explain the paradoxical observation of a balanced co-existence of tumor antigen-specific T cells with their target in a progressively growing tumor mass, several hypotheses have been proposed. Accumulated experience, however, has shown that predictions of biologic phenomena based on these intriguing theories and based on preclinical models but untested in humans frequently deviate from the behavior of human disease, and future investigations should strongly encourage the involvement of physicians in the recruitment of human material to be brought to the bench side to frame such hypotheses according to human reality [2,4].

In this article we emphasize the role that surgeons could play in contributing to the solution of this puzzling observation. In particular, we believe that the analysis of tumor lesions undergoing immunotherapy may shed important insights on the mechanisms that can turn a chronic indolent inflammatory process into an acute reaction that could lead to tumor destruction. We hypothesize that such information not only will lead to the understanding of the mechanisms of tumor rejection by the immune system but also provide a mechanistic explanation for a common pathway followed by immune cells when inducing tissue-specific rejection in the context of autoimmunity and during acute response to pathogens [20].

Heterogeneity of human subjects and their cancers

One of the main reasons why experimental models often do not fit human reality is their intrinsic requirement for the minimization of experimental variance. Although the hypothesis testing approach is required for the validation of a biologic theory, it does not address its relevance to a particular pathologic condition because the question is extracted from human pathology and transferred to an arbitrarily chosen experimental model. This is the reason why most immunotherapy models that show efficacy in animal models do not translate into clinical benefit. This concept particularly applies to the study of tumor immunology, which is a compound discipline in which the complexity of cancer biology is approached through the complexity of immune biology. Human cancer is a heterogeneous disease to the point that each cancer is a separate biologic entity specific for each individual patient [45]. A good example of the heterogeneity of cancer is the mixed response phenomenon. In several cases, patients treated with immunotherapy approaches experience regression of some lesions, whereas other synchronous lesions continue undisturbed in their growth. Considering that a patient's immune responses during that particular treatment are identical, the mixed response phenomenon demonstrates how even within the same patient tumors may display biologic characteristics that are sufficiently disparate to significantly affect the natural history of the disease.

To the individual heterogeneity of cancer biology, the extremely different genetic background of each individual adds a level of complexity that cannot be compensated for by any experimental model. The immune system includes pathways characterized by extreme genetic variability among individuals; this extreme genetic variability might have served evolutionarily the need of the immune system to adapt to the extreme variability of pathogens against which the immune response is primarily aimed [46].

Although cancer heterogeneity and variability in the genetics of the immune response in different individuals may limit our ability to test hypotheses in humans, it may present a powerful model to discern common patterns that may explain specific biologic events despite such heterogeneity. Recent advancements in the study of human disease adopting high-throughput genomic approaches allow for the simultaneous analysis of the whole genome. Signatures for relevant events, such as response to therapy or prediction of disease outcome, may be identified if the collaborations between clinicians and scientists are optimized and relevant material appropriately collected could reach the bench side [43,47,48].

Modulation of the tumor microenvironment by immunotherapy

From a clinical standpoint, several strategies have been implemented to awaken an immune response against cancer. A comprehensive discussion of immunotherapy approaches is beyond our purposes, and we limit our discussion to examples that demonstrate the role of immunotherapy as a modulator of the tumor microenvironment. In particular, we discuss how immunotherapy, when effective in inducing tumor rejection, takes advantage of the natural chronic inflammation that is ongoing at the tumor site but is insufficient to induce tumor regression and turns it into an acute inflammatory process capable of powerfully activating effector immune mechanisms [20,31].

Advances in immunotherapy against cancer include systemic administration of cytokines [49,50], tumor antigen-based vaccines [51], adoptive transfer of tumor antigen-specific T cells [52], and antibody therapy [53,54]. Recently, significant interest had been directed toward the development of dendritic cell (DC)-based vaccinations in which tumor antigens are presented to T cells by cells characterized by "professional" antigen presentation characteristics. DC can concomitantly present antigens (signal one) to CD8-expressing cytotoxic T cells through human leukocyte antigen class I T-cell receptor interactions but also to CD4-expressing helper T cells because they express in abundance human leukocyte antigen class II molecules that target the latter. DCs also express costimulatory molecules capable of increasing the activatory antigen-dependent signals through cell-to-cell interactions (signal 2). More recently, methods have been described for the full activation of DCs that can be educated to produce biologically active IL-12p70, a cytokine with potent activatory effects on effector T cells [55]. Although tumor antigen-directed vaccines with or without DCs have been effective in increasing the number of circulating tumor antigen-specific T cells, they have not produced the desired effects on tumor regression, possibly because the T cells generated do not have the effector properties necessary for killing and destruction of tumor cells [56].

For instance, DCs that are effective in inducing T-cell responses when injected at the vaccine site have different characteristics compared with cells that infiltrate the tumors receiving the vaccine-induced T cells. In the tumor microenvironment, DCs generally are defective in number and are deficient functionally [57]. Such deficiency can be reversed by in vitro expansion and activation [55,58]. These ex vivo manipulations cannot compensate for the in vivo need of activating DCs within the tumor microenvironment, however, because adoptively transferred DCs do not travel there. More recently, several lines of evidence based on animal experimentation and limited information from human trials suggested that homeostatic mechanisms regulate the immune response through the activation of regulatory T cells that can inhibit the effector functions of cytotoxic and helper T cells during the contraction of the immune response. It seems that in cancer, the balance is shifted toward excessive regulatory compensation because cancer tissues generally display a chronic inflammatory profile that does not produce enough proinflammatory stimuli to overcome regulatory mechanisms because they occur during acute pathogen infection. Depletion of Treg prolongs the survival of tumor-bearing mice [59,60]. Treg frequency is associated with outcome of therapy in patients treated with rIL-2, and therapies that aim at the selective depletion of Treg are being considered [61]. Although the existence of Treg in humans is undeniable, their weight in modulating tumor/host interactions remains to be elucidated.

The tumor microenvironment: where progression and regression occur

Most of the studies directed at the analysis of tumor host interactions in human have been performed on circulating lymphocytes to test their ability to recognize and kill cancer cells [62] because of the ease in which blood components can be obtained by venipuncture. We have repeatedly emphasized that tumor immunobiology is better studied within the tumor microenvironment, however, where the active interactions between immune and cancer cells actually occur.

If cancer cells can be recognized by immune cells such as TIL naturally present in the metastases, the biologic reason for their inability to clear tumor cells might be most efficiently tested within the tumor site. Various hypotheses have been raised to explain the inability of TIL to spontaneously induce cancer rejection. Tumor cells can modulate immune response by producing soluble factors that can suppress the immune response [30]. As proposed recently, tumors can be characterized by seven hallmarks: self-sufficiency in growth signals, insensitivity to antigrowth signals, evasion of apoptosis, limitless replicative potential, sustained angiogenesis and tissue invasion and metastasis, and avoidance of immunosurveillance [63]. These processes involve molecules that affect the immune response, such as IL-4 and IL-10 (which induce down-regulation of immune effector mechanisms), IL-6 (which suppresses inflammation), and TGF-β (which inhibits T cell natural killer cell function) while at the same time activating immune regulatory mechanisms. Research also has proposed that tumors protect themselves from T-cell infiltration by constructing a barrier composed of stromal tissues that may prevent efficient T-cell priming and expansion at the tumor site [64,65].

Although these theories are intriguing, they have never been tested in human samples. Each of these theories may contribute an incremental explanation for immune tolerance, whereas the most important question of the mechanisms that can reverse the balances that in natural conditions favor cancer growth into successful tumor rejection remains unanswered. Our contention is that the biology of tumor rejection is simpler than that described by these complex theories and revolves around the acceptance of the concept that tumors in natural conditions do not provide sufficient stimulatory signals to induce the kind of immune reaction capable of destroying a pathogenic process [66], as can be observed during acute infections when an acute inflammatory process in the affected organ sustained by the presence of virus or bacterium is capable of activating immune cells at the receiving end of their effector function [67]. Identification of the natural requirements through the direct study of human tissues during acute clearance of infection and comparison with human tumor samples undergoing immunotherapy provides the information to understand the mechanisms for this switch from an indolent inflammatory process to an acute one. Implementations of strategies that could activate similar pathways in tumors through biologic therapy will lead to successful immune-mediated rejection of cancer [20].

Direct ex vivo study of the tumor microenvironment

Systematic analysis of immune responses indicates that a high frequency of tumor-recognizing T cells in peripheral blood does not correlate with tumor rejection [56,67]. Direct ex vivo monitoring of melanoma patients who are receiving melanoma antigen vaccination characterized a quiescent phenotype of tumor specific CD8+ T cells induced by the immunization. Ex vivo analysis of the CD8+ T cell function demonstrated that they lack expression of effector function related to their cytolytic activity and do not proliferate when exposed to antigen unless secondary costimulation is provided. This quiescent phenotype can be reversed by exposing the T cells in vitro to antigens in a costimulatory environment. This ex vivo model suggests that T cells induced by vaccination physiologically require more than antigen exposure to acquire their anticancer function. We hypothesize that tumor antigen-specific T cells that localize at a tumor site—although exposed to the antigen expressed on the surface of tumor cells—cannot be activated fully simply because the tumor microenvironment does not provide the necessary costimulation [67,68]. This hypothesis could be tested only by studying directly the tumor microenvironment in quiescence and during active immunotherapy [62].

Different strategies can be adopted to study the tumor microenvironment in human samples:

1. Excisional biopsies provide material of sufficient quantity and quality and allow structural investigations because the architecture of the lesion is not disturbed. This strategy does not allow serial sampling of the same lesion or follow its natural history, however. Biologic information obtained from an excised specimen is used with the assumption that the removed lesion is representative of those left in place. Unfortunately, extensive analysis of synchronous melanoma metastases has shown clearly that their phenotype can be different in a significant proportion of cases [69,70] and that it may rapidly change in response to immune manipulation [70,71].

2. Although they provide a limited amount of material and do not allow structural analyses, fine-needle aspirates (FNA) allow repeated sampling of the same lesion, which provides for an accurate estimate of the dynamic changes that occur in time within a lesion undergoing treatment [62,70,72]. FNA also allows the documentation of the natural history of the same lesion or its response to treatment, which avoids inaccuracies related to attempts to link the biology of the excised lesion to the in vivo behavior of those that were left in place [70]. FNA are commonly criticized because blind sampling of a lesion through a needle may not necessarily collect material that represents the whole lesion. Although this theoretical concern is sensible, practical experience has shown that repeated biopsies of the same lesions done at close time points and analyzed with a whole genome approach are representative of each other, particularly when a four-quadrant aspiration is performed [70].

3. Punch biopsies, through-cut biopsies, and other methods that do not require removal of the tumor are similar to FNA but could be used when the lesion is too shallow (punch biopsies) to perform successfully the aspiration, as in the case of basal cell carcinomas [73] or when biopsies are obtained under circumstances in which through-cut biopsies are routinely used for diagnostic purposes. In that case, either an extra passage or a small portion of a clinically required specimen may suffice for the analysis of tumor samples [62].

The use of FNA and other small sample material for the study of the tumor microenvironment was made possible by several biotechnologic breakthroughs during the previous decade. Among them is the ability to amplify up to 1 million-fold the small quantities of mRNA that can be obtained by these noninvasive approaches into sufficient quantities that could be applied to high-throughput studies in which the activation of all human genes could be analyzed simultaneously and with high fidelity using gene expression arrays [43,48,74–77]. According to our experience, FNA is the simplest and least invasive method, and it is well tolerated by patients, which makes it more palatable to the institutional review boards. The obtained material can be used successfully for direct ex vivo studies or in vitro analyses performed after expansion of tumor and immune cells, which can give precious information [68,71,78–80]. FNA are also well suitable for high-throughput gene expression analysis for the identification of biomarkers associated with tumor progression, regression, and prognosis [70,72].

Many techniques can be applied for the study of material derived from FNA, such as immunohistochemistry [69,81], flow cytometry and other immunofluorescence staining procedures [68,82], real-time quantitative polymerase chain reaction [68,71,83], and expansion of tumor cell/TIL pairs [79]. In Fig. 1, we illustrate a simple protocol for the collection of large libraries of relevant clinical samples using the FNA technique [62].

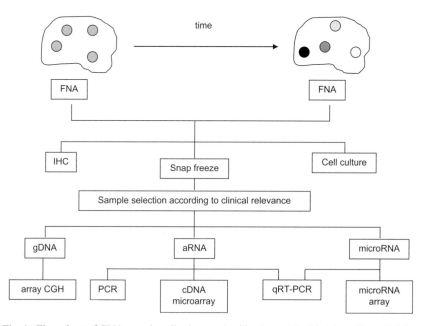

Fig. 1. Flow chart of FNA sample collections and utilizations. (*Modified from* Wang E, Marincola FM. A natural history of melanoma: serial gene expression analysis. Immunol Today 2000;21(12):619–23; with permission.)

FNA is a powerful, cheap, and easy tool that allows noninvasive collection of real-time information relevant to specific time points of the natural or treatment-induced history of a cancer [72,73]. In turn, this approach allows the formulation of novel hypotheses based on direct human observation. With this sampling approach, we could follow the natural history of melanoma metastases before and during immunotherapy [70,72]. We could generate autologous tumor cell lines/TIL pairs that could be used to test their interactions during active specific immunization against cancer [79] or could be cloned to characterize a novel tumor antigen [80].

Most importantly, through mRNA amplification it is possible to apply expression profiling with high-throughput gene arrays. With the advent of such modern high-throughput tools, existing theories based on oligothematic observations can be shaken. By prospectively following the history of melanoma metastases in patients undergoing tumor antigen-specific immunization followed by the systemic administration of IL-2, we could correlate transcriptional patterns with clinical outcome. Ranking of gene expression data from pretreatment samples identified 30 genes predictive of clinical response [70]. Analysis of their function denoted that approximately half of them were related to T-cell regulation, which suggested that immune responsiveness might be predetermined by a tumor microenvironment conducive to immune recognition.

We also studied the mechanism of action of IL-2 by sampling lesions during therapy. Global transcript analysis of melanoma metastases demonstrated that the administration of high-dose IL-2 to cancer patients does not induce migration of T cells within the tumor microenvironment [72] as previously hypothesized to explain the observation that their disappearance from the circulation was associated with increased frequency of tumor regression [84]. In contrast, an unbiased discovery-driven approach demonstrated that IL-2 activates innate immune mechanisms that had not been suspected before and could not have been hypothesized based on available knowledge. This unprecedented opportunity to re-evaluate the basis of human disease through high-throughput observation cannot be dismissed.

Finally, we investigated the mechanism that may be at the basis of tumor rejection through direct activation of immune stimulatory signals within the tumor microenvironment. Toll receptor (TLR)-7 agonists are commonly used to treat skin carcinomas because they selectively destroy cancer cells through an immune-mediated mechanism [85–87]. TLR agonists mimic single-stranded RNA of viruses [88] and activate DCs to secrete type one interferons and induce T-cell and natural killer cell activation, which in turn secretes interferon-γ. Simultaneously, effector mechanisms in activated T and natural killer cells induce destruction of target cells that feed tumor antigens to DCs for presentation to upcoming T and B cells attracted by the inflammatory process [88,89]. The cancer specificity of TLR-7 agonists consists in the preferential attraction of DCs that express TLR-7 to chronically inflamed tissues, including cancer [90]. TLR agonists exemplify how

the missing link between the induction of TA-specific T cells by immunization and their activation at the receiving end could be circumvented by
provoking acute inflammation to overcome regulatory mechanisms. We
recently documented the biologic pathways induced by a TLR-7 agonist
in a placebo-controlled, double-blinded, randomized study [73]. The study
confirmed that regression of basal cell carcinoma mediated by TLR agonists
follows a specific immunologic pattern that can be observed during acute
clearance of pathogen, acute allograft rejection, and flares of autoimmunity.
This process includes the activation of interferon-stimulated genes simultaneously to the activation of innate and adaptive immune effector mechanisms, which outlines the requirements for tissue-specific immune rejection.

With whole genome amplification technology, sufficient and representative genomic DNA also can be amplified from 5 to 10 ng DNA isolated
from FNA sample. Genetic alterations with time can be followed at individual gene levels using array comparative genomic hybridization. Using this
method in combination with gene expression profiling, we recently studied
a unique patient who had melanoma and survived for more than a decade
and completely responded to immunotherapy twice. During her history,
she experienced recurrence five times from which tumor cell lines were established for high-throughput analysis (cDNA microarray, microRNA, array
comparative genomic hybridization). With these methods we could verify
that the different metastases derived were from the same tumor progenitor
cell because they all shared the same signature. These studies may provide
important insights about the dynamics of cancer progression and support
the development of targeted anticancer therapies aimed at stable genetic
factors maintained through the endstage that determine the individuality
of each patient's disease [91].

The recently discovered endogenous noncoding microRNA generated
a new wave of interest in the scientific community. The miRNAome has
an important inhibitory role in posttranscription and translation processes.
Although the genes targeted by each miRNA have not been evaluated fully
yet, a clear difference in miRNA expression between normal and malignant
tissues from the same tissue linage has been documented [92], which suggests
that miRNA could play an important role in human neoplasia. miRNA
profiling has been reported as a sensitive method for disease classification
and prediction of clinical outcome [93–95]. With a valid miRNA amplification method, material isolated from FNA samples could be used for miRNA
analysis to identify treatment susceptibility and prognosis.

Summary

Clinicians, particularly surgeons, have a unique opportunity to contribute to the biomedical enterprise because they have physical access to the
tumor microenvironment on a routine basis and can obtain samples at the
most relevant times. By standing at the front line where the battle between

the host and cancer occurs, they can provide precious reagents that allow observations likely to yield information relevant to human disease. We hope that this article inspires some of the readers to become involved in the study of the tumor microenvironment.

References

[1] Lengauer C, Kinzler KW, Vogelstein B. Genetic instabilities in human cancers. Nature 1998; 396(6712):643–9.

[2] Marincola FM. Translational medicine: a two way road. J Transl Med 2003;1:1.

[3] Jemal A, Tiwari RC, Murray T, et al. Cancer statistics, 2004. CA Cancer J Clin 2004;54(1): 8–29.

[4] Marincola FM. In support of descriptive studies: relevance to translational research. J Transl Med 2007;5:21.

[5] Shan BE, Hao JS, Li QX, et al. Antitumor activity and immune enhancement of murine interleukin-23 expressed in murine colon carcinoma cells. Cell Mol Immunol 2006;3(1): 47–52.

[6] Hao JS, Shan BE. Immune enhancement and anti-tumour activity of IL-23. Cancer Immunol Immunother 2006;55(11):1426–31.

[7] Overwijk WW, De Visser KE, Tirion FH, et al. Immunological and antitumor effects of IL-23 as a cancer vaccine adjuvant. J Immunol 2006;176(9):5213–22.

[8] Langowski JL, Zhang X, Wu L, et al. IL-23 promotes tumour incidence and growth. Nature 2006;442(7101):461–5.

[9] Oniki S, Nagai H, Horikawa T, et al. Interleukin-23 and interleukin-27 exert quite different antitumor and vaccine effects on poorly immunogenic melanoma. Cancer Res 2006;66(12): 6395–404.

[10] Hu J, Yuan X, Belladonna ML, et al. Induction of potent antitumor immunity by intratumoral injection of interleukin 23-transduced dendritic cells. Cancer Res 2006;66(17): 8887–96.

[11] Wang E, Lichtenfels R, Bukur J, et al. Ontogeny and oncogenesis balance the transcriptional profile of renal cell cancer. Cancer Res 2004;64(20):7279–87.

[12] Mischiati C, Natali PG, Sereni A, et al. cDNA-array profiling of melanomas and paired melanocyte cultures. J Cell Physiol 2006;207(3):697–705.

[13] Schreiber K, Rowley DA, Riethmuller G, et al. Cancer immunotherapy and preclinical studies: why we are not wasting our time with animal experiments. Hematol Oncol Clin North Am 2006;20(3):567–84.

[14] Uchi H, Stan R, Turk MJ, et al. Unraveling the complex relationship between cancer immunity and autoimmunity: lessons from melanoma and vitiligo. Adv Immunol 2006;90: 215–41.

[15] Wilcox R, Markovic SN. Tumor immunotherapy in melanoma: on the dawn of a new era? Curr Opin Mol Ther 2007;9(1):70–8.

[16] Old LJ, Chen YT. New paths in human cancer serology. J Exp Med 1998;187(8):1163–7.

[17] Jager D. Potential target antigens for immunotherapy identified by serological expression cloning (SEREX). Methods Mol Biol 2007;360:319–26.

[18] Boon T, Coulie PG, Van den Eynde B. Tumor antigens recognized by T cells. Immunol Today 1997;18(6):267–8.

[19] Boon T, Coulie PG, van den Eynde BJ, et al. Human T cell responses against melanoma. Annu Rev Immunol 2006;24:175–208.

[20] Mantovani A, Romero P, Palucka AK, et al. Tumor immunity: effector response to tumor and the influence of the microenvironment. Lancet, in press.

[21] Shankaran V, Ikeda H, Bruce AT, et al. IFN-g and lymphocytes prevent primary tumour development and shape tumour immunogenicity. Nature 2001;410:1107–11.

[22] Dunn GP, Bruce AT, Ikeda H, et al. Cancer immunoediting: from immunosurveillance to tumor escape. Nat Immunol 2002;3(11):991–8.

[23] Dunn GP, Old LJ, Schreiber RD. The three Es of cancer immunoediting. Annu Rev Immunol 2004;22:329–60.

[24] Andres A. Cancer incidence after immunosuppressive treatment following kidney transplantation. Crit Rev Oncol Hematol 2005;56(1):71–85.

[25] Ippoliti G, Rinaldi M, Pellegrini C, et al. Incidence of cancer after immunosuppressive treatment for heart transplantation. Crit Rev Oncol Hematol 2005;56(1):101–13.

[26] Vallejo GH, Romero CJ, de Vicente JC. Incidence and risk factors for cancer after liver transplantation. Crit Rev Oncol Hematol 2005;56(1):87–99.

[27] Ghelani D, Saliba R, Lima M. Secondary malignancies after hematopoietic stem cell transplantation. Crit Rev Oncol Hematol 2005;56(1):115–26.

[28] Taylor AL, Marcus R, Bradley JA. Post-transplant lymphoproliferative disorders (PTLD) after solid organ transplantation. Crit Rev Oncol Hematol 2005;56(1):155–67.

[29] Dunn GP, Old LJ, Schreiber RD. The immunobiology of cancer immunosurveillance and immunoediting. Immunity 2004;21(2):137–48.

[30] Marincola FM, Jaffe EM, Hicklin DJ, et al. Escape of human solid tumors from T cell recognition: molecular mechanisms and functional significance. Adv Immunol 2000;74:181–273.

[31] Marincola FM, Wang E, Herlyn M, et al. Tumors as elusive targets of T cell-based active immunotherapy. Trends Immunol 2003;24(6):335–42.

[32] Mocellin S, Panelli MC, Wang E, et al. The dual role of IL-10. Trends Immunol 2002;24(1):36–43.

[33] Gordon S. Alternative activation of macrophages. Nat Rev Immunol 2003;3:23–35.

[34] Mantovani A, Sica A, Sozzani S, et al. The chemokine system in diverse forms of macrophage activation and polarization. Trends Immunol 2004;25(12):677–86.

[35] Banchereau J, Steinman RM. Dendritic cells and the control of immunity. Nature 1998;392(6673):245–52.

[36] Wynn TA. Fibrotic disease and the T(H)1/T(H)2 paradigm. Nat Rev Immunol 2004;4(8):583–94.

[37] Coussens LM, Werb Z. Inflammation and cancer. Nature 2002;420(6917):860–7.

[38] De Visser KE, Korets LV, Coussens LM. De novo carcinogenesis promoted by chronic inflammation is B lymphocyte dependent. Cancer Cell 2005;7(5):411–23.

[39] Mantovani A. Cancer: inflammation by remote control. Nature 2005;435(7043):752–3.

[40] Wolfel T, Klehmann E, Muller C, et al. Lysis of human melanoma cells by autologous cytolytic T cell clones: identification of human histocompatibility leukocyte antigen A2 as a restriction element for three different antigens. J Exp Med 1989;170:797–810.

[41] Marincola FM, Rivoltini L, Salgaller ML, et al. Differential anti-MART-1/MelanA CTL activity in peripheral blood of HLA-A2 melanoma patients in comparison to healthy donors: evidence for in vivo priming by tumor cells. J Immunother 1996;19(4):266–77.

[42] van der Bruggen P, Traversari C, Chomez P, et al. A gene encoding an antigen recognized by cytolytic T lymphocytes on a human melanoma. Science 1991;254:1643–7.

[43] Wang E, Panelli MC, Marincola FM. Gene profiling of immune responses against tumors. Curr Opin Immunol 2005;17(4):423–7.

[44] Wang E, Panelli M, Marincola FM. Autologous tumor rejection in humans: trimming the myths. Immunol Invest 2006;35(3–4):437–58.

[45] Wang E, Voiculescu S, Le Poole IC, et al. Clonal persistence and evolution during a decade of recurrent melanoma. J Invest Dermatol 2006;126(6):1372–7.

[46] Jin P, Wang E. Polymorphism in clinical immunology: from HLA typing to immunogenetic profiling. J Transl Med 2003;1:8.

[47] Wang E, Marincola FM. cDNA microarrays and the enigma of melanoma immune responsiveness. Cancer J Sci Am 2001;7(1):16–23.

[48] Wang E, Panelli MC, Marincola FM. Genomic analysis of cancer. Principle and Practice of Oncology Updates 2003;17(9):1–16.

[49] Atkins MB, Lotze MT, Dutcher JP, et al. High-dose recombinant interleukin-2 therapy for patients with metastatic melanoma: analysis of 270 patients treated between 1985 and 1993. J Clin Oncol 1998;17(7):2105–16.

[50] Atkins MB, Regan M, McDermott D. Update on the role of interleukin 2 and other cytokines in the treatment of patients with stage IV renal carcinoma. Clin Cancer Res 2004;10(18 Pt 2):6342S–6S.

[51] Slingluff CL Jr, Speiser DE. Progress and controversies in developing cancer vaccines. J Transl Med 2005;3:18.

[52] Dudley ME, Wunderlich JR, Robbins PF, et al. Cancer regression and autoimmunity in patients after clonal repopulation with antitumor lymphocytes. Science 2002;298(5594): 850–4.

[53] Grillo-Lopez AJ, White CA, Varns C, et al. Overview of the clinical development of rituximab: first monoclonal antibody approved for the treatment of lymphoma. Semin Oncol 1999;26(5 Suppl 14):66–73.

[54] Hortobagyi GN. Trastuzumab in the treatment of breast cancer. N Engl J Med 2005;353(16): 1734–6.

[55] Zobywalski A, Javorovic M, Frankenberger B, et al. Generation of clinical grade dendritic cells with capacity to produce biologically active IL-12p70. J Transl Med 2007;5:18.

[56] Monsurro' V, Wang E, Yamano Y, et al. Quiescent phenotype of tumor-specific CD8+ T cells following immunization. Blood 2004;104(7):1970–8.

[57] Gabrilovich D. Mechanisms and functional significance of tumour-induced dendritic-cell defects. Nat Rev Immunol 2004;4(12):941–52.

[58] Figdor CG, de Vries IJ, Lesterhuis WJ, et al. Dendritic cell immunotherapy: mapping the way. Nat Med 2004;10(5):475–80.

[59] El Andaloussi A, Han Y, Lesniak MS. Prolongation of survival following depletion of CD4+CD25+ regulatory T cells in mice with experimental brain tumors. J Neurosurg 2006;105(3):430–7.

[60] Comes A, Rosso O, Orengo AM, et al. CD25+ regulatory T cell depletion augments immunotherapy of micrometastases by an IL-21-secreting cellular vaccine. J Immunol 2006; 176(3):1750–8.

[61] Cesana GC, DeRaffele G, Cohen S, et al. Characterization of CD4+CD25+ regulatory T cells in patients treated with high-dose interleukin-2 for metastatic melanoma or renal cell carcinoma. J Clin Oncol 2006;24(7):1169–77.

[62] Wang E, Marincola FM. A natural history of melanoma: serial gene expression analysis. Immunol Today 2000;21(12):619–23.

[63] Zitvogel L, Tesniere A, Kroemer G. Cancer despite immunosurveillance: immunoselection and immunosubversion. Nat Rev Immunol 2006;6(10):715–27.

[64] Singh S, Ross SR, Acena M, et al. Stroma is critical for preventing or permitting immunological destruction of antigenic cancer cells. J Exp Med 1992;175(1):139–46.

[65] Ochsenbein AF, Klenerman P, Karrer U, et al. Immune surveillance against a solid tumor fails because of immunological ignorance. Proc Natl Acad Sci U S A 1999;96:2233–8.

[66] Fuchs EJ, Matzinger P. Is cancer dangerous to the immune system? Semin Immunol 1996; 8(5):271–80.

[67] Monsurro' V, Wang E, Panelli MC, et al. Active-specific immunization against cancer: is the problem at the receiving end? Semin Cancer Biol 2003;13:473–80.

[68] Kammula US, Lee K-H, Riker A, et al. Functional analysis of antigen-specific T lymphocytes by serial measurement of gene expression in peripheral blood mononuclear cells and tumor specimens. J Immunol 1999;163:6867–79.

[69] Cormier JN, Hijazi YM, Abati A, et al. Heterogeneous expression of melanoma-associated antigens (MAA) and HLA-A2 in metastatic melanoma in vivo. Int J Cancer 1998; 75:517–24.

[70] Wang E, Miller LD, Ohnmacht GA, et al. Prospective molecular profiling of subcutaneous melanoma metastases suggests classifiers of immune responsiveness. Cancer Res 2002;62: 3581–6.

[71] Ohnmacht GA, Wang E, Mocellin S, et al. Short term kinetics of tumor antigen expression in response to vaccination. J Immunol 2001;167:1809–20.

[72] Panelli MC, Wang E, Phan G, et al. Genetic profiling of peripheral mononuclear cells and melanoma metastases in response to systemic interleukin-2 administration. Genome Biol 2002;3(7):RESEARCH0035.

[73] Panelli MC, Stashower M, Slade HB, et al. Sequential gene profiling of basal cell carcinomas treated with Imiquimod in a placebo-controlled study defines the requirements for tissue rejection. Genome Biol 2006;8(1):R8.

[74] Wang E, Miller L, Ohnmacht GA, et al. High fidelity mRNA amplification for gene profiling using cDNA microarrays. Nat Biotechnol 2000;17(4):457–9.

[75] Wang E, Marincola FM. Amplification of small quantities of mRNA for transcript analysis. In: Bowtell D, Sambrook J, editors. DNA arrays: a molecular cloning manual. Cold Spring Harbor (NY): Cold Spring Harbor Laboratory Press; 2002. p. 204–13.

[76] Feldman AL, Costouros NG, Wang E, et al. Advantages of mRNA amplification for microarray analysis. Biotechniques 2002;33(4):906–14.

[77] Wang E. RNA amplification for successful gene profiling analysis. J Transl Med 2005;3:28.

[78] Lee K-H, Panelli MC, Kim CJ, et al. Functional dissociation between local and systemic immune response following peptide vaccination. J Immunol 1998;161:4183–94.

[79] Panelli MC, Riker A, Kammula US, et al. Expansion of tumor/T cell pairs from fine needle aspirates (FNA) of melanoma metastases. J Immunol 2000;164(1):495–504.

[80] Panelli MC, Bettinotti MP, Lally K, et al. Identification of a tumor infiltrating lymphocyte recognizing MAGE-12 in a melanoma metastasis with decreased expression of melanoma differentiation antigens. J Immunol 2000;164:4382–92.

[81] Cormier JN, Abati A, Fetsch P, et al. Comparative analysis of the in vivo expression of tyrosinase, MART-1/Melan-A, and gp100 in metastatic melanoma lesions: implications for immunotherapy. J Immunother 1998;21(1):27–31.

[82] Mocellin S, Fetsch PA, Abati A, et al. Laser scanner cytometer evaluation of MART-1, gp100 and HLA-A2 expression in melanoma metastases. J Immunother 2001;24(6):447–58.

[83] Mocellin S, Ohnmacht GA, Wang E, et al. Kinetics of cytokine expression in melanoma metastases classifies immune responsiveness. Int J Cancer 2001;93:236–42.

[84] Rosenberg SA, Yang JC, Schwartzentruber D, et al. Immunologic and therapeutic evaluation of a synthetic tumor associated peptide vaccine for the treatment of patients with metastatic melanoma. Nat Med 1998;4(3):321–7.

[85] Richwald GA. Imiquimod. Drugs Today (Barc) 2003;35(7):497–511.

[86] Urosevic M, Maier T, Benninghoff B, et al. Mechanisms underlying imiquimod-induced regression of basal cell carcinoma in vivo. Arch Dermatol 2003;139(10):1325–32.

[87] Dahl MV. Imiquimod: a cytokine inducer. J Am Acad Dermatol 2002;47(Suppl 4):S205–8.

[88] Iwasaki A, Medzhitov R. Toll-like receptor control of the adaptive immune responses. Nat Immunol 2004;5(10):987–95.

[89] Hemmi H, Kaisho T, Takeuchi O, et al. Small anti-viral compounds activate immune cells via the TLR7 MyD88-dependent signaling pathway. Nat Immunol 2002;3(2): 196–200.

[90] Urosevic M, Dummer R, Conrad C, et al. Disease-independent skin recruitment and activation of plasmacytoid predendritic cells following imiquimod treatment. J Natl Cancer Inst 2005;97(15):1143–53.

[91] Sabatino M, Zhao Y, Voeculesceu S, et al. Conservation of genetic alterations in recurrent melanoma supports the melanoma stem cell hypothesis. Submitted for publication.

[92] Lu J, Getz G, Miska EA, et al. MicroRNA expression profiles classify human cancers. Nature 2005;435(7043):834–8.

[93] Cummins JM, Velculescu VE. Implications of micro-RNA profiling for cancer diagnosis. Oncogene 2006;25(46):6220–7.

[94] Murakami Y, Yasuda T, Saigo K, et al. Comprehensive analysis of microRNA expression patterns in hepatocellular carcinoma and non-tumorous tissues. Oncogene 2006;25(17): 2537–45.

[95] Bottoni A, Zatelli MC, Ferracin M, et al. Identification of differentially expressed micro-RNAs by microarray: a possible role for microRNA genes in pituitary adenomas. J Cell Physiol 2007;210(2):370–7.

Surg Oncol Clin N Am
16 (2007) 755–774

SURGICAL
ONCOLOGY CLINICS
OF NORTH AMERICA

Tumor Microenvironment and Immune Escape

Soldano Ferrone, MD, PhD*,
Theresa L. Whiteside, PhD

*Hillman Cancer Center, University of Pittsburgh Cancer Institute,
5117 Centre Avenue, Pittsburgh, PA 15213-1863, USA*

In recent years the treatment of malignant diseases has changed dramatically because of novel combined modality therapy and improvement in surgical and radiotherapeutic techniques. Survival of patients with locally advanced disease and distant metastasis continues to be poor, however. These disappointing results have highlighted the need to develop and apply alternative therapeutic strategies. Among them, immunotherapy with a special emphasis on T-cell–based immunotherapy has attracted much attention, because mouse models have provided convincing evidence that T-cell–based immunotherapy can control tumor growth [1]. The molecular characterization of T-cell–defined tumor antigens (TAs) and the major progress in our ability to modulate the immune system have facilitated the development and application of immunotherapeutic strategies in clinical trials [2,3]. Results derived from the analysis of many immunized patients have shown convincingly that a significant proportion of these patients develop or enhance a TA-specific immune response [4,5]. Unfortunately, the immune responses have not been paralleled by clinical responses. Regression of malignant lesions has been documented in a limited number of patients. Finally, although many trials performed in one center have reported a beneficial impact of active specific immunotherapy on the clinical course of malignant diseases [4,5], four phase III multicenter clinical trials using different immunization strategies have detected no significant clinical benefit [6].

These disappointing clinical results, which are in sharp contrast to the well-documented ability of antibody-based immunotherapy [7] and the

This work was supported by PHS grants RO1CA67108, RO1CA110249 and PO1CA109688 awarded by the National Cancer Institute, DHHS.

* Corresponding author.

E-mail address: ferrones@upmc.edu (S. Ferrone).

potential of adaptive immunotherapy [8] to control tumor growth, have stimulated interest in defining the mechanisms underlying the lack of clinical efficacy of active specific immunotherapy. Growing evidence indicates that a major obstacle to the successful clinical application of T-cell–based immunotherapy is caused by the multiple escape mechanisms used by tumor cells to avoid immune recognition and destruction by the host's immune system. This topic has been reviewed extensively by us and other investigators. We refer interested readers to recently published reviews for a detailed discussion [9–15].

In this article, the authors first briefly describe the multiple escape mechanisms used by tumor cells to avoid T-cell–mediated recognition and destruction. Next we focus our discussion on escape mechanisms that may result from changes at the level of TA-specific cytotoxic T lymphocytes (CTLs) and tumor cells in the tumor microenvironment. These changes reflect the ability of tumor cells to alter and activate their adjacent stroma to promote the formation of a growth-permissive microenvironment required for full neoplastic manifestation [16,17]. Specifically, the authors discuss the negative impact of regulatory T cells (T_{reg}) and T-cell apoptosis on the TA-specific CTL immune response. The authors also discuss changes in the expression of histocompatibility antigens by tumor cells, which may affect tumor cell–immune cell interactions.

Tumor growth, disease progression, and disease recurrence despite the presence of tumor antigen–specific immune responses

Malignant transformation of cells may be associated with changes in their antigenic profile. The changes that are of interest to tumor immunologists include those that affect the expression of immunologically relevant molecules, such as histocompatibility antigens, costimulatory molecules, and TAs. In recent years the successful application of molecular biology, T-cell cloning, and hybridoma technology has led to the identification and structural characterization of many different types of TAs. These TAs have distinct structural profiles, have different expression patterns in tumor cells and in normal tissues, and use different signaling pathways. Based on their pattern of distribution in various tumor types, TAs can be classified as shared or unique antigens.

Unique TAs that are expressed only by one or a few tumors result from somatic point mutations that occur in many proteins expressed by tumor cells or from alterations in RNA splicing. They are tumor specific and are not detected in normal cells [18]. Shared TAs, on the other hand, are expressed by a variable percentage of tumors within a tumor type and may be expressed by various tumors types. They are not tumor specific, because they are expressed by a variable number of normal tissues. Shared TAs include those encoded by cancer-germline genes, genes overexpressed in malignant cells, and differentiation genes [19].

Convincing evidence indicates that the host can mount a TA-specific cellular or humoral immune response spontaneously or after immunizations with vaccines [20–22]. The latter have been created using whole tumor cells, tumor cell lysates, purified TA, and defined epitope peptides derived from TA. The potential role of these immune responses in the control of tumor growth, which is taken as evidence to support the tumor immunosurveillance theory [23,24], is supported by several lines of experimental and clinical evidence. Briefly, the frequency of tumors is increased in immunodeficient mice [25,26] and in immunosuppressed patients [26–28], which supports the contention that the host's immune system plays an important role in the control of tumor growth. Transmission of a donor-derived tumor to a transplanted immunosuppressed recipient also has been described, although in a limited number of patients [27,28]. On the other hand, infiltration of malignant lesions by T cells, natural killer (NK) cells, or NK T cells is associated with an improved prognosis in several tumor types, including breast, gastric, colorectal, and ovarian cancer and malignant melanoma [26]. The type, density, and location of immune cells in colorectal carcinoma lesions recently were found to have a prognostic value that is superior to and independent of the UICC-TNM classification [29].

The data we have summarized raise the question of why tumors develop and progress in patients given the ability of their immune system to recognize TA expressed by tumor cells and to develop TA-specific immune responses. The available evidence indicates that this dichotomy is caused, at least in part, by the escape mechanisms tumor cells use to interfere with one or more of the events that occur at different sites, which lead to a TA-specific immune response. As shown in Fig. 1, they include activation/induction of T cells, expansion, trafficking/homing to tumor sites, recognition of tumor cells, and effector activity at tumor sites. Studies performed in animal model systems and in tumor-bearing patients have shown that the encounter of T cells with TA may not lead to their priming but may generate anergy, tolerance to TA, TA-specific T cells with an impairment of some of their effector functions, and TA-specific T_{reg} [30]. Analysis of the cellular and molecular mechanisms underlying these abnormalities has pointed to TA capture by dendritic cells (DC) in the absence of inflammatory mediators as a contributing factor to T-cell unresponsivness [31]. Additional factors that have a negative influence on DC maturation and function include immunosuppressive molecules provided by tumors in their microenvironment, such as gangliosides, interleukin (IL)-6, IL-10, transforming growth factor (TGF)-β, and vascular endothelial growth factor (VEGF) [30]. At least for gangliosides the molecular basis of the induced functional changes has been defined: it is caused by down-regulation of some of the antigen-processing machinery components that play a crucial role in the recognition of target cells by antigen-specific CTLs [32]. Tumor cells also may interfere with the homing of TA-specific

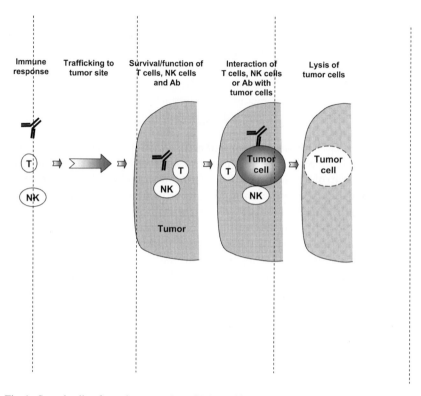

Fig. 1. Steps leading from the generation of TA-specific CTL to distinction of tumor cells. The TA-specific CTLs generated spontaneously or induced by immunization have to traffic to the tumor site, maintain their functional properties in the tumor microenvironment, recognize tumor cells, and lyse them. Tumor cells may interfere with each of these steps and escape from T-cell–mediated recognition and destruction.

T cells to the tumor microenvironment, as exemplified by the lack of tumor-infiltrating lymphocytes (TIL) in most metastases.

Scant information is available about the signals crucial for the recruitment of T cells to the tumor microenvironment. Adhesion molecules, such as E-selectin, ICAM-1, and VCAM-1, which are expressed on endothelial cells of peritumoral and intratumoral microvessels and chemokines, are likely to play an important role. Adhesion molecules have been reported to be poorly expressed on endothelial cells of intratumoral microvessels. This phenotype has been suggested to reflect the inhibitory activity of angiogenic factors, such as b fibroblast growth factor (bFGF), hepatocyte growth factor (HGF), VEGF-C and VEGF-D, and anti-inflammatory cytokines, such as IL-10 and TGF-β, present in the tumor microenvironment [33,34]. The effect of chemokines may be influenced by their level in the tumor microenvironment, because in an animal model system the chemokine CXCL12 serves as a T-cell chemoattractant at low concentration but induces TA-specific T-cell chemorepulsion at high concentration [33].

Additional escape mechanisms include T-cell dysfunction caused by alterations in signal transduction molecules, TA loss, stimulation of the inhibitory receptor CTLA-4 on T cells, overproduction of indoleamine 2,3-dioxygenase, and induction of tumor infiltration by T_{reg} and certain types of NK cells, which inhibit tumor immune destruction [3,9,35–37].

Suppression of T-cell responses by regulatory T cells

T_{reg} cells are a subset of CD4+ T lymphocytes, which are currently considered to be key mediators of peripheral tolerance [37,38]. They mediate tolerance to self-antigens by suppressing expansion of autoreactive effector cells. As a result, T_{reg} cells play a beneficial role in preventing autoimmunity in healthy individuals but represent one of the most potent suppressive mechanisms of TA-specific cellular immunity. In healthy individuals, T_{reg} cells, defined as CD4+CD25^{high}FOXP3+ T cells, represent less than 1% of peripheral circulating CD4+ T lymphocytes [39,40]. The number of T_{reg} cells is increased in patients who have cancer, because they may account for up to 10% to 15% of CD4+ T cells in blood, malignant effusions, tumor microenvironment (Fig. 2), and lymph nodes [40,41]. Suppressor function of

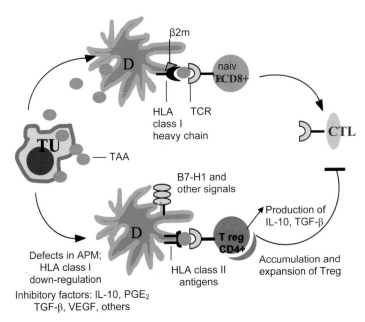

Fig. 2. Mechanisms underlying the generation of T_{reg} in the tumor microenvironment. In the tumor microenvironment, an excess of immunoinhibitory factors favors generation and expansion of T_{reg}, which accumulate and interfere with functions of TA-specific effector cells (CTLs). It is unclear in humans whether suppression of effector cells is tumor antigen specific or represents global functional suppression of all CD8+ T cells in the tumor microenvironment. Suppression may be partial or complete, and it involves various subsets of T_{reg}.

T_{reg} cells in patients who have cancer is markedly augmented relative to that mediated by normal donors' T_{reg} cells [39,41,42].

In humans, at least four subtypes of T_{reg} cells have been identified to date: (1) naturally occurring CD4+CD25^{high}FoxP3+ T cells (nT$_{reg}$), which arise in the thymus and can suppress responses of CD4+CD25(−) and CD8+CD25(−) T cells in a contact-dependent, cytokine-independent, antigen-nonspecific manner [42–44]; (2) CD4$^+$CD25^{low} FoxP3^{low}, known as type 1 regulatory (Tr1) T cells, which arise in the periphery upon encountering Ag in a tolerogenic environment via an IL-10/TGF-β1–dependent process [45]; (3) IL-4–dependent Th3 T cells [46]; and (4) adoptively induced, antigen-specific T_{reg} cells [47].

The characteristics and functional attributes of T_{reg} cells responsible for cancer-related suppression in humans have not been completely defined so far, although nT$_{reg}$ and Tr1 cells are postulated to play a critical role in suppressing TA-specific immunity [37,41,48–50] and are present in tumors, malignant effusions, and peripheral blood of patients who have cancer [42,51–54]. nT$_{reg}$ cells are a heterogeneous population of cells with the memory T-cell phenotype (CD45RO+/CD45RA(−)) differentially expressing CTLA-4, glucocorticoid-induced tumor necrosis factor receptor (GITR), and CD62L [40]. They are endowed with the ability to down-regulate mitogen- or antigen-driven proliferation of responder T cells [39,40,42]. nT$_{reg}$ cells that accumulate in human tumors have a unique phenotype, which is distinct from that of nT$_{reg}$ cells present in the peripheral circulation [54]. nT$_{reg}$ cells isolated from TIL are FoxP3^{high} GITR+FASL+IL-10+TGF-β1+ and suppress CD3/anti-CD28 antibody-driven proliferation of autologous CD4+CD25(−) responder T cells even at the ratio of one stimulator to ten responders in carboxyfluorescein succinimidyl ester (CFSE)-based suppression assays. In contrast, nT$_{reg}$ isolated from the same cancer patients' peripheral circulation have lower FoxP3 expression, do not express GITR, FASL, IL-10, or TGF-β1, and mediate only modest suppression [54].

Our data suggest that nT$_{reg}$ that accumulate in human solid tumors are powerful suppressor cells using inhibitory cytokines (IL-10 and TGF-β1) and the FAS/FASL pathway to suppress function of autologous effector T cells responsible for TA-specific immunity [54]. Tr1 cells are derived from CD4+CD25(−) precursors, which upon encountering antigens presented by immature DC are induced to differentiate and expand in a microenvironment enriched in inhibitory cytokines, notably IL-10 [45,55]. We have shown that Tr1 cells can be generated in vitro by co-incubating naïve CD4+ T cells with tumor cells, autologous immature DC, and a mix of cytokines containing IL-2, IL-10, and IL-15 [56]. The Tr1 cells present in human TIL are CD4+CD25−FoxP3$^{low/neg}$ CD132^{high}IL10+TGF-β1+ and thus are a clearly distinct subset of suppressor cells from nT$_{reg}$ [52]. Although Tr1 cells are induced via IL-10–dependent mechanisms, their characteristic feature is secretion of immunoinhibitory cytokines, such as IL-10 and TGF-β1, which mediate suppression by a contact-independent process [45,52]. We also have shown that tumor-derived prostaglondin E_2 (PGE$_2$) controls the induction and expansion of Tr1 cells, which are responsible for TA-specific immune responses [55]. CD4+ Th3 cells, also defined by the production of TGF-β, are yet another subset of regulatory CD4+ T cells, which may be of special significance in oral tolerance [46]. Apart from CD4+ cells, CD8+ regulatory T cells have been reported recently [57]. CD8+CD28− T cells can be generated in vitro after stimulation of human PBMC with either allogeneic or xenogeneic antigen-presenting cells. CD8+CD28−T cells induce antigen-specific tolerance by increasing the expression of inhibitory receptor ILT3 and ILT4 on antigen-presenting cells rather than by IL-10 production [58].

Currently, the nature of human T$_{reg}$ cells is only partially defined, and it is not clear how the various subsets of T$_{reg}$ cells function in vivo. The phenotype, functions (ie, antigen specificity, stability, trafficking, or survival), lineage, differentiation, and relationship among the various T$_{reg}$ cell subsets are a focus of intense investigation. No single specific marker has emerged that can distinguish T$_{reg}$ cells from other T-cell subpopulations. Even FoxP3, widely considered a T$_{reg}$ cell marker, may be up-regulated on effector cells after activation [59,60], and it has been reported to be expressed by tumor cells in culture and in situ [61]. The lack of a specific marker represents a major limitation in the analysis of the phenotype and functional properties of T$_{reg}$ cells, which are expanded in the circulation and tumor sites of patients who have cancer, including head and neck squamous cell carcinoma, breast cancer, lung cancer, colorectal cancer, pancreatic cancer, ovarian cancer, and melanoma [52–54,62–67]. It has been reported recently that expression of CD127, the α chain of the IL-7 receptor, discriminates between CD127^{low} T$_{reg}$ and CD127^{high} conventional T cells in human peripheral blood and lymph nodes [68,69]. The differential expression of this marker does not provide a solid distinction, however, because effector T cells that do not differentiate into CD127^{high} memory T cells after activation down-regulate CD127 [70]. We were unable to detect CD127 on human T$_{reg}$ purified by sorting from TIL or peripheral blood of patients who have cancer [44,54]. The inability to reliably identify T$_{reg}$ cells by phenotyping makes the assessment of their role in the regulation of TA-specific immune responses especially difficult. It is also important to distinguish T$_{reg}$ cells from activated CD4+CD25+ effector T cells. Our preliminary data suggest that in contrast to the latter, T$_{reg}$ cells are resistant to spontaneous and drug-induced apoptosis [42].

The clinical significance of T$_{reg}$ cell accumulation in the tumor microenvironment and in the circulation of patients who have cancer has been investigated by correlating T$_{reg}$ numbers and function with disease activity and known prognostic factors. Curiel and colleagues [53] have shown that infiltration of functional T$_{reg}$ cells in ovarian tumors is associated with shorter survival. These results have been corroborated by our own findings in patients who have head and neck squamous cell carcinoma in whom we have examined the association of Tr1 cell number and suppressor activity in peripheral blood mononuclear cells with disease activity, tumor stage, and nodal involvement. Although Tr1 number and function did not correlate with lymph node involvement, Tr1 precursors and differentiated Tr1 cells showed a significantly higher expression of FoxP3, IL-10, and TGF-β1 in patients who had late-stage disease (T3/T4) relative to patients with early-stage disease (T1/T2) at the time of surgery. In another cohort of patients who had head and neck squamous cell carcinoma, we observed that T_{reg} and Tr1 cell populations were significantly expanded in the peripheral circulation of patients who had no evident disease after oncologic therapy relative to patients who had active disease. The expanded T_{reg} in patients who had no evident disease significantly increased suppressor function, which remained elevated for months after termination of oncologic therapy [42]. These data derived from a cross-sectional study are paralleled by our preliminary follow-up results. The frequency and function of T_{reg} remained significantly elevated for at least 12 months in patients who had head and neck squamous cell carcinoma who were followed longitudinally.

These data have provided the rationale for removal or inactivation of T_{reg} as a therapeutic strategy for patients who have cancer. Therapeutic options for control of T_{reg}-mediated immune suppression include various agents, among them Abs to CD25, which have been used in animal models with some success for depletion of CD25+ T cells [71]. Because T_{reg} express CTLA-4, antibody-mediated CTLA-4 blockade might be effective in reducing their suppressive activity [72]. Application of this strategy to patients who have cancer introduced the specter of substantial autoimmune side effects that accompany significant antitumor responses and even tumor regressions, however [73]. Treatment with anti-CTLA-4 antibody did not significantly decrease T_{reg} levels or function in patients [73]. Alternatively, treatment of patients who have cancer with IL-2 diphtheria toxin fusion protein (denileukin diftitox, Ontak) has shown efficacy in clinical trials initially targeted to treat tumors that express CD25, including cutaneous T cell leukemia [74], although it seems that this drug also ablates $CD25^{high}$ T_{reg} [75,76]. Current TA immunization protocols are beginning to combine depletion of T_{reg} using Ontak with a subsequent immunization to allow for expansion of immunization-induced TA-specific immunity [75]. Clinical evidence indicates that in vivo depletion of CD4+CD25+ T_{reg} with Ontak can enhance immunization-induced TA-specific immune responses [76–78]. Concerns exist, however, that activated CD4+ helper and effector T cells are ablated by this therapy. Recent data suggest that it may be possible to establish a therapeutic window to preferentially eliminate T_{reg} without affecting $CD25^{low}$ effector T cells [75]. Some reports suggest that therapy with Ontak fails to eliminate T_{reg} in patients who have cancer [79]. The effects of this strategy for elimination of T_{reg} are not entirely clear, and additional clinical studies are necessary to confirm its therapeutic benefit in cancer [80].

IL-10 and TGF-β1–specific antibodies could be considered for blocking T_{reg} activity; however, clinical grade IL-10–specific antibodies have been used only for treatment of patients who have systemic lupus erythematosus [81], and safety clinical trials are necessary before this therapy can be used in patients who have cancer for blocking T_{reg} activity. Finally, various pharmacologic agents might be used to reduce numbers of T_{reg}. For example, in vivo administration of low-dose cyclophosphamide is effective in this respect, presumably by selectively inducing apoptosis in T_{reg} [82]. Patients receiving the chemotherapeutic agent fludarabine have been reported to have lower T_{reg} frequencies and activity because of preferential apoptosis of T_{reg} [83]. A reduction of T_{reg} activity can be achieved through altering signaling via CpG motifs from toll-like receptor (TLR) 9 to 8 and enhancing the efficacy of cancer vaccines [84]. Recent reports indicate that analogs of thalidomide, a drug used in therapy for multiple myeloma, are effective in reducing suppressive activities of T_{reg} [85]. Some drugs used in transplantation, such as rapamycin, can promote selective in vivo and in vitro expansion of T_{reg} from CD4+CD25(−) precursors [39,86] and offer a possibility for ex vivo production and adoptive transfer of autologous T_{reg} to patients with autoimmune disorders or after hematopoietic stem cell transplantation to mitigate graft-versus-host disease. Overall, T_{reg} are a target for numerous novel therapies designed to up-regulate TA-specific immune responses [80,87].

Apoptosis and rapid turnover of CD8+ effector T cells

Among the less known but clearly important immunosuppressive effects that tumors mediate is the induction of T-cell apoptosis [88]. Apoptosis of circulating CD8+ T cells has been described in patients who have head and neck, breast, and ovarian cancers and melanoma [89]. Studies involving TUNEL staining of TIL and Annexin V binding to circulating T cells suggest that CD8+ rather than CD4+ T cells selectively undergo apoptosis at the tumor site and in the peripheral circulation of patients who have cancer [88,89]. The proportion of CD8+FAS+ T cells that bind Annexin V and yet are 7-AA(−) or PI(−) is significantly increased in the circulation of patients who have cancer relative to age-matched normal controls [88,89]. The fate of CD8+ and CD4+ T-cell subsets may differ because of their divergent sensitivity to apoptosis. The effector subpopulations of CD8+ T cells (eg, CD8+CD45RO+CD27− and CD8+CD28−) seem to be preferentially targeted for apoptosis in patients who have cancer (Fig. 3) [90,91]. Absolute numbers of circulating T-cell subsets are low in patients who have cancer [92]. Examination of the proliferative history of T-cell subsets using the T-cell receptor excision circle polymerase chain reaction–based analysis confirms aberrant lymphocyte homeostasis characterized by a rapid turnover of T cells in cancer patients [93]. Circulating Vβ-restricted CD8+ T cells [94] and tetramer+CD8+ T cells are especially sensitive to apoptosis

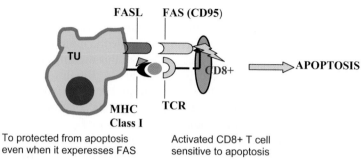

Fig. 3. Mechanisms underlying apoptosis of TA-specific CD8+ effector T cells in the tumor microenvironment. In the tumor microenvironment, CD8+ effector T cells recognize TA (an activation signal) and up-regulate FAS (CD95). Epithelial tumor cells express FASL on their surface. FAS/FASL interactions result in activation of the death pathway and apoptosis of tumor-infiltrating CD8+ T cells. Although tumor cells express FAS, they are protected from FASL-induced apoptosis by various mechanisms.

(T. Whiteside, unpublished data, 2006). Taken together, these findings suggest that a loss of effector T-cell function through targeted apoptosis might severely compromise antitumor functions of the host immune system and contribute to tumor progression [88,89].

The clinical significance of spontaneous apoptosis of CD8+ effector cells in cancer is not currently known. It seems that the level of spontaneous apoptosis can discriminate between patients who have cancer and healthy controls [95]. The percentage of T cells undergoing spontaneous apoptosis is also higher at the tumor site than in the periphery [96]. It is often—but not always—higher in patients with active disease compared with patients with no evident disease [95]. In combination with the assessment of T-cell signaling (ie, ζ chain expression in T cells) and CD95 expression on the T-cell surface, spontaneous apoptosis correlated with the nodal involvement in patients with head and neck cancer [96,97]. This correlation suggests that these immune markers might have a prognostic value and could be used in the future for the assessment of tumor aggressiveness and as predictors of patient survival. It seems that T lymphocytes and monocytes/macrophages isolated from tumor sites, lymph nodes, peripheral blood mononuclear cells, and body fluids of such subjects are dysfunctional but not all irreversibly damaged. Earlier limiting-dilution studies with human TIL have indicated that a subset of TIL T cells retains or recovers the ability to proliferate in response to IL-2 in culture [89,98]. These results suggest that some T cells or their precursors resist tumor-induced dysfunction and can be rescued and expanded after removal from the tumor site or upon exposure to exogenous cytokines ex vivo. This mechanism might account for the objective clinical responses observed in a few patients who have melanoma or ovarian carcinoma after the administration of ex vivo expanded TIL [99]. On the other hand, CD8+ T cells that are targeted for or are in the process of apoptosis are unlikely to recover and are deleted.

Protection of effector T cells from apoptosis, extension of their survival, and changes in lymphocyte turnover must be considered as therapeutic strategies aimed at preventing tumor escape via the extension of lymphocyte survival and normalization of their turnover in the circulation of subjects who have cancer. This goal may be achieved by therapy with survival cytokines, including IL-7, -12, -15, or -21 [100–105]. Protection of T cells from apoptosis or untimely activation-induced cell death and the normalized immune cell turnover also could be achieved by increasing expression of "survival" or antiapoptotic proteins in T cells. For example up-regulated or normalized expression of survivin, Mcl-1, the Bcl2 family of antiapoptotic factors, or cFLIP in T cells could afford protection, as indicated by ex vivo and animal experiments [106–108]. The inhibitor of apoptotic pathway family is another target for selective therapy [109]. These molecular targets are expressed in T cells as well as in tumor and normal tissue cells, however, and selective therapy—whether with specific drugs or cytokines—is likely to have multiple and often undesirable consequences, including promotion of tumor growth. For this reason, targets such as certain chemokine receptors expressed only on subsets of lymphocytes may be of greater therapeutic significance than previously anticipated. Our data suggest, for example, that expression of CCR7 on CD8+ T cells is associated with their resistance to spontaneous apoptosis in the peripheral circulation of patients who have squamous cell carcinoma of the head and neck [110]. This chemokine receptor could be an interesting target for therapy aimed at correcting lymphocyte homeostasis [111], because its expression is known to be associated with T-cell differentiation and trafficking to lymph nodes.

Changes in histocompatibility antigen expression by tumor cells

The major role played by human leukocyte antigen (HLA) class I antigens in the interactions of tumor cells with immune cells has stimulated several studies to characterize the expression of these molecules by tumor cells and assess the functional significance and clinical relevance of changes in their expression. Analysis of cell lines in long-term culture has provided convincing evidence that changes in the expression of histocompatibility antigens may take place when cells undergo malignant transformation [12]. They include down-regulation or loss of classic HLA class I antigens and appearance of the nonclassic HLA class I antigen, HLA-G, and NK cell–activating ligands. In vitro evidence clearly indicates that these abnormalities may affect the interactions of tumor cells with immune cells. Classic HLA class I antigen down-regulation or loss may cause escape of tumor cells from recognition by HLA class I antigen-restricted CTLs. On the other hand, the expression of HLA-G antigens on tumor cells may inhibit the cytotoxic activity of CTL and NK cells, CD4+ T cell proliferation and cytokine release, and cell cycle progression in alloreactive T cells, may generate a new type of regulatory T cells through the mechanism of "trogocytosis," and may induce a "Th2" cytokine profile at the tumor site [112]. Finally, the expression of NK cell activating ligands on tumor cells in combination with the released soluble forms may cause internalization and lysosomal degradation of their receptor NKG2D. Its resulting down-regulation on effector cells may lead to defective NK cell–mediated cytotoxicity [15].

The frequency of abnormalities in histocompatibility antigen expression, which is generally higher in metastatic than in primary lesions (at least for classic HLA class I antigens), differs among the various types of tumors analyzed. Classic HLA class I antigen loss or down-regulation has been found in approximately 50% of primary breast and prostate carcinoma but in approximately 20% of primary renal cell carcinoma lesions. This variability is likely to reflect the extent of genetic instability of tumor cells, the level of selective pressure imposed by the patient's immune response on the tumor cell population analyzed, and the length of time tumor cells have been exposed to selective pressure in the patient [11]. HLA-G has been found to be expressed in approximately 40% of clear renal cell carcinoma and ovarian carcinoma but has not been detected in uveal melanoma and laryngeal carcinoma [25]. Information about the expression of the stress-inducible MHC class I chain-related surface glycoproteins MICA and MICB and the UL16-binding proteins ULBP1, ULBP2, ULBP3, and ULBP4 in malignant tumors is more limited, because only a limited number of tumors has been analyzed. The available information indicates that MICA and MICB are expressed by many types of epithelial and neuroectodermal tumors and have a higher frequency than ULBP molecules [113]. The expression of the latter and the MIC molecules by malignant cells is not coordinated with that of classic and nonclassic HLA class I antigens.

Growing evidence indicates that tumor cells often harbor multiple abnormalities that affect the expression of distinct types of histocompatibility antigens or multiple alleles within a histocompatibility antigenic system [11,114]. Given the role of immunoselective pressure in the outgrowth of cells with histocompatibility antigen defects in a tumor cell population [114], the presence of multiple defects in tumor cells has been taken as evidence that a host's immune system adapts its immune response to changes that take place in the antigenic phenotype of tumor cells. As a result, when tumor cells acquire the ability to escape from the immune response developed by the host, the immune system changes its attack mechanisms or the target of its response. To illustrate these possibilities we can envision two scenarios, which are schematically shown in Fig. 4. In the early response against cancer, the immune system may use NK cells. The selective pressure imposed by these cells may lead to the outgrowth of a tumor cell population that has become resistant to NK cell–mediated recognition and lysis because of defects in NK cell–activating ligand expression. At this stage in the course of the disease, the immune system may develop a TA-specific CTL response. The selective pressure imposed on the tumor cell populations by HLA class I antigen-restricted CTL may favor the outgrowth of tumor cells with defects

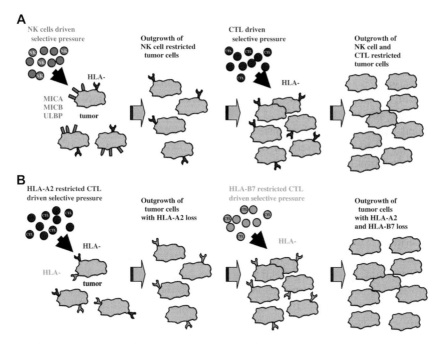

Fig. 4. Role of immunoselection in the generation of multiple defects in histocompatibility antigens in tumor cells.

in classic HLA class I antigen expression. As a result, malignant lesions are populated by tumor cells with defects in NK cell–activating ligand and classic HLA class I antigen expression or function. Similar mechanisms may be envisioned to account for the sequential loss by tumor cells of two of the classic HLA class I antigenic systems, which are used as restricting elements by TA-specific CTLs.

Changes in histocompatibility antigen expression by tumor cells seem to have clinical significance because they may be associated with the histopathologic characteristics of the lesions, disease progression, disease-free survival, or overall survival. To mention a few examples [9,11], the frequency of classic HLA class I antigen defects is higher in primary cervical carcinoma lesions than in premalignant cervical intraepithelial neoplasia but lower than in metastases. HLA class I antigen down-regulation in primary melanoma lesions is associated with reduced disease-free survival and overall survival. Similar findings have been described for the nonclassic HLA class I antigen, HLA-G, in colorectal carcinoma. HLA-G expression in colorectal lesions is significantly correlated with the depth of invasion, histologic grade, lymph node metastasis, and clinical stage of the disease. HLA-G expression in tumors is associated with a reduced survival; the latter association is independent of other prognostic markers, suggesting that

HLA-G expression in colorectal carcinoma lesions may serve as an independent prognostic marker [114]. Finally, an association has been found between MICA loss and disease progression in melanoma [11].

These topics and the molecular mechanisms underlying changes in the expression of histocompatibility antigens associated with malignant transformation of cells recently were reviewed by us. We refer interested readers to these reviews [9,11,15,25,112,114]. Here we discuss the potential functional changes induced in histocompatibility antigens expressed by tumor cells by cytokines present in the tumor microenvironment and the impact of histocompatibility antigens released by tumor cells in the microenvironment on immune cells.

IL-10 is present in the tumor microenvironment because it may be secreted by tumor cells and tumor-infiltrating mononuclear cells. The latter include plasmacytoid DCs, myeloid suppressor cells, and T_{reg}. In vitro experiments with mouse and human cell lines have shown that IL-10 down-regulates components of the antigen-processing machinery [113]. This machinery plays a crucial role in the generation of HLA class I antigen-derived peptide complexes, which mediate the recognition of target cells by CTL. Specifically, peptides generated from mostly—although not exclusively—endogenous proteins are transported into the endoplasmic reticulum by the transporter associated with antigen processing. Here peptides are loaded on β_2 microglobulin (β_2m)-HLA class I heavy chain complexes, which are properly folded with the assistance of the chaperones, BiP, calnexin, calreticulin, and endoplasmic reticulum p57. Trimeric HLA class I heavy chain-β_2m-peptide complexes are then transported to the cell surface, where they are recognized by T cells expressing cognate T-cell receptors. The available evidence raises the possibility that IL-10 present in the tumor microenvironment may affect the function of antigen-processing machinery in tumor cells. As a result, the generation and expression of HLA class I antigen TA-derived peptides may be defective, providing tumor cells with an escape mechanism from CTL recognition and destruction. Another cytokine present in the tumor microenvironment that may affect the expression of histocompatibility by tumor cells is represented by TGF-β, which is produced by tumor cells, normal stromal cells, and infiltrating mononuclear cells. TGF-β may down-regulate the expression of classic HLA class I antigens and some of the NK cell–activating ligands [113]. These changes are likely to have a negative impact on the recognition of tumor cells not only by TA-specific CTLs but also by NK cells.

Histocompatibility antigens released by tumor cells in the microenvironment may affect interactions with immune cells. Classic HLA class I antigens and HLA-G may induce apoptosis of activated T cells [113]. This mechanism may account for the presence of apoptotic T cells in the tumor microenvironment. NK cell–activating ligands released from tumor cells may have a negative impact on tumor immunosurveillance, because they may promote down-regulation of NKG2D on NK and CD8 T cells and may reduce the expression of NK cell–activating ligands on tumor cells [113]. These changes impair the cytotoxic activity of NK cells and TA-specific CTLs.

Summary

The data we have reviewed clearly indicate that the multiple mechanisms that tumor cells use to avoid immune recognition and destruction represent a major obstacle to the successful application of T-cell–based immunotherapy for the treatment of malignant diseases. A major challenge in oncology is the development of strategies to counteract the escape mechanisms used by tumor cells. These strategies must be combined with immunization approaches to enhance the clinical efficacy of T-cell–based immunotherapy.

Acknowledgments

We would like to thank Dr. Cristina R. Ferrone, Department of Surgery, Massachusetts General Hospital, Boston, MA, for constructive comments to the manuscript.

References

[1] Ostrand-Rosenberg S. Animal models of tumor immunity, immunotherapy and cancer vaccines. Curr Opin Immunol 2004;16:143–50.

[2] Rosenberg SA. Progress in human tumour immunology and immunotherapy. Nature 2001; 411:380–4.

[3] Peggs KS, Quezada SA, Korman AJ, et al. Principles and use of anti-CTLA4 antibody in human cancer immunotherapy. Curr Opin Immunol 2006;18:206–13.

[4] Schuler G, Schuler-Thurner B, Steinman RM. The use of dendritic cells in cancer immunotherapy. Curr Opin Immunol 2003;15:138–47.

[5] Coulie PG, van der Bruggen P. T-cell response of vaccinated cancer patients. Curr Opin Immunol 2003;15:131–7.

[6] Srivastava PK. Therapeutic cancer vaccines. Curr Opin Immunol 2006;18:201–5.

[7] Waldmann TA, Morris JC. Development of antibodies and chimeric molecules for cancer immunotherapy. Adv Immunol 2006;90:83–131.

[8] June CH. Adoptive T cell therapy for cancer in the clinic. J Clin Invest 2007;117:1466–76.

[9] Marincola FM, Jaffee EM, Hicklin DJ, et al. Escape of human solid tumors from T-cell recognition: molecular mechanisms and functional significance. Adv Immunol 2000;74: 181–273.

[10] Khong HT, Restifo NP. Natural selection of tumor variants in the generation of "tumor escape" phenotypes. Nat Immunol 2002;3:999–1005.

[11] Chang CC, Campoli M, Ferrone S. Classical and non-classical HLA class I antigen and NK cell activating ligand changes in malignant cells: current challenges and future directions. Adv Cancer Res 2005;93:189–234.

[12] Ferris R, Whiteside TL, Ferrone S. Immune escape associated with functional defects in antigen processing machinery in head and neck cancer. Clin Cancer Res 2006;12:3890–5.

[13] Rivoltini L, Canese P, Huber V, et al. Escape strategies and reasons for failure in the interaction between tumour cells and the immune system: how can we tilt the balance towards immune-mediated cancer control? Expert Opin Biol Ther 2005;5:463–76.

[14] Zitvogel L, Tesniere A, Kroemer G. Cancer despite immunosurveillance: immunoselection and immunosubversion. Nat Rev Immunol 2006;6:715–27.

[15] Ferrone S, Whiteside TL. Histocompatibility antigens, tumor microenvironment and escape mechanisms utilized by tumor cells. Springer Science, in press.

[16] Bhowmick NA, Moses HL. Tumor-stroma interactions. Curr Opin Genet Dev 2005;15: 97–101.

[17] Kalluri R, Zeisberg M. Fibroblasts in cancer. Nat Rev Cancer 2006;6:392–401.

[18] Parmiani G, De Filippo A, Novellino L, et al. Unique human tumor antigens: immunobiology and use in clinical trials. J Immunol 2007;178:1975–9.

[19] Boon T, Coulie PG, Van den Eynde B. Tumor antigens recognized by T cells. Immunol Today 1997;18:267–8.

[20] Boon T, Coulie PG, Van den Eynde BJ, et al. Human T cell responses against melanoma. Annu Rev Immunol 2006;24:175–208.

[21] Mittelman A, Chen ZJ, Yang H, et al. Human high molecular weight melanoma-associated antigen (HMW-MAA) mimicry by mouse anti-idiotypic monoclonal antibody MK2-23: induction of humoral anti-HMW-MAA immunity and prolongation of survival in patients with stage IV melanoma. Proc Natl Acad Sci U S A 1992;89:466–70.

[22] Old LJ, Chen YT. New paths in human cancer serology. J Exp Med 1998;187:1163–7.

[23] Thomas L. Discussion. In: Lawrence HS, editor. Cellular and humoral aspects of the hypersensitive states. New York: Hoeber-Harper; 1959.

[24] Burnet FM. Immunological factors in the process of carcinogenesis. Br Med Bull 1970;20:154.

[25] Chang C-C, Ferrone S. Immune selective pressure and HLA class I antigen defects in malignant lesions. Cancer Immunol Immunother 2007;56:227–36.

[26] Kim R, Emi M, Tanabe K, et al. Potential functional role of plasmacytoid dendritic cells in cancer immunity. Immunology 2007;121:149–57.

[27] Desoize B, editor. Immunosuppressive treatment and induction of cancer. Crit Rev Oncol Hematol, 56. p. 1–178.

[28] Wimmer CD, Rentsch M, Crispin A, et al. The janus face of immunosuppression: de novo malignancy after renal transplantation. The experience of the Transplantation Center Munich. Kidney Int 2007;71:1271–8.

[29] Galon J, Costes A, Sanchez-Cabo F, et al. Type, density, and location of immune cells within human colorectal tumors predict clinical outcome. Science 2006;313:1960–4.

[30] Rabinovich GA, Gabrilovich D, Sotomayor EM. Immunosuppressive strategies that are mediated by tumor cells. Annu Rev Immunol 2007;25:267–96.

[31] Steinman RM, Hawiger D, Nussenzweig MC. Tolerogenic dendritic cells. Annu Rev Immunol 2003;21:685–711.

[32] Tourkova IL, Shurin GV, Chatta GS, et al. Restoration by IL-15 of MHC class I antigen processing machinery in human dendritic cells inhibited by tumor-derived gangliosides. J Immunol 2005;175:3045–52.

[33] Fisher DT, Chen Q, Appenheimer MM, et al. Hurdles to lymphocyte trafficking in the tumor microenvironment: implications for effective immunotherapy. Immunol Invest 2006; 35:251–77.

[34] Vianello F, Papeta N, Chen T, et al. Murine B16 melanomas expressing high levels of the chemokine stromal-derived factor-1/CXCL12 induce tumor-specific T cell chemorepulsion and escape from immune control. J Immunol 2006;176:2902–14.

[35] Uyttenhove C, Pilotte L, Theate I, et al. Evidence for a tumoral immune resistance mechanism based on tryptophan degradation by indoleamine 2,3-dioxygenase. Nat Med 2003;9: 1269–74.

[36] Terabe M, Matsui S, Noben-Trauth N, et al. NK T cell-mediated repression of tumor immunosurveillance by IL-13 and the IL-4R-STAT6 pathway. Nat Immunol 2000;1:515–20.

[37] Sakaguchi S, Sakaguchi N, Shimizu J, et al. Immunologic tolerance maintained by CD25+CD4+ regulatory T cells: their common role in controlling autoimmunity, tumor immunity, and transplantation tolerance. Immunol Rev 2001;182:18–32.

[38] Shevach EM. CD4+ CD25+ suppressor T cells: more questions than answers. Nat Rev Immunol 2002;2:389–400.

[39] Strauss L, Whiteside TL, Knights A, et al. Selective *in vitro* expansion of naturally occurring human CD4+CD25+FOXP3+ regulatory T cells with rapamycin. J Immunol 2006;178: 320–9.

[40] Strauss L, Bergmann C, Whiteside TL. Functional and phenotypic characteristics of CD4+CD25^{high}FoxP3+ T$_{reg}$ clones obtained from peripheral blood of patients with cancer. Int J Cancer 2007;121:2473–83.

[41] Beyer M, Schultze JL. Regulatory T cells in cancer. Blood 2006;108:804–11.

[42] Strauss L, Bergmann C, Gooding W, et al. The frequency and suppressor function of CD4+ CD25^{high}Foxp3+ T cells in the circulation of patients with squamous cell carcinoma of the head and neck (HNSCC). Clin Cancer Res, in press.

[43] Dieckmann D, Plottner H, Berchtold S, et al. Ex vivo isolation and characterization of CD4(+)CD25(+) T cells with regulatory properties from human blood. J Exp Med 2001; 193:1303–10.

[44] Jonuleit H, Schmitt E, Stassen M, et al. Identification and functional characterization of human CD4(+)CD25(+) T cells with regulatory properties isolated from peripheral blood. J Exp Med 2001;193:1285–94.

[45] Roncarolo MG, Gregori S, Battaglia M, et al. Interleukin-10-secreting type 1 regulatory T cells in rodents and humans. Immunol Rev 2006;212:28–50.

[46] Weiner HL. Induction and mechanism of action of transforming growth factor-beta-secreting Th3 regulatory cells. Immunol Rev 2001;182:207–14.

[47] Wang HY, Lee DA, Peng G. Tumor-specific human CD4+ regulatory T cells and their ligands: implications for immunotherapy. Immunity 2004;20:107–18.

[48] Ng WF, Duggan PJ, Ponchel F, et al. Human CD4(+)CD25(+) cells: a naturally occurring population of regulatory T cells. Blood 2001;98:2736–44.

[49] Woo EY, Yeh H, Chu CS, et al. Regulatory T cells from lung cancer patients directly inhibit autologous T cell proliferation. J Immunol 2002;168:4272–6.

[50] Larmonier N, Marron M, Zeng Y, et al. Tumor-derived CD4(+)CD25 (+) regulatory T cell suppression of dendritic cell function involves TGF-beta and IL-10. Cancer Immunol Immunother 2007;56:48–59.

[51] Shevach EM. Fatal attraction: tumors beckon regulatory T cells. Nat Med 2004;10:900–1.

[52] Liyanage UK, Moore TT, Joo H-G, et al. Prevalence of regulatory T cells is increased in peripheral blood and tumor microenvironment of patients with pancreas or breast adenocarcinoma. J Immunol 2002;169:2756–61.

[53] Curiel TJ, Coukos G, Zou L, et al. Specific recruitment of regulatory T cells in ovarian carcinoma fosters immune privilege and predicts reduced survival. Nat Med 2004;10:942–9.

[54] Strauss L, Bergmann C, Szczepanski M, et al. A unique subset of CD4+ CD25^{high}Foxp3+ T cells secreting IL-10 and TGF- β1 mediates suppression in the tumor microenvironment. Clin Cancer Res 2007;13:4345–54.

[55] Bergmann C, Strauss L, Zeidler R, et al. Expansion of human T regulatory type 1 cells in the microenvironment of COX-2 overexpressing head and neck squamous cell carcinoma. Cancer Res 2007;67:8865–73.

[56] Bergmann C, Strauss L, Zeidler R, et al. Expansion and characteristics of human regulatory type 1 cells in co-cultures simulating tumor microenvironment. Cancer Immunol Immunother 2007;56:1429–42.

[57] Bisikirska B, Colgan J, Luban JA, et al. TCR stimulation with modified anti-CD3 mAb expands CD8+ T cell population and induces CD8+CD25+ T regs. J Clin Invest 2005; 115:2904–13.

[58] Chang CC, Ciubotariu R, Manavalan JS, et al. Tolerization of dendritic cells by T(S) cells: the crucial role of inhibitory receptors ILT3 and ILT4. Nat Immunol 2002;3:237–43.

[59] Allan SE, Crome SQ, Crellin NK, et al. Activation-induced Foxp3 in human T effector cells does not suppress proliferation of or cytokine production. Int Immunol 2007;79:345–54.

[60] Wang J, Ioan-Facsinay A, van der Voort EI, et al. Transient expression of Foxp3 in human activated nonregulatory CD4+ T cells. Eur J Immunol 2007;37:129–38.

[61] Pagerols-Raluy L, Hinz S, Oberg H-H, et al. Foxp3 expression in pancreatic carcinoma cells as a novel mechanism of immune evasion in cancer [abstract PR8]. Presented at the AACR Special Conference on Tumor Immunology: an integrated perspective. Miami (FL), November 29–December 2, 2006.

[62] Woo EY, Chu CS, Goletz TJ, et al. Regulatory CD4(+)CD25(+) T cells in tumors from patients with early-stage non-small cell lung cancer and late-stage ovarian cancer. Cancer Res 2001;61:4766–72.

[63] Ichihara F, Kono K, Takahashi A, et al. Increased populations of regulatory T cells in peripheral blood and tumor-infiltrating lymphocytes in patients with gastric and esophageal cancers. Clin Cancer Res 2003;9:4404–8.

[64] Albers AE, Kim GG, Ferris RL, et al. Immune responses to p53 in patients with cancer enrichment in tetramer+ p53 peptide-specific T cells and regulatory CD4+CD25+ cells at tumor sites. Cancer Immunol Immunother 2005;54:1072–81.

[65] Schaefer C, Kim GG, Albers A, et al. Characteristics of CD4+CD25+ regulatory T cells in the peripheral circulation of patients with head and neck cancer. Br J Cancer 2005;92: 913–20.

[66] Hiraoka N, Onozato K, Kosuge T, et al. Prevalence of FOXP3+ regulatory T cells increases during the progression of pancreatic ductal adenocarcinoma and its premalignant lesions. Clin Cancer Res 2006;12:5423–34.

[67] Liyanage UK, Goedegebuure PS, Moore TT, et al. Increased prevalence of regulatory T cells (Treg) is induced by pancreas adenocarcinoma. J Immunother 2006;29:416–24.

[68] Liu W, Putnam AL, Xu-Yu Z, et al. CD127 expression inversely correlates with FoxP3 and suppressive function of human CD4+ T reg cells. J Exp Med 2006;203:1701–11.

[69] Seddiki N, Santner-Nanan B, Martinson J, et al. Expression of interleukin (IL)-2 and IL-7 receptors discriminates between human regulatory and activated T cells. J Exp Med 2006; 203:1693–700.

[70] Kaech SM, Tan JT, Wherry EJ, et al. Selective expression of the interleukin 7 receptor identifies effector CD8 T cells that give rise to long-lived memory cells. Nat Immunol 2003;4(12): 1191–8.

[71] Nishikawa H, Kato T, Tawara I, et al. Accelerated chemically induced tumor development mediated by CD4+CD25+ regulatory T cells in wild-type hosts. Proc Natl Acad Sci U S A 2005;102:9253–7.

[72] Hurwitz AA, Yu TF, Leach DR, et al. CTLA-4 blockade synergizes with tumor-derived granulocyte-macrophage colony stimulating factor for treatment of an experimental mammary carcinoma. Proc Natl Acad Sci U S A 1998;95:10067–71.

[73] Maker AV, Attia P, Rosenberg SA. Analysis of the cellular mechanism of antitumor responses and autoimmunity in patients treated with CTLA-4 blockade. J Immunol 2005; 175:7746–54.

[74] Talpur R, Jones DM, Alencar AJ, et al. CD25 expression is correlated with histological grade and response to denileukin diftitox in cutaneous T-cell lymphoma. J Invest Dermatol 2006;126:575–83.

[75] Dannull J, Su Z, Rizzieri D, et al. Enhancement of vaccine-mediated antitumor immunity in cancer patients after depletion of regulatory T cells. J Clin Invest 2005;115:3623–33.

[76] Knutson KL, Dang Y, Lu H, et al. IL-2 immunotoxin therapy modulates tumor-associated regulatory T cells and leads to lasting immune-mediated rejection of breast cancers in neu-transgenic mice. J Immunol 2006;177:84–91.

[77] Barnett B, Kryczek I, Cheng P, et al. Regulatory T cells in ovarian cancer: biology and therapeutic potential. Am J Reprod Immunol 2005;54:369–77.

[78] Litzinger MT, Fernando R, Curiel TJ, et al. The IL-2 immunotoxin denileukin diftitox reduces regulatory T cells and enhances vaccine-mediated T-cell immunity. Blood, in press.

[79] Attia P, Maker AV, Haworth LR, et al. Inability of a fusion protein of IL-2 and diphtheria toxin (denileukin diftitox, DAB389IL-2, ONTAK) to eliminate regulatory T lymphocytes in patients with melanoma. J Immunother 2005;28:582–92.

[80] Curiel TJ. Tregs and rethinking cancer immunotherapy. J Clin Invest 2007;117:1167–74.

[81] Llorrente L, Richaud-Patin Y, Garcia-Padilla C, et al. Clinical and biologic effects of anti-interleukin-10 monoclonal antibody administration in systemic lupus erythematosus. Arthritis Rheum 2000;43:1790–800.

[82] Lutsiak ME, Semnani RT, De Pascalis R, et al. Inhibition of CD4+CD25+ T regulatory cell function implicated in enhanced immune response by low-dose cyclophosphamide. Blood 2005;105:2862–8.

[83] Beyer M, Kochanek M, Darabi K, et al. Reduced frequencies and suppressive function of CD4+CD25hi regulatory T cells in patients with chronic lymphocytic leukemia after therapy with fludarabine. Blood 2005;106:2018–25.

[84] Peng G, Guo Z, Kiniwa Y, et al. Toll-like receptor 8-mediated reversal of CD4+ regulatory T cell function. Science 2005;309:1380–4.

[85] Galustian C, Klaschka DC, Meyer B, et al. Lenalidomide (Revlimid, CC-5013) and Actimid (CC-4047) inhibit the function and expansion of T regulatory (Treg) cells in vitro: implications for anti-tumor activity in vivo [abstract #1147]. Presented at the AACR Annual Meeting. Los Angeles (CA), April 14–18, 2007.

[86] Battaglia M, Stabilini A, Migliavacca B, et al. Rapamycin promotes expansion of functional CD4+CD25+FOXP3+ regulatory T cells of both healthy subjects and type 1 diabetic patients. J Immunol 2006;177:8338–47.

[87] Betts GJ, Clarke SL, Richards HE, et al. Regulating the immune response to tumors. Adv Drug Deliv Rev 2006;58:948–61.

[88] Whiteside TL. Immune suppression in cancer: effects on immune cells, mechanisms and future therapeutic intervention. Semin Cancer Biol 2006;16:3–15.

[89] Whiteside TL. Tumor-induced death of immune cells: its mechanisms and consequences. Semin Cancer Biol 2002;12:43–50.

[90] Kuss I, Donnenberg A, Gooding W, et al. Effector CD8+CD45RO-CD27- T cells have signaling defects in patients with head and neck cancer. Br J Cancer 2003;88:223–30.

[91] Tsukishiro T, Donnenberg AD, Whiteside TL. Rapid turnover of the CD8+CD28- T cell subset of effector cells in the circulation of patients with head and neck cancer. Cancer Immunol Immunother 2003;52:599–507.

[92] Kuss I, Hathaway B, Ferris RL, et al. Decreased absolute counts of T lymphocyte subsets and their relation to disease in squamous cell carcinoma of the head and neck. Clin Cancer Res 2004;10:3755–62.

[93] Kuss I, Schaefer C, Godfrey TE, et al. Recent thymic emigrants and subsets of naïve and memory T cells in the circulation of patients with head and neck cancer. Clin Immunol 2005;116:27–36.

[94] Albers AE, Visus C, Tsukishiro T, et al. Alterations in the T cell receptor variable gene β-restricted profile of CD8+ T lymphocytes in the peripheral circulation of patients with squamous cell carcinoma of the head and neck. Clin Cancer Res 2006;12: 2394–2303.

[95] Kim J-W, Tsukishiro T, Johnson JT, et al. Expression of pro- and anti-apoptotic proteins in circulating CD8+ T cells of patients with squamous cell carcinoma of the head and neck (SCCHN). Clin Cancer Res 2004;10:5101–10.

[96] Reichert TE, Strauss L, Wagner EM, et al. Signaling abnormalities and reduced proliferation of circulating and tumor-infiltrating lymphocytes in patients with oral carcinoma. Clin Cancer Res 2002;8:3137–45.

[97] Kuss I, Saito T, Johnson JT, et al. Clinical significance of decreased zeta chain expression in peripheral blood lymphocytes of patients with head and neck cancer. Clin Cancer Res 1999; 5:329–34.

[98] Miescher S, Whiteside TL, Carrell S, et al. Functional properties of tumor-infiltrating and blood lymphocytes in patients with solid tumors: effects of tumor cells and their supernatants on proliferative responses of lymphocytes. J Immunol 1986;136:1899–1807.

[99] Chang AE, Aruga A, Cameron MJ, et al. Adoptive immunotherapy with vaccine-primed lymph node cells secondarily activated with anti-CD3 and interleukin-2. J Clin Oncol 1997;15:796–807.

[100] Berard M, Brandt K, Bulfone Paus S, et al. IL-15 promotes the survival of naive and memory phenotype CD8+ T cells. J Immunol 2003;170:5018–26.

[101] Schluns KS, Lefrancois L. Cytokine control of memory T-cell development and survival. Nat Rev Immunol 2003;3:269–79.

[102] Trinchieri G. Interleukin-12 and the regulation of innate resistance and adaptive immunity. Nat Rev Immunol 2003;3:133–46.

[103] Gattatoni L, et al. Removal of homeostatic cytokine sinks by lemphodepletion enhances the efficacy of adoptively transferred tumor-specific CD8+ T cells. J Exp Med 2005;202: 907–12.

[104] Speiser DE, Romero P. Toward improved immunocompetence of adoptively transferred CD8+ T cells. J Clin Invest 2005;115:1467–9.

[105] Di Carlo E, de Totero D, Piazza T, et al. Role of IL-21 in immune regulation and tumor immunotherapy. Cancer Immunol Immunother 2007;56:1323–34.

[106] Hemmings BA. Akt signaling: linking membrane events to life and death decisions. Science 1997;275:628–30.

[107] Craig RW. MCL1 provides a window on the role of the BCL2 family in cell proliferation, differentiation and tumorigenesis. Leukemia 2002;16:444–54.

[108] Altieri DC. T cell expansion: the survivin interface between cell proliferation and cell death. Immunity 2005;22:534–5.

[109] Deveraux QL, Reed JC. IAP family proteins: suppressors of apoptosis. Genes Dev 1999; 13(3):239–52.

[110] Kim J-W, Ferris RL, Whiteside TL. Chemokine receptor 7 (CCR7) expression and protection of circulating CD8+ T lymphocytes from apoptosis. Clin Cancer Res 2005;11:7901–10.

[111] Parmiani G, Castelli C, Rivoltini L. Chemokine receptor 7, a new player in regulating apoptosis of CD8+ T cells in cancer patients. Clin Cancer Res 2005;11:7587–8.

[112] Pistoia V, Morandi F, Wang X, et al. Soluble HLA-G: are they clinically relevant? Semin Cancer Biol, in press.

[113] Rouas-Freiss N, Moreau P, Ferrone S, et al. HLA-G proteins in cancer: do they provide tumor cells with an escape mechanism? Cancer Res 2005;66:10139–44.

[114] Ye SR, Yang H, Li K, et al. Human leukocyte antigen G expression: as a significant prognostic indicator for patients with colorectal cancer. Mod Pathol 2007;20:375–83.

ELSEVIER
SAUNDERS

Surg Oncol Clin N Am
16 (2007) 775–792

SURGICAL
ONCOLOGY CLINICS
OF NORTH AMERICA

Monoclonal Antibodies in Therapy of Solid Tumors

David M. Heimann, MD[a], Louis M. Weiner, MD[b],*

[a]Department of Surgical Oncology, Fox Chase Cancer Center, 333 Cottman Avenue,
Philadelphia, PA 19111, USA
[b]Department of Medical Oncology, Fox Chase Cancer Center, 333 Cottman Avenue,
Philadelphia, PA 19111, USA

Monoclonal antibodies have emerged as effective therapeutic agents for a number of solid organ tumors. These antibodies have shown efficacy alone and in conjunction with known effective therapies for an increasing number of malignancies. Although monoclonal antibodies were discovered in 1975, it took approximately 20 years before they began to become standard therapy for common cancers.

During the past two decades, numerous advances in molecular biology have made possible the identification, genetic manipulation, and recombinant production of the monoclonal antibodies that are being used in clinical practice. An unconjugated anti-HER2/*neu* antibody is used alone and in combination with chemotherapy agents in breast cancer [1]. Antibodies directed against the epidermal growth factor receptor exhibit activity in advanced cancer [2]. Antibodies that inhibit T-cell activation by blocking the function of the CTLA-4 co-receptor on T cells continue to undergo clinical evaluation [3].

There have been many success stories, but useful antibodies have not been developed to effectively target many of the common solid tumors, which comprise more than 85% of human malignancies. This illustrates the challenges that remain in developing effective antibody-based therapeutics for solid tumors. A number of potential obstacles have been identified, including (1) overly rapid pharmacokinetics that restrict antibody access to tumors, (2) the induction of host immune responses that rapidly clear circulating therapeutic antibodies and may cause hypersensitivity reactions, (3) the inadequate recruitment of host effector mechanisms to clear

---

* Corresponding author.
E-mail address: lm_weiner@fccc.edu (L.M. Weiner).

surgonc.theclinics.com

antibody-coated tumor cells, (4) the treatment of patients whose tumor biologies are not likely to respond to signaling perturbation properties of the antibody used, and (5) the difficulty of obtaining effective concentrations in solid tumors. An "anti-cancer" monoclonal antibody must reach its binding sites on tumor cells. It then needs to penetrate the tumor to maximize potential therapeutic efficacy. A strong molecular attraction of the antibody for its antigen target on tumor cells (eg, high affinity) tends to restrict efficient tumor penetration because the antibody is sequestered by the first tumor antigen reservoirs it encounters upon leaving the circulation. It thus follows that rapid and thorough tumor penetration is associated with suboptimal retention within the tumor. In designing monoclonal antibodies to be used in the treatment of solid tumors, a suitable balance must be found between promoting tumor penetration and retention. Therapeutic monoclonal antibodies are drugs, and thus their structural properties influence their antitumor effects.

Factors regulating monoclonal antibody therapy

Antibody structure and size

Molecular size is a major determinant of speed of diffusion through tumors [4–6]. The rate of diffusion is inversely proportional to the molecular radius, or approximately to the cube root of molecular weight [4,7]. Single-chain Fv molecules (eg, scFv fragments) contain only the variable-heavy and variable-light chains of the immunoglobulin molecule and thus recapitulate an intact antibody binding site with only one sixth the mass of a conventional immunoglobulin (Ig)G molecule. Because they are smaller, scFv diffuse approximately six times faster than IgG [8]. Loss of the effector functions naturally associated with the Fc portion means that any desired cytotoxic agent would have to be added and thus negate the benefit of smaller size. Moreover, scFv with only one binding domain lose the advantages associated with multivalent binding to a target antigen.

Valence/charge

Molecular charge and shape affect tumor distribution. Slowing the dissociation of antibody–antigen complexes can increase tumor targeting of antibody fragments. This can be accomplished by increasing the valence of the molecules to impart an avidity effect to the binding [9,10]. If the size issue is compromised, then stability conferred by bivalent binding can increase the functional affinity for antigen up to 1000-fold higher for IgG versus Fab. One approach is to make multivalent scFvs that covalently associate to force dimerization of the scFv [11]. Another approach is to fuse a specific scFv at the carboxy terminus of another antibody with a different specificity. This fusion protein would have two different specificities and maintain some effector function of an Ig molecule along with a longer half-life and Fc receptor binding [12].

Affinity

Affinity for the target antigen is an important variable affecting tumor distribution. Modeling has shown that tighter binding results in increased retention of antibody at the periphery of 0.3-mm tumor nodules [13]. The term "binding site barrier" is used to describe the phenomenon of poor tumor penetration by high-affinity antibodies [14].

Work by Jain and Baxter [15] suggests that larger, higher-affinity antibodies take longer to reach a central necrotic core but ultimately have increased retention. Baxter and Jain [16] concluded that in the setting of antibody excess, higher affinity is better; however, when there is an excess of antigen, high-affinity antibodies are hindered by getting "stuck" at the periphery. These models were experimentally validated by a series of studies that used scFv with widely varying affinities for an identical epitope on the extracellular domain of the HER2/*neu* antigen; all the affinity variants were derived from a single scFv parent and differed by no more than a handful of amino acids [17]. These observations have been validated using other tumor models [18].

Tumor exposure to antibody is governed by two kinetic phases: the loading phase and the retention phase. During the loading phase, a shell of bound antibody expands until the entire amount of antigen on the tumor surface is occupied. The bound antibody moves toward the tumor core only as long as the concentration of free antibody at the tumor surface remains high. Low-affinity antibodies penetrate more deeply into the tumor than higher-affinity antibodies. In the retention phase, antigen internalization, which may be associated with antitumor effect or shedding, results in the depletion of antigen–antibody complexes. This can be accomplished by cellular internalization of a toxic substance conjugated to the antibody or by elimination of the antigen as a cellular signaling receptor. As the affinity increases, more antigen–antibody complexes internalize. To avoid competition with each other, retention in the tumor and maximization of intratumoral exposure requires antigen–antibody complex dissociation rates that are no greater than the rate of elimination or internalization of the antigen–antibody complex. Thus, the optimal binding affinity balances two goals: (1) there must be sufficiently rapid diffusion to enable penetration into the solid tumor, and (2) retention must be long enough to enable signaling inhibition, internalization, or other events required for a pharmacologic effect. Hence, this effect is not only controlled by the characteristics of the antibody, but also by the antigen and the requirements for therapeutic efficacy.

Species of origin

The normal physiologic response to the presence of an antigen is the production of polyclonal antibodies. The heterogeneity of this immune response poses safety concerns that limit the application of polyclonal antibodies [19]. Hybridoma technology has led to the ability to produce antibodies that are the products of a single-antibody-producing cell and have a single variable region associated with one constant region [20]. These antibodies are highly specific with a high affinity but have short half-lives in humans, leading to difficulty in maintaining therapeutic levels [19]. Also, the human immune system recognizes the mouse monoclonal antibody as a foreign protein, thus leading to the formation of human-antimouse antibodies that further decrease the circulating half-life and can lead to severe allergic reactions [21,22].

To overcome problems associated with the administration of murine monoclonal antibodies, mouse–human chimeric antibodies are produced by genetically fusing the mouse variable domain to human constant domains. Although chimeric antibodies possess reduced immunogenicity, they can elicit human-antichimeric-antibody responses. To address this issue, the complementary regions within the variable regions, which are responsible for antigen binding, have been transferred to a human Ig backbone, thereby creating humanized antibodies [23]. Trastuzumab is an example of a humanized monoclonal antibody [24].

The production of fully human monoclonal antibodies, using transgenic mouse technology, has essentially circumvented the problems associated with murine protein immunogenicity. The reduced immunogenicity of these antibodies improves the efficacy and safety of their use in humans for the treatment of cancer or chronic diseases. Panitumumab is an example of a fully humanized monoclonal antibody approved by the United States Food and Drug Administration (FDA).

Solid tumor antigens

Tumor-associated antigens

Tumor-associated antigens are expressed not only by cancer cells but are also presented by at least one subset of normal adult cells. Thus, these antigens are not cancer specific, though the extent of their expression by normal cells can vary greatly. Most tumor-associated antigens are lineage specific and represent differentiation antigens. Malignant cells can express a given antigen at levels much higher than a normal cell. For example, MAGE, an antigen expressed on melanoma cells, is also expressed on primary spermatocytes of the testis. Other examples of tumor-associated antigens included CEA, HER-2/neu, AFP, and PSA.

Tumor-specific antigens

Unique tumor antigens were discovered over 40 years ago, yet the molecular basis for the diversity of these antigens has become elucidated in the past decade. Three mechanisms can lead to the appearance of these antigens: (1) mutations, (2) clonal amplification, and (3) gene activation. In the last 10 years, the genetic origins of several T-cell–recognized tumor antigens from cancers have been identified. In each case the antigen was caused by a somatic mutation that creates a truly tumor-specific target. The locations of these mutations are not random but seem to occur in the regions that encode for important components of the overexpressed protein. Examples of this phenomenon include β-catenin and p53. A large deletion in the extracellular domain of the epidermal growth factor receptor leads to a constitutively activated receptor and also creates a tumor-specific epitope that can be targeted by monoclonal antibodies. One such antibody has been conjugated to radionuclides [25] or catalytic toxins [26] and used for therapy of experimental and clinical cancers.

Tumor physiology

Numerous obstacles to transport exist within solid tumors. Solid tumors differ from normal tissue with regard to vasculature, interstitial fluid pressure, cell density, tissue structure, tissue composition, and extracellular matrix (ECM) components [27]. Tumor ECM is richer in collagen, the primary determinant of tissue resistance to macromolecular transport, compared with normal tissue [28]. Measurements within murine solid tumors showed that macromolecular diffusion slowed 2-fold within 200 μm of the surface of the tumor and more than 10-fold beyond 500 μm, correlating with increasing density of ECM and tighter collagen organization near the core of the tumor [29]. ECM composition differs among tumor types [6,28] and changes in response to radiation therapy [30].

Tumor blood vessels are unlike normal blood vessels. Blood vessels associated with tumors are more heterogeneous in distribution, more tortuous in their path, larger in size, and more permeable [31,32]. The blood supply of tumors has a much higher viscosity due to cells and large molecules drained from the interstitium [27]. This results in greater blood flow resistance and lower blood flow relative to normal tissues, especially when the increased tortuosity of the tumor blood vessels is included [33].

Vascularity is an important determinant of tumor biodistribution of antibodies. To uniformly penetrate a tumor, an antibody must penetrate half the distance to the nearest vessel with an average intervessel distance ranging from 40 μm to 100 μm [4,7]. In some areas this distance can range as high as 1 cm [5]. Likewise, areas of functional hypoperfusion can exist due to local elevations in interstitial pressure [15]. The therapeutic relevance of penetrating these extremely hypoperfused areas depends on whether they contain viable tumor cells despite the hypoperfusion.

Retention of macromolecules elevates oncotic pressure [34] and raises interstitial pressure compared with normal tissues. Interstitial fluid pressure is elevated uniformly throughout a tumor and drops precipitously to normal values in the tumor's periphery or in the immediately surrounding tissue [35]. An elevated interstitial pressure correlates with an increased tumor size, a decreased oxygenation level, and a decreased radiosensitivity [36–38]. Antibodies must diffuse against this pressure gradient to penetrate tumors. Because tumor size affects the distance that antibodies must diffuse to uniformly penetrate tumor and the interstitial pressure, larger tumors may be more difficult to treat with monoclonal antibody therapies.

Mechanisms of action

Complement

The complement system is a complex system of proteolytic enzymes, regulatory and inflammatory proteins, cell surface receptors, and proteins capable of inducing cell lysis. The system, via the classical or alternative pathway, leads to the activation of the third component of complement (C3). C3 releases proteins that are critical for opsonization and engages the third set of proteins that produce cell death through osmotic lysis. Fragments generated from some of the complement components (C3a and C5a) possess potent inflammatory activities (Fig. 1).

The classical pathway is initiated by the formation of complexes of antigen with IgM or IgG antibodies. This leads to the binding of the first component of complement (C1) and subsequently cleaves C4 and C2. This leads to the activation of C3 and to cell lysis. The alternative pathway seems to be

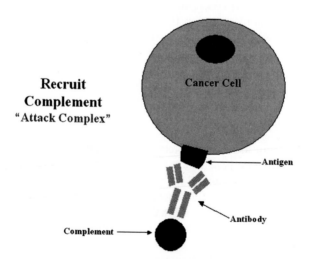

Fig. 1. The complement system is a complex system of proteolytic enzymes, regulatory and inflammatory proteins, cell surface receptors, and proteins capable of inducing cell lysis. The system leads to the activation of the third component of complement, which releases proteins that are critical for opsonization and engages proteins that produce cell death through osmotic lysis.

evolutionary more ancient and can be regarded as a primitive type of non-specific immune system. It can be activated by a variety of agents. The alternative pathway also plays a role in amplifying the activity of the classical pathway.

Antibody-dependent cell-mediated cytotoxicity

Antibody-dependent cell-mediated cytotoxicity (ADCC) is useful in host defenses against pathogens when antibodies are bound to pathogen surfaces, leading to the killing of the pathogen. The process can be mediated by neutrophils, mononuclear phagocytes, or human natural killer cells. When the antibody engages its target antigen, the antibody Fc domain is able to engage activating or inhibitory effector cell Fc receptors, thus sending signals to those cells that can culminate in target destruction through phagocytosis or perforin/granzyme B–related killing mechanisms (Fig. 2) [39]. It has been shown that the anticancer properties of at least one clinically active antibody, rituximab, are critically dependent upon interactions of that antibody with the activating human Fc receptor expressed by human natural killer cells, implying that ADCC is an important, clinically relevant mechanism of action for this antibody [40,41].

Current clinical applications for solid tumors

Trastuzumab

HER-2/*neu* (c-erbB-2), a member of the epidermal growth factor receptor (EGFR) family, has been targeted for antibody therapy because it is overexpressed on a quarter of breast cancers and on adenocarcinomas of the ovary, prostate, lung, and gastrointestinal tract. Trastuzumab is a humanized

ADCC

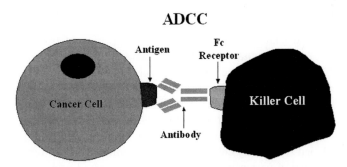

Fig. 2. ADCC is useful in host defenses against pathogens when antibodies are bound to pathogen surfaces, leading to the killing of the pathogen. When the antibody engages its target antigen, the antibody Fc domain is able to engage activating or inhibitory effector cell Fc receptors, thus sending signals to those cells that can culminate in target destruction through phagocytosis or perforin/granzyme B–related killing mechanisms.

antibody that recognizes an epitope on the extracellular domain of HER-2/ *neu* [24,42]. A phase II trial in women who had metastatic breast cancer reported an objective response rate of 11.6%, with responses seen in the liver, mediastinum, lymph nodes, and chest wall. None of the women developed an antibody response against trastuzumab despite the fact that they received at least 10 treatments with the antibody. In a second phase II study, 222 women who had metastatic breast cancer were treated with trastuzumab weekly, with an objective response rate of 16% [24]. The median response duration was 9.1 months, with a median overall survival of 13 months, both of which are superior to outcomes reported for second-line chemotherapy in metastatic disease. Long-term stabilization of disease of at least 5 months was seen in about 30% of patients in both trials. Overexpression of HER-2/*neu* that is associated with gene amplification correlates with a clinical response to trastuzumab, which is why earlier studies that used variable criteria to define HER-2 positivity demonstrate differences in the response rates [43].

A large, randomized, phase III trial evaluating cytotoxic chemotherapy alone or with trastuzumab has shown the efficacy of combination therapy [1]. Patients receiving initial therapy for metastatic breast cancer were treated with cyclophosphamide plus doxorubicin or epirubicin or with paclitaxel if they had received an anthracycline in the adjuvant setting. Patients were randomized to receive this chemotherapy alone or in combination with weekly trastuzumab. Response rates for combination therapy with an anthracycline regimen increased from 43% to 52% with the addition of trastuzumab. Using paclitaxel, response rates increased from 16% to 42% with the addition of trastuzumab. There was evidence that the addition of trastuzumab to chemotherapy improved survival at 1 year by 16% [44] and improved survival at 29 months by 25% [45]. Myocardial dysfunction was observed more commonly in patients receiving doxorubicin or epirubicin when trastuzumab was added. This led to trastuzumab not being recommended in conjunction with anthracycline therapy.

These clinical trial trials led to regulatory approval of trastuzumab for women who have metastatic breast cancer with HER-2/*neu* overexpression, given alone or in combination with paclitaxel. Trastuzumab also has activity in combination with other chemotherapeutic agents [46,47]. Breast cancer patients who have lymph node involvement whose cancers overexpressed HER-2/*neu* were evaluated in a randomized phase III trial studying standard adjuvant chemotherapy with or without trastuzumab. Interim analysis of this study led to its early closure because a significant improvement in disease free survival of patients in the trastuzumab arm had been observed [48]. Trastuzumab has clearly shown a benefit in breast cancer therapy, but, despite the overexpression of Her2/*neu* in other solid tumors, no significant clinical benefit has been seen in patients who have other cancers treated with trastuzumab.

Bevacizumab

Many cancers produce or provoke the production of vascular endothelial growth factor (VEGF) to stimulate the growth of new blood vessels. In some studies, VEGF expression at tumor sites is correlated with risk for metastases; thus, these tumor sites are potentially important targets for antibody therapy. VEGF, which resides in the vasculature that feeds tumor cells, is the first antiangiogenic target to be targeted. Bevacizumab is a humanized monoclonal antibody that blocks binding of VEGF to its receptor on vascular endothelium. A phase I clinical study of bevacizumab tested doses of 0.1 to 10 mg/kg infused on days 1, 28, 35, and 42 [49]. No severe toxicities were found. In a phase II study of bevacizumab combined with carboplatin and paclitaxel in patients who had non–small-cell lung cancer, 6 of 66 patients developed pulmonary hemorrhage, and 4 of the 6 died [50]. Patients who had squamous cell lung cancers and tumors with evidence of cavitation or squamous cell histology seemed to be at higher risk of hemoptysis.

In a randomized trial involving 813 patients who had previously untreated metastatic colorectal cancer, 402 patients received irinotecan, bolus fluorouracil, and leucovorin (IFL) plus bevacizumab (5 mg/kg every 2 weeks), and 411 received IFL plus placebo [51]. The median survival was 20.3 months in the bevacizumab arm versus 15.6 months in the placebo arm. The overall response rates were higher in the antibody treated arm (44.8% versus 34.8%; $P = .004$). The most common side effect was grade 3 hypertension during treatment with IFL plus bevacizumab (11% versus 2.3%), but this was easily managed. This study has led to the regulatory approval of bevacizumab for the treatment of patients who have metastatic colorectal cancer.

In 2006, the combination of carboplatin, paclitaxel, and bevacizumab was approved by the FDA for the initial treatment of patients who have unresectable, locally advanced, recurrent, or metastatic nonsquamous, non-small cell lung cancer. In a trial of more than 800 chemotherapy naive patients, the median survival was 12.3 months in those receiving chemotherapy therapy with bevacizumab compared with 10.3 months in patients receiving chemotherapy alone. Significant, including fatal, toxicities were noted with bevacizumab, including gastrointestinal perforation, bleeding, and thrombosis [52].

Bevacizumab has also been used in the treatment of metastatic breast cancer. Early studies of bevacizumab monotherapy in anthracycline and taxane refractory metastatic breast cancer showed response rates of up to 15% [53]. Bevacizumab has also been evaluated in combination with chemotherapy. A treatment regimen of docetaxel with bevacizumab as first- or second-line therapy observed a response rate of 52% [53]. In a recent phase III trial of 462 women who were previously treated with anthracycline- and taxane-based chemotherapy, patients were randomized to capecitabine or capecitabine with bevacizumab. There was significant improvement in response rates from 9.1% to 19.8% in the combination arm, but there was no significant change in progression-free survival [54]. Another phase III randomized trial investigating paclitaxel versus paclitaxel with bevacizumab as first-line therapy for metastatic breast cancer showed a significant improvement in the combination arm with regard to response rate (14.2% versus 28.2%; $P < .0001$) and progression-free survival (6.1 months versus 11.4 months; $P < .001$) [55]. This finding has led to the increased use of bevacizumab as first-line therapy in metastatic breast cancer.

Cetuximab and panitumumab

The role of EGFR overexpression in tumor growth and development is best studied in colorectal cancers [56] because EGFR overexpression is found in up to 70% of colorectal carcinomas [57]. The anti-EGFR monoclonal antibodies competitively bind to the EGF receptor and thus block the ligand from binding and prevent downstream events. Cetuximab is a chimeric monoclonal antibody directed against the extracellular domain of the EGF receptor. Panitumumab is a fully human monoclonal antibody against the EGF receptor. Unlike cetuximab, it lacks functional mouse immunoglobulin sequences but instead was derived by immunizing a mouse that was transgenic for human immunoglobulin genes to obtain fully human monoclonal antibodies [56]. Both of these antibodies are capable of inhibiting the growth of EGFR expressing cell lines in vitro and in vivo [45,58].

Cetuximab is capable of enhancing the antitumor effects of chemotherapy and radiation therapy in clinical studies. This agent has been used alone or in combination with radiotherapy or various chemotherapeutic agents primarily in patients who had head and neck or colorectal cancers. The most common side effects seen with this agent are rash and occasional allergic reactions. In a phase II study of 120 patients who had EGFR-positive colorectal tumors refractory to 5-FU or irinotecan, the combination of cetuximab and irinotecan had a response rate of 22.5% [59]. A subsequent randomized phase III trial involving 329 patients who had EGFR-positive, irinotecan refractory colorectal cancers was conducted. The participants were randomized to receive cetuximab alone (400 mg/m^2 loading dose followed by 250 mg/m^2 weekly) or cetuximab with irinotecan. There was a significantly higher response rate (22.9% versus 10.8%) and median time to progression in the combination arm [60]. Cetuximab has been approved by the FDA for the treatment of advanced or refractory colorectal cancers, in conjunction with irinotecan.

Colorectal cancer patients who have EGFR-negative tumors seem to have the potential to respond to cetuximab-based therapies. A review of 16 patients who had EGFR-negative colorectal cancers at Memorial Sloan-Kettering Cancer Center treated with cetuximab alone (two patients) or in combination with irinotecan (14 patients) revealed a 25% response rate

(95% confidence interval, 4%–46%) [61]. Thus, EGFR analysis using current immunohistochemical techniques does not have predictive value and should therefore not be used as a basis for offering or excluding cetuximab therapy to these patients.

Panitumumab more recently obtained regulatory approval for the treatment of metastatic colorectal cancer that has failed standard chemotherapy regimens. The approval was based on a trial of 463 patients who had metastatic colorectal cancer after treatment with 5-FU, irinotecan, or oxaliplatin and who were randomly assigned to receive panitumumab (6 mg/kg every 2 weeks) with best supportive care (BSC) or BSC alone. Progression-free survival was significantly prolonged in the panitumumab group ($P<.0001$). After 1-year minimum follow-up, objective response rates were significantly improved in the panitumumab group (10% versus 0% in BSC group; $P<.0001$). No difference was observed in overall survival; however, this is confounded by the fact that 76% of the patients in the BSC group crossed over to receive panitumumab. The treatment was well tolerated [62].

Ipilimumab

Cytotoxic T-lymphocyte–associated antigen 4 (CTLA-4) is an immunomodulatory molecule expressed on T cells. By decreasing T-cell responsiveness and raising the threshold for T-cell activation, CTLA-4 plays a critical role in the maintenance of peripheral T-cell tolerance. Blockade of CTLA-4 function provides a compelling means of enhancing antitumor immunity because tumors primarily express self-antigens. Anti-CTLA-4 antibody has been shown in multiple murine models to induce tumor regression. Likewise, recent clinical trials demonstrated that the administration of a fully human CTLA-4 blocking antibody resulted in objective responses in 21% of patients who had metastatic melanoma [63]. Significant grade 3 or 4 autoimmune toxicities were associated with this treatment in over 40% of patients. Further studies examining higher doses of antibodies did not display improvement in objective responses but were associated with greater number of grade 3 or 4 toxicities [64]. Ongoing clinical trials are studying the antibody in the treatment of renal cell cancer, sarcoma, prostate cancer, and breast cancer.

Toxicities of monoclonal antibodies

Monoclonal antibodies are associated with a number of toxicities that are related to their structural features (eg, hypersensitivity to murine protein components) or to their mechanisms of action (eg, EGFR blockade-related rash, trastuzumab-induced cardiotoxicity). These side effects play a significant role in the ability to treat patients. This is especially true because most monoclonal antibodies are used in conjunction with other therapies, such as chemotherapy or radiotherapy, which have their own inherent side effects (Table 1).

Future directions

Radioimmunotherapy

The FDA has approved two radioimmunoconjugates that combine a monoclonal antibody with a radioisotope for use in clinical practice: ibritumomab tiuxetan and tositumomab. These agents are approved for use in patients who have recurrent or refractory non-Hodgkin's lymphoma. Although the use of radioimmunotherapy has proven useful in the treatment of lymphomas, patients who have solid tumors have not benefited from this type of approach. The reasons for this inefficacy could be related to a lack of tumor penetration. Also, because only a small fraction of antibody localizes at tumor sites, the radioactive particles are deposited widely throughout normal organs, some of which are sensitive to the effects of radiation. Advances in antibody engineering to improve tumor targeting and reduce antibody residence time in the blood may address this challenge. Another potential reason for the inefficacy is incomplete tumor targeting by currently available monoclonal antibodies. To counter this problem, many investigators are targeting the vascular endothelium of solid tumors. This is a means of interrupting the tumor blood supply with antibodies against specific tumor endothelial markers that might prove beneficial in treatment of solid

Table 1
Monoclonal antibody toxicities

Monoclonal antibody	Target antigen	Toxicities
Trastuzumab	HER-2/*neu*	Cardiomyopathy
		Pulmonary
		Respiratory failure
		Pneumonitis
		Diarrhea
Bevacizumab	VEGF	Gastrointestinal perforations
		Hemorrhage
		Arterial thromboembolic events
		Hypertension
		Nephrotic syndrome
		CHF
Cetuximab/panitumumab	EGF receptor	Acneiform rash
		Malaise
		Diarrhea (when used with irinotecan)
		Hypersensitivity (cetuximab)
Ipilimumab	CTLA-4	Autoimmunity
		Enterocolitis
		Hypopituitarism

tumors. Radiolabeled antibodies directed against solid tumor vasculature thus could provide additional treatment by directing radiation toward the solid tumor.

Drug conjugates

Coupling of drugs to tumor-binding monoclonal antibodies can direct the cytotoxic drug to the tumor. An example is an anti-CD33 monoclonal antibody that is linked to calicheamicin, an antibiotic that cleaves DNA [65]. The resulting drug, gemtuzumab, binds to the CD33 antigen, and, after internalization of the conjugated monoclonal antibody, the antibiotic can mediate its toxic effect, leading to tumor-specific cell death [66]. This immunoconjugate has received FDA approval to treat patients who have acute myelogenous leukemia.

Strategies have been developed to take advantage of the specificity of antibody-based targeting without subjecting the host to the potentially toxic side effects associated with the systemic delivery of an active chemotherapeutic drug. In pretargeted antibody therapy, an antibody–enzyme or antibody–ligand conjugate is administered and over time localizes in the solid tumor. After it has cleared from the circulation and normal tissues, a cytotoxic agent is administered that can only be activated by the pretargeted antibody in the tumor. In this manner, the cytotoxic effects are further focused on the tumor.

Immunotoxins

Monoclonal antibodies that are not capable of directly eliciting antitumor effects by themselves can be effective against tumors by delivering cytotoxic agents [67]. Immunotoxins are antibodies that are conjugated to a toxin and are designed to deliver the toxin to the cell surface [68]. Toxins can be derived from plants or bacteria. The goal is to deliver the toxin to the surface of the cancer cells via antibody binding to an antigen target and, after internalization of the toxin, to cause cell death. The clinical and therapeutic benefits are more likely if the antigen is only expressed on cancer cells compared with normal cells. The more potent the toxin is, the fewer immunotoxin molecules are needed to achieve a therapeutic benefit. These toxic agents are potent due to their catalytic nature, which allows as few as one toxin molecule to kill a cell. The most commonly used toxins are derived from plants, such as ricin, or microorganisms, such as pseudomonas or diphtheria. The key in constructing an immunotoxin is that an antibody replaces the toxin's natural translocation domain to limit its internalization to cells that express the target antigen. Immunotoxins have demonstrated significant antitumor effects in preclinical models, but in clinical trials the use of immunotoxins has been associated with significant neurotoxicity and life-threatening vascular leak syndrome [69,70]. Despite such limitations, several immunotoxins show significant clinical activity [71,72].

Modifications of monoclonal antibody structure

Monoclonal antibodies can be engineered to mediate improved ADCC. This could greatly improve antigen presentation and subsequently T-cell activation, so that ADCC-competent antibodies directly promote tumor destruction and act as cancer vaccines. One method to accomplish this would be to increase monoclonal antibody affinity to tumor antigens. An alternative would be by modifying the Fc domain to increase the affinity for the Fc receptor [73,74]. Monoclonal antibodies can be combined with other agents that promote antigen presentation or T-cell expansion and activation, such as cytokines. Research is ongoing to improve and maintain the internalization of monoclonal antibodies in target tumor cells. One area of interest is in the area of recombinant antibody fragments, which are smaller than monoclonal antibodies and have increased clearance and increased tumor penetration. These fragments consist of minibodies, diabodies, and scFv fragments, all of which can be customized to possess any one of a number of desired properties.

Summary

As biology and technology have converged to overcome many obstacles, monoclonal antibodies have become increasingly used therapeutic agents for the treatment of solid cancer. Many are now being tested as components of adjuvant or first-line therapies to assess their efficacy in improving or prolonging survival. Selected unconjugated antibodies can exert clinically significant antitumor effects in many cancers. Antibody conjugates have been used to deliver toxic principles, such as radioactive particles, chemotherapeutic agents, and catalytic toxins, with increasing success in clinical trails. Much work has been done, but much remains, and the next few years should lead to significant improvements in the number and type of monoclonal antibodies in the armamentarium of the treatment of solid tumors.

References

[1] Slamon DJ, Leyland-Jones B, Shak S, et al. Use of chemotherapy plus a monoclonal antibody against HER2 for metastatic breast cancer that overexpresses HER2. N Engl J Med 2001;344(11):783–92.
[2] Robert F, Ezekiel MP, Spencer SA, et al. Phase I study of anti–epidermal growth factor receptor antibody cetuximab in combination with radiation therapy in patients with advanced head and neck cancer. J Clin Oncol 2001;19(13):3234–43.
[3] Egen JG, Kuhns MS, Allison JP. CTLA-4: new insights into its biological function and use in tumor immunotherapy. Nat Immunol 2002;3(7):611–8.
[4] Nugent LJ, Jain RK. Extravascular diffusion in normal and neoplastic tissues. Cancer Res 1984;44(1):238–44.
[5] Clauss MA, Jain RK. Interstitial transport of rabbit and sheep antibodies in normal and neoplastic tissues. Cancer Res 1990;50(12):3487–92.

[6] Pluen A, Boucher Y, Ramanujan S, et al. Role of tumor-host interactions in interstitial diffusion of macromolecules: cranial vs. subcutaneous tumors. Proc Natl Acad Sci USA 2001; 98(8):4628–33.

[7] Gerlowski LE, Jain RK. Microvascular permeability of normal and neoplastic tissues. Microvasc Res 1986;31(3):288–305.

[8] Graff CP, Wittrup KD. Theoretical analysis of antibody targeting of tumor spheroids: importance of dosage for penetration, and affinity for retention. Cancer Res 2003;63(6): 1288–96.

[9] Adams GP, McCartney JE, Tai MS, et al. Highly specific in vivo tumor targeting by monovalent and divalent forms of 741F8 anti-c-erbB-2 single-chain Fv. Cancer Res 1993;53(17): 4026–34.

[10] Tai MS, McCartney JE, Adams GP, et al. Targeting c-erbB-2 expressing tumors using single-chain Fv monomers and dimers. Cancer Res 1995;55(23 Suppl):5983S–9S.

[11] Pack P, Plückthun A. Miniantibodies: use of amphipathic helices to produce functional, flexibly linked dimeric FV fragments with high avidity in Escherichia coli. Biochemistry 1992; 31(6):1579–84.

[12] Coloma MJ, Morrison SL. Design and production of novel tetravalent bispecific antibodies. Nat Biotechnol 1997;15(2):159–63.

[13] Weinstein JN, van Osdol W. Early intervention in cancer using monoclonal antibodies and other biological ligands: micropharmacology and the "binding site barrier". Cancer Res 1992;52(9 Suppl):2747S–51S.

[14] Fujimori K, Covell DG, Fletcher JE, et al. A modeling analysis of monoclonal antibody percolation through tumors: a binding-site barrier. J Nucl Med 1990;31(7):1191–8.

[15] Jain RK, Baxter LT. Mechanisms of heterogeneous distribution of monoclonal antibodies and other macromolecules in tumors: significance of elevated interstitial pressure. Cancer Res 1988;48(24):7022–32.

[16] Baxter LT, Jain RK. Transport of fluid and macromolecules in tumors: IV. A microscopic model of the perivascular distribution. Microvasc Res 1991;41(2):252–72.

[17] Adams GP, Schier R, McCall AM, et al. High affinity restricts the localization and tumor penetration of single-chain fv antibody molecules. Cancer Res 2001;61:4750–5.

[18] Swers JS, Widom A, Phan U, et al. A high affinity human antibody antagonist of P-selectin mediated rolling. Biochem Biophys Res Commun 2006;350(3):508–13.

[19] Penichet ML, Morrison SL. Design and engineering human forms of monoclonal antibodies. Drug Dev Res 2004;61(3):121–36.

[20] Kohler G, Milstein C. Continuous cultures of fused cells secreting antibody of predefined specificity. Nature 1975;256(5517):495–7.

[21] Abramowicz D, Crusiaux A, Goldman M. Anaphylactic shock after retreatment with OKT3 monoclonal antibody. N Engl J Med 1992;327(10):736.

[22] Bajorin DF, Chapman PB, Wong GY, et al. Treatment with high dose mouse monoclonal (anti-GD3) antibody R24 in patients with metastatic melanoma. Melanoma Res 1992; 2(5–6):355–62.

[23] Wright A, Shin SU, Morrison SL. Genetically engineered antibodies: progress and prospects. Crit Rev Immunol 1992;12(3–4):125–68.

[24] Cobleigh M, Vogel CL, Tripathy D, et al. Multinational study of the efficacy and safety of humanized anti-HER2 monoclonal antibody in women who have HER2-overexpressing metastatic breast cancer that has progressed after chemotherapy for metastatic disease. J Clin Oncol 1999;17(9):2639–48.

[25] Reist CJ, Archer GE, Kurpad SN, et al. Tumor-specific anti-epidermal growth factor receptor variant III monoclonal antibodies: use of the tyramine-cellobiose radioiodination method enhances cellular retention and uptake in tumor xenografts. Cancer Res 1995; 55(19):4375–82.

[26] Pastan I, Beers R, Bera TK. Recombinant immunotoxins in the treatment of cancer. Methods Mol Bio 2004;248:503–18.

[27] Jang SH, Wientjes MG, Lu D, et al. Drug delivery and transport to solid tumors. Pharm Res 2003;20(9):1337–50.

[28] Netti PA, Berk DA, Swartz MA, et al. Role of extracellular matrix assembly in interstitial transport in solid tumors. Cancer Res 2000;60(9):2497–503.

[29] Thiagarajah JR, Kim JK, Magzoub M, et al. Slowed diffusion in tumors revealed by micro-fiberoptic epifluorescence photobleaching. Nat Methods 2006;3(4):275–80.

[30] Znati CA, Rosenstein M, McKee TD, et al. Irradiation reduces interstitial fluid transport and increases the collagen content in tumors. Clin Cancer Res 2003;9(15):5508–13.

[31] Tannock IF, Steel GG. Quantitative techniques for study of the anatomy and function of small blood vessels in tumors. J Natl Cancer Inst 1969;42(5):771–82.

[32] Heuser LS, Miller FN. Differential macromolecular leakage from the vasculature of tumors. Cancer 1986;57(3):461–4.

[33] Jain RK. Physiological barriers to delivery of monoclonal antibodies and other macromolecules in tumors. Cancer Res 1990;50(3 Suppl):814S–9S.

[34] Baxter LT, Jain RK. Transport of fluid and macromolecules in tumors: I. Role of interstitial pressure and convection. Microvasc Res 1989;37(1):77–104.

[35] Boucher Y, Baxter LT, Jain RK. Interstitial pressure gradients in tissue-isolated and subcutaneous tumors: implications for therapy. Cancer Res 1990;50(15):4478–84.

[36] Roh HD, Boucher Y, Kalnicki S, et al. Interstitial hypertension in carcinoma of uterine cervix in patients: possible correlation with tumor oxygenation and radiation response. Cancer Res 1991;51(24):6695–8.

[37] Gutmann R, Leunig M, Feyh J, et al. Interstitial hypertension in head and neck tumors in patients: correlation with tumor size. Cancer Res 1992;52(7):1993–5.

[38] Less JR, Posner MC, Boucher Y, et al. Interstitial hypertension in human breast and colorectal tumors. Cancer Res 1992;52(22):6371–4.

[39] Adams GP, Weiner LM. Monoclonal antibody therapy of cancer. Nat Biotechnol 2005; 23(9):1147–57.

[40] Cartron G, Dacheux L, Salles G, et al. Therapeutic activity of humanized anti-CD20 monoclonal antibody and polymorphism in IgG Fc receptor FcgammaRIIIa gene. Blood 2002;99(3):754–8.

[41] Weng WK, Levy R. Expression of complement inhibitors CD46, CD55, and CD59 on tumor cells does not predict clinical outcome after rituximab treatment in follicular non-Hodgkin lymphoma. Blood 2001;98(5):1352–7.

[42] Baselga J, Tripathy D, Mendelsohn J, et al. Phase II study of weekly intravenous recombinant humanized anti-p185HER2 monoclonal antibody in patients with HER2/neu-overexpressing metastatic breast cancer. J Clin Oncol 1996;14(3):737–44.

[43] von Mehren M, Adams GP, Weiner LM. Monoclonal antibody therapy for cancer. Annu Rev Med 2003;54:343–69.

[44] Norton L, Slamon D, Leyland-Jones B. Overall survival (OS) advantage to simultaneous chemotherapy (CRx) plus the humanized anti-HER2 monoclonal antibody HerceptinR (H) in HER2-everexpressing (HER2+) metastatic breast cancer (MBC) [abstract]. In: Proceedings of the American Society of Clinical Oncology Annual Meeting 1999;18:A483.

[45] Baselga J. Clinical trials of Herceptin^R (trastuzumab). Eur J Cancer 2001;37(Suppl 1): 18S–24S.

[46] Burstein HJ, Kuter I, Campos SM, et al. Clinical activity of trastuzumab and vinorelbine in women with HER2-overexpressing metastatic breast cancer. J Clin Oncol 2001;19(10): 2722–30.

[47] Pegram M, Lipton A, Hayes DF, et al. Phase II study of receptor-enhanced chemosensitivity using recombinant humanized anti-p185HER2/neu monoclonal antibody plus cisplatin in patients with HER2/neu-overexpressing metastatic breast cancer refractory to chemotherapy treatment. J Clin Oncol 1998;16(8):2659–71.

[48] Tuma RS. Trastuzumab trials steal show at ASCO meeting. J Natl Cancer Inst 2005;97(12): 870–1.

[49] Gordon MS, Margolin K, Talpaz M, et al. Phase I safety and pharmacokinetic study of re-combinant human anti-vascular endothelial growth factor in patients with advanced cancer. J Clin Oncol 2001;19(3):843–50.

[50] Johnson DH, Fehrenbacher L, Novotny W, et al. Randomized phase II trial comparing bev-acizumab plus carboplatin and paclitaxel with carboplatin and paclitaxel alone in previously untreated locally advanced or metastatic non-small-cell lung cancer. J Clin Oncol 2004; 22(11):2184–91.

[51] Hurwitz H, Fehrenbacher L, Novotny W, et al. Bevacizumab plus irinotecan, fluorouracil, and leucovorin for metastatic colorectal cancer. N Engl J Med 2004;350(23):2335–42.

[52] Sandler A, Gray R, Perry MC, et al. Paclitaxel-carboplatin alone or with bevacizumab for non-small-cell lung cancer. N Engl J Med 2006;355(24):2542–50.

[53] Mayer EL, Lin NU, Burstein HJ, et al. Novel approaches to advanced breast cancer: beva-cizumab and lapatinib. J Natl Compr Canc Netw 2007;5(3):314–23.

[54] Miller KD, Chap LI, Holmes FA, et al. Randomized phase III trial of capecitabine com-pared with bevacizumab plus capecitabine in patients with previously treated metastatic breast cancer. J Clin Oncol 2005;23(4):792–9.

[55] Miller KD, Wang M, Grawlow J, et al. A randomized phase III trial of paclitaxel versus pac-litaxel plus bevacizumab as first-line therapy for locally recurrent or metastatic breast cancer: a trial coordinated by the Eastern Cooperative Oncology Group (E2100). Breast Cancer Res Treat 2005;94:S6.

[56] Lockhart AC, Berlin JD. The epidermal growth factor receptor as a target for colorectal can-cer therapy. Semin Oncol 2005;32(1):52–60.

[57] Messa C, Russo F, Caruso MG, et al. EGF, TGF-alpha, and EGF-R in human colorectal adenocarcinoma. Acta Oncol 1998;37(3):285–9.

[58] Yang XD, Jia XC, Corvalan JR, et al. Development of ABX-EGF, a fully human anti-EGF receptor monoclonal antibody, for cancer therapy. Crit Rev Oncol Hematol 2001;38(1): 17–23.

[59] Saltz L, Rubin J, Hochster N, et al. Cetuximab (IMC-C225) plus irinotecan (CPT-11) is active in cpt-11-refractory colorectal cancer (CRC) that expresses epidermal growth factor receptor (EGFR) [abstract 7]. Proceedings of the American Society of Clinical Oncology An-nual Meeting 2001;20:3A.

[60] Cunningham D, Humblet Y, Siena S, et al. Cetuximab monotherapy and cetuximab plus iri-notecan in irinotecan-refractory metastatic colorectal cancer. N Engl J Med 2004;351(4): 337–45.

[61] Chung KY, Shia J, Kemeny NE, et al. Cetuximab shows activity in colorectal cancer patients with tumors that do not express the epidermal growth factor receptor by immunohistochem-istry. J Clin Oncol 2005;23(9):1803–10.

[62] Van Cutsem E, Peeters M, Siena S, et al. Open-label phase III trial of panitumumab plus best supportive care compared with best supportive care alone in patients with chemotherapy-refractory metastatic colorectal cancer. J Clin Oncol 2007;25(13):1658–64.

[63] Phan GQ, Yang JC, Sherry RM, et al. Cancer regression and autoimmunity induced by cy-totoxic T lymphocyte-associated antigen 4 blockade in patients with metastatic melanoma. Proc Natl Acad Sci USA 2003;100(14):8372–7.

[64] Maker AV, Yang JC, Sherry RM, et al. Intrapatient dose escalation of anti-CTLA-4 anti-body in patients with metastatic melanoma. J Immunother 2006;29(4):455–63.

[65] Zein N, Sinha AM, McGahren WJ, et al. Calicheamicin gamma 1I: an antitumor antibiotic that cleaves double-stranded DNA site specifically. Science 1988;240(4856):1198–201.

[66] Gatto B. Monoclonal antibodies in cancer therapy. Curr Med Chem Anticancer Agents 2004;4(5):411–4.

[67] Allen TM. Ligand-targeted therapeutics in anti-cancer therapy. Nature Reviews Cancer 2002;2(10):750–63.

[68] Presta LG. Engineering antibodies for therapy. Curr Pharm Biotechnol 2002;3(3):237–56.

[69] Pai LH, Bookman MA, Ozols RF, et al. Clinical evaluation of intraperitoneal Pseudomonas exotoxin immunoconjugate OVB3-PE in patients with ovarian cancer. J Clin Oncol 1991; 9(12):2095–103.

[70] Baluna R, Vitetta ES. Vascular leak syndrome: a side effect of immunotherapy. Immunopharmacology 1997;37(2–3):117–32.

[71] Kreitman RJ, Pastan I. Immunotoxins in the treatment of refractory hairy cell leukemia. Hematol Oncol Clin North Am 2006;20(5):1137–51.

[72] Herrera L, Yarbrough S, Ghetie V, et al. Treatment of SCID/human B cell precursor ALL with anti-CD19 and anti-CD22 immunotoxins. Leukemia 2003;17(2):334–8.

[73] Shields RL, Namenuk AK, Hong K, et al. High resolution mapping of the binding site on human IgG1 for Fc gamma RI, Fc gamma RII, Fc gamma RIII, and FcRn and design of IgG1 variants with improved binding to the Fc gamma R. J Biol Chem 2001;276(9): 6591–604.

[74] Rankin CT, Veri MC, Gorlatov S, et al. CD32B, the human inhibitory Fc-gamma receptor IIB, as a target for monoclonal antibody therapy of B-cell lymphoma. Blood 2006;108(7): 2384–91.

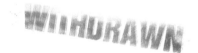

ELSEVIER
SAUNDERS

Surg Oncol Clin N Am
16 (2007) 793–818

SURGICAL
ONCOLOGY CLINICS
OF NORTH AMERICA

Cytokine Therapy for Cancer

Seunghee Kim-Schulze, PhD, Bret Taback, MD,
Howard L. Kaufman, MD*

*The Tumor Immunology Laboratory, Division of Surgical Oncology, 622 West
168th Street, P-S 17-508, Columbia University, New York, NY 10032, USA*

The central goal of cancer immunotherapy is to eradicate established tumors or prevent tumor recurrence through potent, specific, and long-lasting antitumor immune responses. Cytokines play a critical role in regulating the process of tumor recognition and eradication by the immune system. Although host immunity is complex and involves many different cellular and molecular players, the use of single-agent cytokine therapy has thus far been one of the most successful forms of immunotherapy for human cancer. The role of cytokines in tumor immunosurveillance has also been suggested through murine knock-out studies. In fact, mice that are deficient in expression of interferon (IFN)-γ, the type I or type II IFN receptors, or portions of their downstream signal transduction intermediates all have a higher frequency of tumors compared with control mice [1–5].

The most widely evaluated cytokines for human cancer have been members of the IFN and interleukin (IL) families. IFNα and IL-2 have achieved US Food and Drug Administration (FDA) approval for the treatment of melanoma and renal cell carcinoma [4], two tumors that seem to be highly sensitive to immunotherapeutic approaches. IL-2 and other member of the IL-2–related family of T-cell growth factors (ie, IL-4, IL-7, IL-9, IL-15, IL-18, IL-21) provide necessary signaling for activation and expansion of CD4+ and CD8+ T cells. The IL-12–related cytokines have also shown promise in preclinical tumor models, although the effects seem to be complex. More recently, the regulatory nature of IL-2 has been demonstrated through IL-2 knock-out mice, which exhibit a loss of self-tolerance and development of severe autoimmune disease [6]. The induction of inhibitory T cells, termed *regulatory T cells* (Tregs), by IL-2 may suggest a dual role for

* Corresponding author. Division of Surgical Oncology, Columbia University, 177 Fort Washington Avenue, MHB-7Sk, New York, NY 10032.
E-mail address: hlk2003@columbia.edu (H.L. Kaufman).

1055-3207/07/$ - see front matter © 2007 Elsevier Inc. All rights reserved.
doi:10.1016/j.soc.2007.07.011
surgonc.theclinics.com

this cytokine in the management of patients who have cancer. Our new understanding of these pleiotropic effects for IL-2 has resulted in new insights into cytokine biology and regulation of the immune response. This information is being translated into clinical practice through innovative strategies aimed at stimulating effector T cells while blocking suppressive Tregs.

This review provides a review of the basic biology of the major cytokines under consideration for use in tumor immunotherapy. The authors also describe the clinical role of cytokine therapy for human tumors, with a focus on melanoma and renal cell carcinoma. Finally, they present details of new cytokines and suggest possible direction for future clinical investigation using new cytokines or combinations of biologic agents. A better understanding of cytokine biology, coupled with new insights into the role of immunoregulation and the microenvironment in patients who have cancer, has provided new therapeutic targets for the treatment of human cancer.

Classification of cytokines and their receptors

Cytokines are secreted proteins that have pleiotropic effects, including regulation of innate immunity, adaptive immunity, and hematopoiesis. In the immune system, cytokines function in cascades and with a level of redundancy. The first cytokines identified were the IFNs; subsequently, new cytokines were referred to as ILs because they were produced by and acted on leukocytes. Because of their pleiotropic effects, multiple classification systems for cytokines have been devised. A functional classification system has been proposed, which segregates cytokines based on whether they affect innate immunity, adaptive immunity, or hematopoiesis [7]. Given that several cytokines affect the innate and adaptive immune systems, however, a more practical classification system based on the homology of their cognate receptors may be more appropriate. Overall, there are five cytokine receptor families (Fig. 1): type I cytokine receptors, type II cytokine receptors, immunoglobulin superfamily receptors, tumor necrosis factor (TNF) receptors, and G-protein–coupled receptors. The type I cytokine receptors are characterized by a common signaling subunit that complexes with a cytokine-specific subunit or units to initiate intracellular signals. Type I cytokine receptor family members include IL-2, IL-4, IL-7, IL-9, IL-15, and IL-21, and all share the common γ chain. Additional type I cytokine receptor subgroups include the granulocyte macrophage colony-stimulating factor (GM-CSF) and IL-6 receptor families. Similar to the IL-2–related cytokines, IL-6, IL-11, and IL-12 share GP130 as a common subunit. Likewise, IL-3, IL-5, and GM-CSF are members of the GM-CSF receptor subfamily and share a common β chain that complexes with the cytokine-specific α chain. The effects of IFNα, IFNβ, IFNγ, and IL-10 are mediated by type II cytokine receptors, which are composed of a signaling chain and

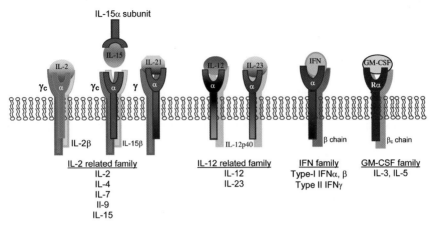

Fig. 1. Diagram of major cytokine receptor families showing selected receptors and how they share common subunits among family members. Biologic activity is distinguished by spatial and temporal expression of the receptors.

a ligand-binding chain. The immunoglobulin superfamily receptors contain extracellular immunoglobulin domains and include the receptors for IL-1, IL-18, stem cell factor, and monocyte CSF.

These cytokines are intimately involved in the induction of active immune responses against tumors and also negatively regulate immune responses to maintain homeostasis and self-tolerance. This self-tolerance is mediated by Tregs, and these cells are currently the focus of intense scrutiny by tumor immunologists. In recent years, tremendous progress has been made in identifying different types of Tregs and in understanding how cytokines regulate the generation and maintenance of Tregs [8]. An IL-10–dependent type I T-regulatory (Tr1) cell arises in the periphery on encountering antigen in a tolerogenic environment and mediates immune suppression. In contrast, a naturally occurring CD4+ CD25high FOXP3+ T-cell population (nTreg) mediates immune suppression in a contact-dependent, cytokine-independent, and antigen-nonspecific manner [9]. Cytokines help to maintain the number and functional characteristics of these cells and of the effector cells that help to clear pathogens and tumors. The balance between effector cells and Tregs may be critical for influencing the rejection or acceptance of tumors. IL-2, transforming growth factor (TGF)-β, and IL-10 have been shown to mediate the generation of Tregs and may be involved in the fine balance between effector and regulatory populations [10,11].

Biology of cytokines: focus on interleukins and interferons

Cytokines are critical in the development of the immune system, in host defense, and tumor immunobiology. Therefore, defining their biologic activities and understanding their mechanisms of action are key elements in the development of cytokine-based immunotherapy for the treatment of cancer. Impaired T-cell effector function at the tumor site is an important obstacle in spontaneous and vaccine-induced T-cell immunity for cancer. Cytokines act through direct stimulation of immune effector cells and stroma cells at the tumor site, enhancing tumor cell recognition by or susceptibility to cytotoxic effector T cells. Studies of cytokines in animal tumor models suggested that they would have broad antitumor activity and have resulted in translation into a large number of cytokine-based approached for cancer therapy. To date, only two cytokines have achieved approval for cancer: IL-2 for the treatment of metastatic melanoma and renal cell carcinoma and IFNα for the adjuvant therapy of stage III melanoma. The authors therefore describe the basic biology of these two cytokines.

Interleukin-2

The biologic effects of IL-2 are mediated by the IL-2 receptor, which belongs to a type I cytokine receptor [12]. The IL-2 receptor is a trimeric complex composed of three subunits: α, β, and γ chains. The β and γ chains are involved in signaling, whereas the α chain is only involved in cytokine binding. These subunits form a high-, intermediate-, or low-affinity receptor, depending on which of the chains are in the receptor complex. The high-affinity receptor complex is composed of all three subunits, whereas the intermediate affinity receptor is composed of the β and γ chains. The α subunit (CD25) does not initiate intracellular signaling [13]. Although the β and γ chains are expressed on T cells, B cells, and natural killer (NK) cells, the α chain (CD25) is inducible and its expression is restricted to T cells. IL-2 has a multitude of effects on the immune system. When T-cells recognize their cognate antigen, IL-2 is produced, resulting in autocrine and paracrine effects on the activated T cell.

In contrast to T cells, NK cells express the intermediate-affinity IL-2 receptor [14]. Exposure of NK cells to IL-2 results in proliferation, enhanced cytolytic activity, and secretion of other cytokines. B cells also express intermediate-affinity IL-2 receptors and can secrete IL-2 in cooperation with other cytokines, resulting in B-cell proliferation and differentiation [15].

IL-2 also plays a critical role in suppressing immune responses. A subpopulation of CD4+ T cells, characterized by high levels of CD25 and the forkhead/winged helix transcription factor FOXP3, function to suppress self-reactive T cells [16]. These Tregs likely maintain tolerance and prevent autoimmunity after activation of effector T-cell responses. This is supported by data demonstrating that depletion of CD4+CD25+ Tregs breaks tolerance to self-antigens and can lead to increased autoimmunity [16]. Furthermore, in murine models, depletion of CD4+CD25+ Tregs enhances tumor rejection and improves response to cancer vaccines by promoting the function of CD8+ cytotoxic T-cell lymphocytes (CTLs) [17]. The mechanisms by which CD4+CD25+ T cells inhibit the function of CD8+ CTLs is poorly understood. Mice with targeted deletion of IL-2 or the IL-2 receptor develop a generalized inflammatory syndrome and often die of autoimmune colitis [18–21]. These data suggest that IL-2 not only activates immune responses but participates in a negative feedback loop to limit immune responses. This view of IL-2 as a regulatory cytokine rather than a purely stimulatory T-cell growth factor suggests that the use of IL-2 in the clinical setting needs to be re-evaluated. An important area of further investigation is likely to be a more careful analysis of the dosing, schedule, and kinetics of IL-2 administration on specific T-cell subsets.

Interferons

The IFNs can be classified on their ability to bind to specific IFN receptors. The type I and type II IFN receptors are a subset of the type II cytokine receptors [22]. IFNα and IFNβ are predominantly involved in cellular immune responses to viral infections [23–25]. IFNα and IFNβ, representing more than 20 molecules, activate the type I IFN receptor and are referred to as type I IFNs [22–25]. IFNγ, the only type II IFN, is also important in cell-mediated immunity and activates the type II IFN receptor [26].

Although a great deal of murine experimentation has suggested the importance of IFNγ in tumor immunity, the type I IFNs have emerged as the most clinically useful IFNs for treatment of malignancy. The type I IFNs consist of at least five classes in human beings, of which IFNα and IFNβ have been used the most clinically [22]. These IFNs induce the expression of major histocompatibility complex (MHC) class I molecules on tumor cells and induce maturation of a subset of dendritic cells (DCs) [27–29]. Type I IFNs also activate CTLs, NK cells, and macrophages [30–33]. In addition to their immunologic effects, the type I IFNs can have a cytostatic effect on tumor cells and may also promote tumor cell apoptosis [34]. When administered at lower doses, they also have antiangiogenic effects on tumor neovasculature [35]. Mice with targeted deletion of the type I IFN receptor have a higher rate of carcinogen-induced cancer, and this results in enhanced tumor development in transplantable tumor models, supporting the hypothesis that the type I IFNs are important in immunosurveillance [36,37].

IFNα is composed of a group of at least 12 distinct proteins [22]. Recombinant IFNα-2a, IFNα-2b, and IFNα-2c differ by one or two amino acids and have been the isoforms most commonly used in the clinic [22]. Because IFNα and IFNβ signal through the same receptor, they would be expected to have similar biologic effects and to have overlapping indications. This is not always the case, however. The mechanism of antitumor activity in vivo is not completely defined for the IFNs; however, to date, the most widely used IFN is IFNα.

IFNγ is secreted by NK cells, NK T cells, T helper (Th) 1 CD4+ T cells, CD8+ T cells, antigen-presenting cells (APCs), and B cells [38–40]. IFNγ activates macrophages and stimulates upregulation of MHC class I, MHC class II, and costimulatory molecules on APCs [41–43]. Additionally, IFNγ induces changes in the proteosome, leading to enhanced antigen presentation [44,45]. IFNγ also promotes Th1 differentiation of CD4+ T cells and blocks IL-4–dependent isotype switching in B cells [41,46]. Mice with targeted deletion of IFNγ or the type II IFN receptor have an increased risk for spontaneous and chemically induced tumors compared with controls [1,3,37,47]. IFNγ is cytotoxic to some malignant cells and has modest antiangiogenic activity [48–50].

The antitumor effects of IFNγ in murine models suggested that it would be effective against a wide spectrum of malignancies. In reality, IFNγ has demonstrated limited clinical utility for the treatment of human cancer but may play a critical role in the in vivo effects of other cytokines [51,52].

Cytokine treatment of melanoma

Malignant melanoma is a tumor of melanocytes, and the natural history of this tumor suggests that it can be recognized by the immune system. An important observation has been that many primary cutaneous melanomas exhibit histologic regression at the time of clinical detection [53]. Further, in up to 5% of patients who have melanoma with metastatic disease, no obvious primary lesion can be identified, and most experts believe that this is because the melanoma was completely eradicated by the immune system [54,55]. The incidence of melanoma is increasing at a faster rate than any other cancer and is responsible for more years of productive life lost than any other cancer except childhood malignancies and testicular cancer. The success of surgical resection for thin lesions is offset by the dismal prognosis for patients who have metastatic melanoma. Once distant metastases occur, the median survival for most patients is less than 9 months. In general, melanoma has not been responsive to cytotoxic chemotherapy. Thus, early work focused on the generation of effective immune responses in patients who have melanoma. The pioneering work of Steve Rosenberg in the Surgery Branch of the National Cancer Institute (NCI) found that adoptively transferred T cells supported with concomitant administration of IL-2 resulted in significant tumor regression in selected patients [56]. Further investigation of these encouraging results suggested that most of the therapeutic activity was related to the high doses of IL-2 being given to the patients.

High-dose IL-2 induces objective clinical responses in 15% to 20% of patients and durable complete responses in a 10% of these patients [57,58]. Importantly, those patients with any response seem to have increased survival, and most complete responses are durable [59]. In fact, with prolonged follow-up data now available, it is clear that complete responders can be cured of metastatic melanoma. The toxicity associated with IL-2 administration, however, can be considerable and requires expertise in physician and nursing care, thus limiting the broader application of IL-2 for patients who have melanoma. To reduce the IL-2–related side effects, a variety of IL-2–containing regimens have been tested in patients who have melanoma. These have included continuous infusion of lower doses, delivery of low doses by subcutaneous and intravenous routes, and altered dosing schedules. To date, only the high-dose bolus regimen has shown consistent benefit for melanoma.

The toxicity profile of IL-2 is largely associated with a capillary leak syndrome, which is characterized by hypotension, tachycardia, and peripheral edema secondary to third space fluid accumulation. In addition, IL-2 can cause constitutional symptoms (eg, fever, chill, fatigue) and gastrointestinal side effects (eg, nausea, vomiting, anorexia, transaminitis, cholestasis, diarrhea) [60]. In addition to hypotension, IL-2 may induce pulmonary edema, cardiac arrhythmias, myocarditis, reversible renal and hepatic dysfunction, pruritus, electrolyte abnormalities, thrombocytopenia, anemia, and coagulopathy. Rarely, IL-2 may also induce confusion, disorientation, or visual hallucinations. Although early studies with IL-2 reported a 2% mortality rate that was generally related to gram-positive sepsis, current IL-2 centers that routinely use prophylactic antibiotics report no mortality [61]. In experienced centers, IL-2–related toxicity can usually be easily managed and all side effects are reversible on cessation of treatment.

To improve the clinical effectiveness of IL-2, studies combining IL-2 with other agents have been widely evaluated. In one study, a gp100 peptide vaccine administered with high-dose IL-2 was initially shown to induce an objective clinical response rate of 42%, although subsequent multi-institutional studies failed to confirm these findings [62–64]. Clinical trials combining Il-2 with IFNα also had encouraging results in phase II studies that could not be verified in later phase III randomized trials [62,65]. The combination of low doses of IL-2 with cytotoxic chemotherapy has been extensively studied with early-phase clinical trials reporting response rates in excess of 40% and selected durable responses [58,59,66–69]. Once again, subsequent randomized trials failed to show any survival advantage when compared with chemotherapy alone [69–72].

Interferon-α

IFNα has been investigated in patients who have metastatic melanoma and, to an even greater extent, in patients who have stage III melanoma. Multiple dose levels and schedules have been tested, and the overall response rate for single-agent IFNα in patients who have metastatic melanoma is approximately 15% [73–83]. Although there is no obvious "best regimen" in terms of response rate, IFNα is typically administered three times a week at a range of doses because of an improved toxicity profile [84,85]. A survival advantage has not been demonstrated because no prospective randomized trials have been conducted in patients who have metastatic melanoma [86].

In contrast to the patient who has stage IV melanoma, IFNα is an important agent in stage III adjuvant therapy of melanoma. IFNα was approved by the FDA for adjuvant therapy in patients who have high-risk melanoma based on data from a cooperative group multi-institutional clinical trial [80]. In this trial, patients who had primary lesions greater than 4 mm or those who had regional lymph node involvement after lymph node dissection were treated with 1 year of IFNα-2b. The regimen consisted of 20 million $U/m^2/d$ for 5 days per week for 4 weeks, followed by 10 million $U/m^2/d$ for three times per week for 48 weeks. An overall improvement in median relapse-free survival from 1 to 1.7 years and in median overall survival from 2.8 to 3.8 years was reported [80]. A follow-up intergroup clinical trial also reported an improvement in median and overall relapse-free survival but failed to demonstrate any improvement in overall survival [87]. The reason for these disparate outcomes is not entirely clear but may be related to improved patient selection, the advent of sentinel node technology, or the crossover of patients on the observation arm to receive IFNα off protocol [88]. Another large cooperative group trial compared a novel ganglioside GM2 vaccine with standard 1-year IFNα therapy and was halted prematurely because patients receiving IFNα alone demonstrated a significant increase in relapse-free and overall survival [88].

These studies established IFNα as the standard of care for patients who have high-risk stage III melanoma. Nonetheless, there is significant controversy as to the overall effectiveness of IFNα as an adjuvant in melanoma. Patients should understand the issues surrounding the benefits and risks of IFNα and the alternative treatment options before deciding against IFNα therapy.

The toxicity profile of IFNα is usually dose related, and most side effects can be managed without discontinuation of treatment. Experience with IFNα administration has resulted in well-established guidelines for recognition and management of adverse side effects. Constitutional symptoms are quite common and are likely to occur in 80% or more of patients. These typically consist of fever, fatigue, headaches, and myalgias [89,90]. Most of these symptoms can be controlled with acetaminophen or nonsteroidal anti-inflammatory drugs, although severe fatigue may necessitate an interruption in treatment or dose reduction. More serious are the neuropsychiatric issues, which include depression (45%), confusion (10%), and mania (<1%) [89–91].

In some studies of IFNα, the depression was highly significant and rare suicides were reported [92]. Currently, close monitoring of patient mental status or prophylactic use of antidepressants can reduce the risk for these side effects [92]. Gastrointestinal side effects are also common and consist of nausea, vomiting, anorexia, and diarrhea. These symptoms can usually be controlled with antiemetics and antidiarrheals. IFNα also produces increases in the hepatic enzymes in some patients, and serial monitoring of liver function test results is recommended. A significant elevation of hepatic enzymes may necessitate dose reduction or cessation of therapy. Thrombocytopenia, leukopenia, and neutropenia are common and can also be readily managed with dose reductions; rarely, transfusion may be required [89,90].

An interesting side effect that occurs in a subset of patients is related to alteration in immune function and often manifests as autoimmunity. Most commonly, autoimmune hyperthyroidism or hypothyroidism develops; therefore, thyroid function should be routinely monitored in patients receiving IFN therapy [93]. Other rare forms of autoimmune disease in patients who are receiving IFNα include sarcoidosis, vitiligo, lupus, rheumatoid arthritis, polymyalgia rheumatica, and psoriasis [94,95]. Interestingly, those patients who do develop signs of autoimmune vitiligo or autoantibodies have improved relapse-free and overall survival [96].

Experimental cytokine immunotherapy

Interleukin-2–related cytokines

IL-12 consists of 35-kd and 40-kd subunits and functions as a heterodimer. IL-12 stimulates IFNγ production by T cells and NK cells, which, in turn, activate macrophages [97–99]. IL-12 also promotes CD4+ T-cell differentiation into Th1 CD4+ T cells and enhances the cytotoxic activity of CD8+ CTLs [100–102]. IL-12 has demonstrated antitumor activity in murine models of melanoma, colon carcinoma, mammary carcinoma, and sarcoma [49,103–108]. Experimental investigation of the mechanism of IL-12 activity using mice with molecularly targeted defects suggests that different branches of the immune system mediate the antitumor effects. In the B16 murine melanoma model, a significant role for NK cells has been demonstrated in mediating antitumor immunity with high doses of IL-12 [109]. In contrast, antitumor responses at low doses of IL-12 seem to be mediated by NKT cells [110]. IL-12 also exhibits antiangiogenic effects mediated by IFNγ and interferon-8 inducible protein 10 (IP-10) [111].

Based on these preclinical studies, IL-12 has been evaluated in clinical trials as a treatment for melanoma. Preliminary results from these trials suggest that the objective clinical response rates were less than 5% [112]. Although the response rates were low, patients who did respond had sustained serum levels of IFNγ, IL-15, and IL-18, suggesting that sustained IFNγ production might result in better responses. In a phase I trial combining IL-12 with low doses of IL-2, sustained levels of IFNγ and expansion of NK cells were observed; however, only one patient achieved a partial response [113].

IL-15 is closely related to IL-2 and has emerged as an attractive cytokine for cancer immunotherapy based on extensive in vitro T-cell data and in vivo murine tumor models. Although IL-2 and IL-15 both provide initial stimulation for T-cell proliferation of activation, IL-15 acts to block

IL-2–induced apoptosis [114–116]. IL-15 also supports the persistence of CD8+ memory T cells, which may be important for maintaining long-term antitumor immunity [117]. IL-15 has demonstrated significant therapeutic activity in several preclinical murine models of cancer [118]. These effects are mediated through direct activation of CD8+ effector T cells in an antigen-independent manner [119] Importantly, IL-15 must be presented to CD8+ memory T cells by neighboring bone marrow (BM)–derived cells on a high-affinity receptor (IL-15Rα) [120]. With an intense interest in creating the optimal conditions for survival and expansion of tumor antigen-specific CD8+ T cells, several studies are ongoing to induce the optimal lymphopenic conditions to reduce the number of immune-suppressive Tregs, decrease the competition for the available cytokines, and allow a niche for antitumor T-cell expansion. Therefore, the prosurvival effects on CD8+ T cells attributable to IL-15 are a major advantage for tumor immunotherapy. IL-15 has not yet been directly tested in the clinic for metastatic melanoma. The combination of IL-15 and IL-12 gene therapy, however, has been shown to induce tumor rejection in a human transplantable tumor model [121].

IL-18 was initially identified as IFNγ-inducing factor and is structurally related to IL-1 [122]. IL-18 stimulates IFNγ secretion by NK and CD8+ T cells and enhances their cytotoxicity [123–125]. Other functions of IL-18 include macrophage activation, development of Th1 cells, and increased expression of Fas ligand (FasL) on lymphocytes [107,108,126–128]. Phase I clinical trials documented the safety of IL-18 and found increased levels of serum IFNγ and GM-CSF in patients after they received intravenous doses of IL-18 [129–134]. The clinical responses have been modest, with only two objective responses in 26 patients in one trial and in 3 patients who had stable disease in another study [135]. Further trials are expected with IL-18, and combinations of IL-18 with other cytokines have not yet been evaluated.

IL-21 is a member of the IL-2 cytokine family that was isolated using a ligand-receptor pairing method. The IL-21 receptor exists as a heterodimer consisting of the common IL-2 γ subunit and a unique IL-21 subunit [136]. IL-21 is produced by activated CD4+ T cells and has pleiotropic effects [137,138]. IL-21 mediates proliferation CD4+ and CD8+ T cells and also enhances CD8+ T-cell and NK-cell cytotoxicity. Although the role of IL-21 in Th1/Th2 differentiation is unclear, it is required for normal humoral responses [139–158].

IL-21 has demonstrated therapeutic activity in murine tumor models of melanoma and has recently entered phase I clinical trials with modest preliminary results [144,159–161].

IL-23 is a related cytokine composed of two subunits: a unique p19 subunit and the IL-12 p40 subunit. IL-12 and IL-23 are secreted from activated DCs and enhance proliferation of memory T cells and production of IFNγ from activated T cells. IL-23 has shown complex biologic activity in vivo, and contradictory roles in tumor rejection have been reported [162]. Whereas IL-12 promotes T-cell infiltration into tumors, IL-23 blocks local accumulation of tumor-infiltrating lymphocytes. Recently, human tumor tissues showed a significant increase in local IL-23p19 mRNA. In murine models, deletion of the IL-23 gene or use of a neutralizing anti-IL23p19 antibody consistently led to CD8+ T-cell infiltration and protective antitumor immunity [163]. In contrast to these observations, several studies have suggested that IL-23 might modulate certain antitumor immune responses leading to tumor rejection. In a murine melanoma system, systemic IL-23 treatment followed by gp100 peptide vaccination greatly increased the relative and absolute numbers of vaccine-induced CD8+ T cells and enhanced their effector function within the tumor microenvironment. Interestingly, TNF rather than IFNγ was the primary mediator of this activity [162]. Clinical trials have not been initiated with IL-23 to date.

Granulocyte macrophage colony-stimulating factor

GM-CSF was initially identified as a mediator of hematopoiesis. GM-CSF is also a highly pleiotropic cytokine and is closely related to IL-3 and IL-5. The receptors for GM-CSF, like those for IL-3 and IL-5, are composed of two subunits: a ligand-specific α chain and a common β chain. GM-CSF is produced by monocytic cells and T lymphocytes and promotes the attraction and maturation of DCs. This ability suggested that GM-CSF might be a good adjuvant for the induction of an immune response using various vaccine agents. In a murine melanoma model, injection of irradiated melanoma cells expressing GM-CSF provided protection against subsequent tumor challenge in more than 90% of mice [164]. These data have subsequently been validated in other animal model systems using various vaccination strategies. The antitumor activity of GM-CSF seems to be related to its ability to activate macrophages and DCs [165,166]. GM-CSF also matures DCs, leading to upregulation of costimulatory molecules and CD1d receptors [167]. Initial studies suggested that CD4+ and CD8+ T cells mediated GM-CSF tumor immunity, but recent models using CD1d-deficient mice support a critical role for NKT cells in GM-CSF antitumor immune responses [168]. Additional research suggests that GM-CSF may also serve a regulatory role in the induction of DC-mediated T-cell immunity [169].

Clinical trials of single-agent GM-CSF have suggested therapeutic activity in patients who have melanoma when injected intralesionally [170]. Additionally, multiple trials using autologous tumor vaccines engineered to secrete GM-CSF have shown biologic activity with occasional objective clinical responses [171]. GM-CSF has also been used as a subcutaneous injection in patients who have stage III and IV melanoma, with prolonged relapse-free and overall survival compared with that of historic control patients [172]. This observation is being tested in a recent cooperative group clinical trial, and results are expected shortly. GM-CSF has also been tested in combination with IL-2, with a reported complete clinical response rate of 15% in patients who had previously obtained stable disease or better on biochemotherapy [173].

Cytokine treatment of renal cell carcinoma

Tumors of the renal parenchyma have been increasing at a slow but steady rate for the past 30 years. Those tumors that are confined to the kidney can usually be successfully managed by nephrectomy, although 50% of these patients develop recurrent or metastatic disease after surgical resection. Similar to melanoma, renal cell carcinomas have been refractory to standard cytotoxic chemotherapy agents. These tumors, however, are responsive to immunologic manipulation. More recently, molecular targeted inhibitors of the tyrosine kinase pathways have shown significant benefit in patients who have renal cell carcinoma, although long-term durable responses are unusual [174–177]. The immunogenicity of renal cell carcinoma led to extensive clinical testing of IL-2 in the late 1980s, and FDA approval was granted in 1992. At present, IL-2 is the only cytokine approved for treatment of advanced renal cell carcinoma and produces significant objective responses and durable complete responses in a subset of patients.

The biology and rationale for the use of IL-2 have already been reviewed. The response rate with high-dose bolus IL-2 is approximately 20% for patients who have metastatic renal cell carcinoma, similar to that seen in patients who have melanoma. In renal cell carcinoma, lower doses of IL-2 have been evaluated, and although some patients do respond to these lower doses, the frequency of clinical responses is greatest in those receiving the standard high-dose bolus regimen [178]. Using a three-arm randomized trial design, two intravenous bolus regimens of IL-2 (high-dose and low-dose) and one low-dose subcutaneous IL-2 regimen were compared in patients who had metastatic renal cell carcinoma. The objective response rate in the high-dose intravenous arm was twice that of both low-dose arms (21% versus 11% and 10%). The overall clinical responses with high-dose IL-2 have been relatively durable; the median duration of response ranges from 24 to 54 months, with more than 80% of complete responders being long-term survivors [179]. IL-2 should remain in the armamentarium of the clinical oncologist for advanced renal cell carcinoma, although interactions with tyrosine kinase inhibitors need to be better understood, because these agents are likely to be used in most of this population.

Although not approved for renal cell carcinoma, numerous clinical trials have evaluated the effects of single-agent IFNα in patients who have metastatic disease. Overall, there has been a response rate of approximately 10% to 15%. The effective dosing of IFNα in renal cell carcinoma is not firmly established, but there does seem to be a dose-response relation, with a plateau at 10 million $U/m^2/d$ [180]. In a randomized clinical trial that compared

IFNα-2a with medroxyprogesterone, an increase in median overall survival from 6 to 8.5 months was reported in 1999 [181]. Importantly, for the surgical oncologist, cytoreductive nephrectomy has been reported to increase survival in patients subsequently treated with IFNα even in the metastatic setting [182,183]. Thus, all patients who present with metastatic renal cell carcinoma and their primary tumor in place should be considered for nephrectomy before immunotherapy.

Combinations of IL-2 and IFNα, with or without 5-fluorouracil (5FU)–based chemotherapy, have also been tested, and initial reports documented improved response rates with the cytokine combination compared with IFNα alone [184,185]. These initial results, however, were not confirmed in a larger randomized phase III trial for the combination. This trial was complicated by the lack of a placebo control group and instead used high-dose IL-2–treated patients as the comparison population. Although objective responses were observed with the combination of low-dose IL-2 and IFNα, a greater response rate was seen in patients receiving high-dose IL-2 [59,186]. These results suggest that high-dose IL-2 therapy should still be considered the standard of care for patients who have renal cell carcinoma and are able to tolerate treatment.

Cytokine treatment of other tumors

Although IFNα has met with limited success in the treatment of solid tumors, it has been particularly effective as therapy for hematologic malignancies. The best clinical responses have been observed in hairy cell leukemia (HCL) and chronic myelogenous leukemia (CML). IFNα-2b given subcutaneously at a dose of 2 million U/m^2 subcutaneously three times a week for 1 year resulted in an overall response rate of 77%, with a complete response rate of 5% in patients who had HCL [187]. Follow-up study demonstrated a complete response rate of 25% to 35% in patients with an intact spleen, suggesting the importance of early initiation of cytokine therapy [188]. Based on these data, IFNα was approved by the FDA for the treatment of HCL. Despite, the initial enthusiasm, a large number of patients developed relapse after discontinuation of therapy; however, remission could be induced in most by retreating them with IFNα [189]. The introduction of nucleoside analogues, with a complete response rate close to 90%, has relegated IFN therapy to second-line treatment in patients who have refractory disease or in those with contraindications to nucleoside analogues [190].

IFNα has been tested in patients who have CML, and preliminary trials suggested that complete hematologic responses were possible in more than half of patients who had CML, with complete cytogenic responses in nearly 25% [191]. Further prospective randomized trials documented the superiority of IFNα over chemotherapy [192]. Although the mechanism of response to IFNα is not completely established, there is evidence that human leukocyte antigen (HLA) haplotype and induction of immunity to the BCR-Abl translocation are associated with clinical responses in patients who have CML [193]. This supports a role of immune-mediated antitumor activity of IFNα in CML, and this is further supported by the observation that completely responding patients correct abnormalities in Th1 cytokine secretion, which are often present in these patients before treatment. IFNα also exerts direct antiproliferative effects on CML cells by means of DNA polymerase-dependent mechanisms, suggesting that the mechanism of IFNα activity may be more complex.

The lymphomas represent a heterogeneous group of lymphocyte malignancies. Preliminary clinical trials of IFNα in follicular lymphoma documented a 50% objective response rate [194]. Further studies were not as encouraging as this initial report, but several trials have shown significant benefits to using IFNα. In a clinical trial comparing standard chemotherapy with chemotherapy and IFNα (5 million U/m^2/d three times a week for 18 months), an increased response rate (85% versus 69%; $P < .001$) and overall survival (34 months versus 19 months; $P = .02$) were reported in the combination arm. These results resulted in subsequent approval of IFNα for the treatment of follicular lymphoma. A more recent meta-analysis of several IFNα clinical trials continues to support a significant survival advantage for intensive chemotherapy regimens containing IFNα [195].

Kaposi's sarcoma (KS) is a multifocal proliferative vascular tumor associated with HIV and Kaposi's sarcoma herpesvirus (KSHV)/human herpes virus-8 (HHV-8) coinfection [196]. The KS lesions are highly angiogenic, a process that is maintained through specific autocrine and paracrine cytokine loops within the tumor microenvironment. Based on the antiangiogenic activity of IFNα, as in hemangioma therapy, an evaluation of IFNα in patients who had KS was conducted [197]. Overall response rates of 30% to 40% have been reported, and there seems to be a dose-dependent relation between IFNα dose and clinical response [198]. The therapeutic responses may also be somewhat higher when IFNα is combined with antiretroviral drug therapy [199].

Future directions

The observation that single-agent IL-2 and IFNα can induce durable responses in selected patients suggests the potential utility of using cytokines as agents for the treatment of cancer. Despite these clinical observations, little is known about the mechanism used by these cytokines to induce the therapeutic responses. This is highly problematic, because a better understanding of the underlying mechanisms would likely result in more effective application of these agents to a larger number of patients. Recent investigations in cellular immunology and molecular biology have provided new insight into the biologic activity of many cytokines, including IL-2. These findings have fueled intense interest in designing new therapeutic strategies for patients who have cancer.

The potential threat of the immune system to the survival of individual tumor cells has resulted in a variety of tumor escape mechanisms, wherein tumors avoid detection by effector immune cells or mediate the eradication of such cells. The presence of Tregs, defined as CD4+CD25+FOXP3+ T cells, and their inhibitory nature have prompted a search for such cells in patients who have cancer. Perhaps not surprisingly, these cells are found in higher numbers in patients who have established tumors, including pancreas, breast, colon, and renal cell carcinoma and melanoma [200,201]. The unexpected discovery that IL-2 is involved in the regulation of these cells suggested that a possible explanation for the low response rates with IL-2–based immunotherapy may lie in the increase of Tregs compared with effector T cells [202]. Although this may be true in some patients, there is also evidence that clinically responding patients receiving IL-2 exhibit a paradoxical decrease in Tregs after exposure to high-dose IL-2 therapy [201]. These descriptive studies demonstrate the importance in pursuing more mechanistic investigations into the role of cytokines under physiologic and pathologic conditions.

Another area of recent interest has been the local tumor microenvironment. Tumors clearly induce an immunosuppressive microenvironment by multiple mechanisms, and this may block effector T cells from eradicating established tumor cells even when appropriate antigens are present [203]. Tumors secrete several immunosuppressive cytokines, such as IL-10, TGFβ, and IL-6 [204,205]. These cytokines may act to inhibit effector T cells after entrance into the local tumor site. In addition, local release of nutrient-catabolizing enzymes, such as indoleamine 2,3-dioxygenase (IDO) and arginase, further contributes to an immunosuppressive environment through depletion of local tyrosine stores essential for T-cell activity [206–208]. Tumors cells may also be protected from immune detection through loss of costimulatory molecule expression, increased levels of coinhibitory molecules, and accumulation of Tregs, all initiated as a protective mechanism designed to prevent autoimmune disease.

Based on these new insights, future studies likely need to focus on a two-pronged approach to immunotherapy of cancer. This should include agents to stimulate potent effector T-cell immune responses in combination with strategies aimed at blocking the immunoregulatory mechanisms within the host and tumor microenvironment. For example, efforts to deplete Tregs have begun investigation and include the anti-CD25 agent denileukin diftitox (ONTAK), which is composed of a chimeric molecule containing IL-2 and diphtheria toxin. The IL-2 moiety targets CD25, which is expressed at high levels on Tregs. A single dose of ONTAK has been shown to deplete circulating Tregs and enhanced the antitumor responses to DC-based vaccines [209]. Another strategy for deleting Tregs has been the use of nonmyeloablative chemotherapy, and this has been employed before vaccination or adoptive T-cell therapy with dramatic results [210]. The NCI Surgery Branch piloted the use of lymphodepletion using fludarabine and cyclophosphamide to deplete immunoregulatory cells, followed by adoptive transfer of T cells and IL-2 therapy. This regimen produced a response rate of 50% in patients who were previously resistant to IL-2–based immuno-therapy [211]. A phase II study of lymphodepletion followed by high-dose IL-2 is underway within the Cytokine Working Group. The use of anti-bodies to block the activation coinhibitory molecule, such as cytotoxic T-lymphocyte–associated antigen-4 (CTLA-4), has also resulted in dramatic responses in early clinical trials [212–215]. Although these approaches pre-sumably work to deplete Tregs, they may also regulate other processes, and this requires careful study.

Finally, the long-held belief that standard cancer therapy and immuno-therapy could not be mixed may not be true. Several preclinical studies evaluating the effects of combining cytokines with cytotoxic chemotherapy, radiation therapy, and vaccines are yielding clues that these combinations may be superior to single-agent treatment regimens. The inclusion of GM-CSF as a vaccine adjuvant has already shown promise in several vaccine trials, including allogeneic whole-cell, DC, peptide, and viral vaccines [216]. Chemotherapy may lead to tumor necrosis and apoptosis, re-sulting in cross-priming, and may enhance recognition of tumor-associated antigens. Radiation therapy also promotes local tumor apoptosis and alters local cytokine and immune regulatory pathways [217]. These observations have led to several new hypotheses related to how chemotherapy agents or ionizing radiation may enhance the antigenic presentation of tumor anti-gens or improve priming of tumor-specific immunity. These hypotheses are testable, and further preclinical modeling should be accompanied by well-designed clinical trials to optimize the rapid translation of these findings in patients who have cancer.

References

[1] Kaplan DH, Shankaran V, Dighe AS, et al. Demonstration of an interferon gamma-depen-dent tumor surveillance system in immunocompetent mice. Proc Natl Acad Sci U S A 1998; 95:7556–61.

[2] Picaud S, Bardot B, De Maeyer E, et al. Enhanced tumor development in mice lacking a functional type I interferon receptor. J Interferon Cytokine Res 2002;22:457–62.

[3] Shankaran V, Ikeda H, Bruce AT, et al. IFNgamma and lymphocytes prevent primary tumour development and shape tumour immunogenicity. Nature 2001;410:1107–11.

[4] Pure E, Allison JP, Schreiber RD. Breaking down the barriers to cancer immunotherapy. Nat Immun 2005;6:1207–10.

[5] Petrulio CA, Kim-Schulze S, Kaufman HL. The tumour microenvironment and implica-tions for cancer immunotherapy. Expert Opin Biol Ther 2006;6:671–84.

[6] Malek TR, Yu A, Vincek V, et al. CD4 regulatory T cells prevent lethal autoimmunity in IL-2R[beta]-deficient mice. Implications for the nonredundant function of IL-2. Immunity 2002;17:167–78.

[7] Abbas AK, Lichtman AH, Pober PS. Cellular and molecular immunology. 5th edition. Philadelphia: Saunders; 2003.

[8] Curiel TJ. Tregs and rethinking cancer immunotherapy. J Clin Invest 2007;117:1167–74.

[9] Jonuleit H, Schmitt E, Stassen M, et al. Identification and functional characterization of human CD4+CD25+ T cells with regulatory properties isolated from peripheral blood. J Exp Med 2001;193:1285–94.

[10] Asseman C, Mauze S, Leach MW, et al. An essential role for interleukin 10 in the function of regulatory T cells that inhibit intestinal inflammation. J Exp Med 1999;190: 995–1004.

[11] Setoguchi R, Hori S, Takahashi T, et al. Homeostatic maintenance of natural FOXP3+CD25+CD4+ regulatory T cells by interleukin (IL)-2 and induction of autoimmune disease by IL-2 neutralization. J Exp Med 2005;201:723–35.

[12] Waldmann TA. The interleukin-2 receptor on normal and malignant lymphocytes. Adv Exp Med Biol 1987;213:129–37.

[13] Waldmann TA. The biology of interleukin-2 and interleukin-15: implications for cancer therapy and vaccine design. Nat Rev Immunol 2006;6:595–601.

[14] Chan WC, Dahl C, Waldmann T, et al. Large granular lymphocyte proliferation: an analysis of T-cell receptor gene arrangement and expression and the effect of in vitro culture with inducing agents. Blood 1988;71:52–8.

[15] Begley CG, Burton JD, Tsudo M, et al. Human B lymphocytes express the p75 component of the interleukin 2 receptor. Leuk Res 1990;14:263–71.

[16] Sakaguchi S. Regulatory T cells: key controllers of immunologic self-tolerance. Cell 2000; 101:455.

[17] Golgher D, Jones E, Powrie F, et al. Depletion of CD25+ regulatory cells uncovers immune responses to shared murine tumor rejection antigens. Eur J Immunol 2002;32:3267–75.

[18] Thornton AM, Donovan EE, Piccirillo CA, et al. Cutting edge: IL-2 is critically required for the in vitro activation of CD4+CD25+ T cell suppressor function. J Immunol 2004;172: 6519–23.

[19] Shevach EM, Piccirillo CA, Thornton AM, et al. Control of T cell activation by CD4+CD25+ suppressor T cells. Novartis Found Symp 2003;252:24–36 [discussion: 36–44, 106–14].

[20] McHugh RS, Shevach EM, Thornton AM. Control of organ-specific autoimmunity by immunoregulatory CD4(+)CD25(+) T cells. Microbes Infect 2001;3:919–27.

[21] Thornton AM, Shevach EM. CD4+CD25+ immunoregulatory T cells suppress polyclonal T cell activation in vitro by inhibiting interleukin 2 production. J Exp Med 1998;188: 287–96.

[22] Pestka S, Krause CD, Walter MR. Interferons, interferon-like cytokines, and their receptors. Immunol Rev 2004;202:8–32.

[23] Constantinescu SN, Croze E, Wang C, et al. Role of interferon alpha/beta receptor chain 1 in the structure and transmembrane signaling of the interferon alpha/beta receptor complex. Proc Natl Acad Sci U S A 1994;91:9602–6.

[24] Muller U, Steinhoff U, Reis LF, et al. Functional role of type I and type II interferons in antiviral defense. Science 1994;264:1918–21.

[25] Muller M, Ibelgaufts H, Kerr IM. Interferon response pathways—a paradigm for cytokine signalling? J Viral Hepat 1994;1:87–103.

[26] Isaacs A, Lindenmann J. Virus interference. I. The interferon. By A. Isaacs and J. Lindenmann, 1957. J Interferon Res 1987;7:429–38.

[27] Basham TY, Bourgeade MF, Creasey AA, et al. Interferon increases HLA synthesis in melanoma cells: interferon-resistant and -sensitive cell lines. Proc Natl Acad Sci U S A 1982;79:3265–9.

[28] Dolei A, Capobianchi MR, Ameglio F. Human interferon-gamma enhances the expression of class I and class II major histocompatibility complex products in neoplastic cells more effectively than interferon-alpha and interferon-beta. Infect Immun 1983;40:172–6.

[29] Ameglio F, Capobianchi MR, Dolei A, et al. Differential effects of gamma interferon on expression of HLA class II molecules controlled by the DR and DC loci. Infect Immun 1983;42:122–5.

[30] Jones CM, Varesio L, Herberman RB, et al. Interferon activates macrophages to produce plasminogen activator. J Interferon Res 1982;2:377–86.

[31] Herberman RB. Overview on NK cells and possible mechanisms for their cytotoxic activity. Adv Exp Med Biol 1982;146:337–51.

[32] Herberman RB. Overview and perspectives: natural resistance mechanisms. Adv Exp Med Biol 1982;155:799–808.

[33] Brunda MJ, Varesio L, Herberman RB, et al. Interferon-independent, lectin-induced augmentation of murine natural killer cell activity. Int J Cancer 1982;29:299–307.

[34] Wagner TC, Velichko S, Chesney SK, et al. Interferon receptor expression regulates the antiproliferative effects of interferons on cancer cells and solid tumors. Int J Cancer 2004;111:32–42.

[35] Tsuruoka N, Sugiyama M, Tawaragi Y, et al. Inhibition of in vitro angiogenesis by lympho-toxin and interferon-gamma. Biochem Biophys Res Commun 1988;155:429–35.

[36] Dunn GP, Ikeda H, Bruce AT, et al. Interferon-gamma and cancer immunoediting. Immunol Res 2005;32:231–45.

[37] Dunn GP, Bruce AT, Sheehan KC, et al. A critical function for type I interferons in cancer immunoediting. Nat Immun 2005;6:722–9.

[38] Carnaud C, Lee D, Donnars O, et al. Cutting edge: cross-talk between cells of the innate immune system: NKT cells rapidly activate NK cells. J Immunol 1999;163:4647–50.

[39] Lighvani AA, Frucht DM, Jankovic D, et al. T-bet is rapidly induced by interferon-gamma in lymphoid and myeloid cells. Proc Natl Acad Sci U S A 2001;98:15137–42.

[40] Frucht DM, Fukao T, Bogdan C, et al. IFN-gamma production by antigen-presenting cells: mechanisms emerge. Trends Immunol 2001;22:556–60.

[41] Boehm U, Klamp T, Groot M, et al. Cellular responses to interferon-gamma. Annu Rev Immunol 1997;15:749–95.

[42] Freedman AS, Freeman GJ, Rhynhart K, et al. Selective induction of B7/BB-1 on interferon-gamma stimulated monocytes: a potential mechanism for amplification of T cell activation through the CD28 pathway. Cell Immunol 1991;137:429–37.

[43] Yong VW, Moumdjian R, Yong FP, et al. Gamma-interferon promotes proliferation of adult human astrocytes in vitro and reactive gliosis in the adult mouse brain in vivo. Proc Natl Acad Sci U S A 1991;88:7016–20.

[44] Groettrup M, van den Broek M, Schwarz K, et al. Structural plasticity of the proteasome and its function in antigen processing. Crit Rev Immunol 2001;21:339–58.

[45] Groettrup M, Khan S, Schwarz K, et al. Interferon-gamma inducible exchanges of 20S proteasome active site subunits: why? Biochimie 2001;83:367–72.

[46] Snapper CM, Paul WE. Interferon-gamma and B cell stimulatory factor-1 reciprocally regulate Ig isotype production. Science 1987;236:944–7.

[47] Street SE, Trapani JA, MacGregor D, et al. Suppression of lymphoma and epithelial malignancies effected by interferon gamma. J Exp Med 2002;196:129–34.

[48] Coughlin CM, Salhany KE, Gee MS, et al. Tumor cell responses to IFNgamma affect tumorigenicity and response to IL-12 therapy and antiangiogenesis. Immunity 1998;9: 25–34.

[49] Coughlin CM, Salhany KE, Wysocka M, et al. Interleukin-12 and interleukin-18 synergis-tically induce murine tumor regression which involves inhibition of angiogenesis. J Clin Invest 1998;101:1441–52.

[50] Friesel R, Komoriya A, Maciag T. Inhibition of endothelial cell proliferation by gamma-interferon. J Cell Biol 1987;104:689–96.

[51] Elhilali MM, Gleave M, Fradet Y, et al. Placebo-associated remissions in a multicentre, randomized, double-blind trial of interferon gamma-1b for the treatment of metastatic renal cell carcinoma. The Canadian Urologic Oncology Group. BJU Int 2000;86:613–8.

[52] Koziner B, Dengra C, Cisneros M, et al. Double-blind prospective randomized comparison of interferon gamma-1b versus placebo after autologous stem cell transplantation. Acta Haematol 2002;108:66–73.

[53] Barnetson RS, Halliday GM. Regression in skin tumours: a common phenomenon. Australas J Dermatol 1997;38(Suppl 1):S63–5.

[54] Panagopoulos E, Murray D. Metastatic malignant melanoma of unknown primary origin: a study of 30 cases. J Surg Oncol 1983;23:8–10.

[55] Gromet MA, Epstein WL, Blois MS. The regressing thin malignant melanoma: a distinctive lesion with metastatic potential. Cancer 1978;42:2282–92.

[56] Dudley ME, Wunderlich J, Nishimura MI, et al. Adoptive transfer of cloned melanoma-reactive T lymphocytes for the treatment of patients with metastatic melanoma. J Immunother (1997) 2001;24:363–73.

[57] Atkins MB, Regan M, McDermott D. Update on the role of interleukin 2 and other cytokines in the treatment of patients with stage IV renal carcinoma. Clin Cancer Res 2004;10:6342S–6S.

[58] Atkins MB. Interleukin-2: clinical applications. Semin Oncol 2002;29:12–7.

[59] McDermott DF, Regan MM, Clark JI, et al. Randomized phase III trial of high-dose interleukin-2 versus subcutaneous interleukin-2 and interferon in patients with metastatic renal cell carcinoma. J Clin Oncol 2005;23:133–41.

[60] Schwartz R, Stover L, Dutcher J. Managing toxicities of high-dose interleukin-2. Oncology 2002;16:11–20.

[61] Klempner MS, Noring R, Mier JW, et al. An acquired chemotactic defect in neutrophils from patients receiving interleukin-2 immunotherapy. N Engl J Med 1990;322:959–65.

[62] Rosenberg SA, Zhai Y, Yang JC, et al. Immunizing patients with metastatic melanoma using recombinant adenoviruses encoding MART-1 or gp100 melanoma antigens. J Natl Cancer Inst 1998;90:1894–900.

[63] Rosenberg SA, Yang JC, Schwartzentruber DJ, et al. Impact of cytokine administration on the generation of antitumor reactivity in patients with metastatic melanoma receiving a peptide vaccine. J Immunol 1999;163:1690–5.

[64] Gollob JA, Upton MP, DeWolf WC, et al. Long-term remission in a patient with metastatic collecting duct carcinoma treated with taxol/carboplatin and surgery. Urology 2001;58:1058.

[65] Sparano JA, Fisher RI, Sunderland M, et al. Randomized phase III trial of treatment with high-dose interleukin-2 either alone or in combination with interferon alfa-2a in patients with advanced melanoma. J Clin Oncol 1993;11:1969–77.

[66] Feun L, Marini A, Moffat F, et al. Cyclosporine A, alpha-1 interferon and interleukin-2 following chemotherapy with BCNU, DTIC, cisplatin, and tamoxifen: a phase II study in advanced melanoma. Cancer Invest 2005;23:3–8.

[67] Atkins MB, Gollob JA, Sosman JA, et al. A phase II pilot trial of concurrent biochemotherapy with cisplatin, vinblastine, temozolomide, interleukin 2, and IFN-alpha 2B in patients with metastatic melanoma. Clin Cancer Res 2002;8:3075–81.

[68] McDermott DF, Regan MM, Atkins MB. Interleukin-2 therapy of metastatic renal cell carcinoma: update of phase III trials. Clin Genitourin Cancer 2006;5:114–9.

[69] Gollob JA, Veenstra KG, Parker RA, et al. Phase I trial of concurrent twice-weekly recombinant human interleukin-12 plus low-dose IL-2 in patients with melanoma or renal cell carcinoma. J Clin Oncol 2003;21:2564–73.

[70] Eton O, Rosenblum MG, Legha SS, et al. Phase I trial of subcutaneous recombinant human interleukin-2 in patients with metastatic melanoma. Cancer 2002;95:127–34.

[71] Hauschild A, Kleeberg UR. Adjuvant therapy of melanoma. From non-specific immune stimulants into the future. Hautarzt 2006;57:764–72.

[72] Hauschild A, Volkenandt M, Garbe C. Adjuvant drug therapy of malignant melanoma. Current knowledge and multi-center studies in German-speaking countries. Dtsch Med Wochenschr 2000;125:1272–8.

[73] Khor M, Lowrie DB, Coates AR, et al. Recombinant interferon-gamma and chemotherapy with isoniazid and rifampicin in experimental murine tuberculosis. Br J Exp Pathol 1986;67:587–96.

[74] Hersey P, MacDonald M, Hall C, et al. Immunological effects of recombinant interferon alfa-2a in patients with disseminated melanoma. Cancer 1986;57:1666–74.

[75] Coates A, Rallings M, Hersey P, et al. Phase-II study of recombinant alpha 2-interferon in advanced malignant melanoma. J Interferon Res 1986;6:1–4.

[76] Neefe JR, Legha SS, Markowitz A, et al. Phase II study of recombinant alpha-interferon in malignant melanoma. Am J Clin Oncol 1990;13:472–6.

[77] Vlock DR, Andersen J, Kalish LA, et al. Phase II trial of interferon-alpha in locally recurrent or metastatic squamous cell carcinoma of the head and neck: immunological and clinical correlates. J Immunother Emphasis Tumor Immunol 1996;19:433–42.

[78] Sparano JA, Lipsitz S, Wadler S, et al. Phase II trial of prolonged continuous infusion of 5-fluorouracil and interferon-alpha in patients with advanced pancreatic cancer. Eastern Cooperative Oncology Group Protocol 3292. Am J Clin Oncol 1996;19:546–51.

[79] Schiller JH, Pugh M, Kirkwood JM, et al. Eastern Cooperative Group trial of interferon gamma in metastatic melanoma: an innovative study design. Clin Cancer Res 1996;2:29–36.

[80] Kirkwood JM, Strawderman MH, Ernstoff MS, et al. Interferon alfa-2b adjuvant therapy of high-risk resected cutaneous melanoma: the Eastern Cooperative Oncology Group Trial EST 1684. J Clin Oncol 1996;14:7–17.

[81] Franke W, Neumann NJ, Ruzicka T, et al. Adjuvant therapy of malignant melanoma. Schweiz Rundsch Med Prax 2001;90:301–6.

[82] Cole BF, Gelber RD, Kirkwood JM, et al. Quality-of-life-adjusted survival analysis of in-terferon alfa-2b adjuvant treatment of high-risk resected cutaneous melanoma: an Eastern Cooperative Oncology Group study. J Clin Oncol 1996;14:2666–73.

[83] Agarwala SS, Kirkwood JM. Interferons in melanoma. Curr Opin Oncol 1996;8:167–74.

[84] Santhanam S, Decatris M, O'Byrne K. Potential of interferon-alpha in solid tumours: part 2. BioDrugs 2002;16:349–72.

[85] Decatris M, Santhanam S, O'Byrne K. Potential of interferon-alpha in solid tumours: part 1. BioDrugs 2002;16:261–81.

[86] Falkson CI, Ibrahim J, Kirkwood JM, et al. Phase III trial of dacarbazine versus dacarba-zine with interferon alpha-2b versus dacarbazine with tamoxifen versus dacarbazine with interferon alpha-2b and tamoxifen in patients with metastatic malignant melanoma: an Eastern Cooperative Oncology Group study. J Clin Oncol 1998;16:1743–51.

[87] Kirkwood JM, Manola J, Ibrahim J, et al. A pooled analysis of Eastern Cooperative Oncology Group and intergroup trials of adjuvant high-dose interferon for melanoma. Clin Cancer Res 2004;10:1670–7.

[88] Kirkwood JM, Ibrahim JG, Sosman JA, et al. High-dose interferon alfa-2b significantly prolongs relapse-free and overall survival compared with the GM2-KLH/QS-21 vaccine in patients with resected stage IIB-III melanoma: results of intergroup trial E1694/S9512/C509801. J Clin Oncol 2001;19:2370–80.

[89] Jonasch E, Kumar UN, Linette GP, et al. Adjuvant high-dose interferon alfa-2b in patients with high-risk melanoma. Cancer J 2000;6:139–45.

[90] Jonasch E, Haluska FG. Interferon in oncological practice: review of interferon biology, clinical applications, and toxicities. Oncologist 2001;6:34–55.

[91] Greenberg DB, Jonasch E, Gadd MA, et al. Adjuvant therapy of melanoma with inter-feron-alpha-2b is associated with mania and bipolar syndromes. Cancer 2000;89:356–62.

[92] Musselman DL, Lawson DH, Gumnick JF, et al. Paroxetine for the prevention of depres-sion induced by high-dose interferon alfa. N Engl J Med 2001;344:961–6.

[93] Jones TH, Wadler S, Hupart KH. Endocrine-mediated mechanisms of fatigue during treat-ment with interferon-alpha. Semin Oncol 1998;25:54–63.

[94] Brenard R. Practical management of patients treated with alpha interferon. Acta Gastro-enterol Belg 1997;60:211–3.

[95] Dalekos GN, Christodoulou D, Kistis KG, et al. A prospective evaluation of dermatolog-ical side-effects during alpha-interferon therapy for chronic viral hepatitis. Eur J Gastroen-terol Hepatol 1998;10:933–9.

[96] Gogas H, Ioannovich J, Dafni U, et al. Prognostic significance of autoimmunity during treatment of melanoma with interferon. N Engl J Med 2006;354:709–18.

[97] Aragane Y, Riemann H, Bhardwaj RS, et al. IL-12 is expressed and released by human keratinocytes and epidermoid carcinoma cell lines. J Immunol 1994;153:5366–72.

[98] Aste-Amezaga M, D'Andrea A, Kubin M, et al. Cooperation of natural killer cell stimulatory factor/interleukin-12 with other stimuli in the induction of cytokines and cytotoxic cell-associated molecules in human T and NK cells. Cell Immunol 1994;156:480–92.

[99] Kubin M, Chow JM, Trinchieri G. Differential regulation of interleukin-12 (IL-12), tumor necrosis factor alpha, and IL-1 beta production in human myeloid leukemia cell lines and peripheral blood mononuclear cells. Blood 1994;83:1847–55.

[100] Perussia B, Chan SH, D'Andrea A, et al. Natural killer (NK) cell stimulatory factor or IL-12 has differential effects on the proliferation of TCR-alpha beta+, TCR-gamma delta+ T lymphocytes, and NK cells. J Immunol 1992;149:3495–502.

[101] Chehimi J, Starr SE, Frank I, et al. Natural killer (NK) cell stimulatory factor increases the cytotoxic activity of NK cells from both healthy donors and human immunodeficiency virus-infected patients. J Exp Med 1992;175:789–96.

[102] Chan SH, Kobayashi M, Santoli D, et al. Mechanisms of IFN-gamma induction by natural killer cell stimulatory factor (NKSF/IL-12). Role of transcription and mRNA stability in the synergistic interaction between NKSF and IL-2. J Immunol 1992;148:92–8.

[103] Rao JB, Chamberlain RS, Bronte V, et al. IL-12 is an effective adjuvant to recombinant vaccinia virus-based tumor vaccines: enhancement by simultaneous B7-1 expression. J Immunol 1996;156:3357–65.

[104] Strengell M, Lehtonen A, Matikainen S, et al. IL-21 enhances SOCS gene expression and inhibits LPS-induced cytokine production in human monocyte-derived dendritic cells. J Leukoc Biol 2006;79:1279–85.

[105] Li Q, Carr AL, Donald EJ, et al. Synergistic effects of IL-12 and IL-18 in skewing rumor-reactive T-cell responses towards a type 1 pattern. Cancer Res 2005;65:1063–70.

[106] Kaufman HL, Flanagan K, Lee CS, et al. Insertion of interleukin-2 (IL-2) and interleukin-12 (IL-12) genes into vaccinia virus results in effective anti-tumor responses without toxicity. Vaccine 2002;20:1862–9.

[107] Yoshimoto T, Takeda K, Tanaka T, et al. IL-12 up-regulates IL-18 receptor expression on T cells, Th1 cells, and B cells: synergism with IL-18 for IFN-gamma production. J Immunol 1998;161:3400–7.

[108] Yoshimoto T, Nagai N, Ohkusu K, et al. LPS-stimulated SJL macrophages produce IL-12 and IL-18 that inhibit IgE production in vitro by induction of IFN-gamma production from CD3intIL-2R beta+ T cells. J Immunol 1998;161:1483–92.

[109] Smyth MJ, Swann J, Kelly JM, et al. NKG2D recognition and perforin effector function mediate effective cytokine immunotherapy of cancer. J Exp Med 2004;200:1325–35.

[110] Kawamura T, Takeda K, Mendiratta SK, et al. Critical role of NK1+ T cells in IL-12-induced immune responses in vivo. J Immunol 1998;160:16–9.

[111] Boggio K, Nicoletti G, Di Carlo E, et al. Interleukin 12-mediated prevention of spontaneous mammary adenocarcinomas in two lines of Her-2/neu transgenic mice. J Exp Med 1998;188:589–96.

[112] Mahvi DM, Henry MB, Albertini MR, et al. Intratumoral injection of IL-12 plasmid DNA—results of a phase I/IB clinical trial. Cancer Gene Ther 2007.

[113] Gollob JA, Mier JW, Veenstra K, et al. Phase I trial of twice-weekly intravenous interleukin 12 in patients with metastatic renal cell cancer or malignant melanoma: ability to maintain IFN-gamma induction is associated with clinical response. Clin Cancer Res 2000;6:1678–92.

[114] Prlic M, Blazar BR, Farrar MA, et al. In vivo survival and homeostatic proliferation of natural killer cells. J Exp Med 2003;197:967–76.

[115] Waldmann TA, Tagaya Y. The multifaceted regulation of interleukin-15 expression and the role of this cytokine in NK cell differentiation and host response to intracellular pathogens. Annual Review of Immunology 1999;17:19–49.

[116] Marks-Konczalik J, Dubois S, Losi JM, et al. IL-2-induced activation-induced cell death is inhibited in IL-15 transgenic mice. Proc Natl Acad Sci U S A 2000;97:11445–50.

[117] Ku CC, Murakami M, Sakamoto A, et al. Control of homeostasis of CD8+ memory T cells by opposing cytokines. Science 2000;288:675–8.

[118] Waldmann TA. IL-15 in the life and death of lymphocytes: immunotherapeutic implications. Trends in Molecular Medicine 2003;9:517–21.

[119] Meresse B, Chen Z, Ciszewski C, et al. Coordinated induction by IL15 of a TCR-independent NKG2D signaling pathway converts CTL into lymphokine-activated killer cells in celiac disease. Immunity 2004;21:357–66.

[120] Zaft T, Sapoznikov A, Krauthgamer R, et al. CD11high dendritic cell ablation impairs lymphopenia-driven proliferation of naive and memory CD8+ T cells. J Immunol 2005; 175:6428–35.

[121] Di Carlo E, Comes A, Basso S, et al. The combined action of IL-15 and IL-12 gene transfer can induce tumor cell rejection without T and NK cell involvement. J Immunol 2000;165:3111–8.

[122] Okamura H, Tsutsi H, Komatsu T, et al. Cloning of a new cytokine that induces IFN-gamma production by T cells. Nature 1995;378:88–91.

[123] Tsutsui H, Matsui K, Kawada N, et al. IL-18 accounts for both TNF-alpha- and Fas ligand-mediated hepatotoxic pathways in endotoxin-induced liver injury in mice. J Immunol 1997;159:3961–7.

[124] Tomura M, Zhou XY, Maruo S, et al. A critical role for IL-18 in the proliferation and activation of NK1.1+ CD3− cells. J Immunol 1998;160:4738–46.

[125] Tomura M, Maruo S, Mu J, et al. Differential capacities of CD4+ CD8+, and CD4−CD8− T cell subsets to express IL-18 receptor and produce IFN-gamma in response to IL-18. J Immunol 1998;160:3759–65.

[126] Takeda K, Tsutsui H, Yoshimoto T, et al. Defective NK cell activity and Th1 response in IL-18-deficient mice. Immunity 1998;8:383–90.

[127] Okamura H, Tsutsui H, Kashiwamura S, et al. Interleukin-18: a novel cytokine that augments both innate and acquired immunity. Adv Immunol 1998;70:281–312.

[128] Okamura H, Kashiwamura S, Tsutsui H, et al. Regulation of interferon-gamma production by IL-12 and IL-18. Curr Opin Immunol 1998;10:259–64.

[129] Robertson MJ, Mier JW, Logan T, et al. Clinical and biological effects of recombinant human interleukin-18 administered by intravenous infusion to patients with advanced cancer. Clin Cancer Res 2006;12:4265–73.

[130] Park CC, Morel JC, Amin MA, et al. Evidence of IL-18 as a novel angiogenic mediator. J Immunol 2001;167:1644–53.

[131] Morel JC, Park CC, Woods JM, et al. A novel role for interleukin-18 in adhesion molecule induction through NF kappa B and phosphatidylinositol (PI) 3-kinase-dependent signal transduction pathways. J Biolumin Chemilumin 2001;276:37069–75.

[132] Morel JC, Park CC, Kumar P, et al. Interleukin-18 induces rheumatoid arthritis synovial fibroblast CXC chemokine production through NFkappaB activation. Lab Invest 2001; 81:1371–83.

[133] Kaser A, Novick D, Rubinstein M, et al. Interferon-alpha induces interleukin-18 binding protein in chronic hepatitis C patients. Clin Exp Immunol 2002;129:332–8.

[134] Amin MA, Mansfield PJ, Pakozdi A, et al. Interleukin-18 induces angiogenic factors in rheumatoid arthritis synovial tissue fibroblasts via distinct signaling pathways. Arthritis Rheum 2007;56:1787–97.

[135] Lee JK, Kim SH, Lewis EC, et al. Differences in signaling pathways by IL-1beta and IL-18. Proc Natl Acad Sci U S A 2004;101:8815–20.

[136] Parrish-Novak J, Dillon SR, Nelson A, et al. Interleukin 21 and its receptor are involved in NK cell expansion and regulation of lymphocyte function. Nature 2000;408:57–63.

[137] Brandt K, Bulfone-Paus S, Jenckel A, et al. Interleukin-21 inhibits dendritic cell-mediated T cell activation and induction of contact hypersensitivity in vivo. J Invest Dermatol 2003;121:1379–82.

[138] Brandt K, Bulfone-Paus S, Foster DC, et al. Interleukin-21 inhibits dendritic cell activation and maturation. Blood 2003;102:4090–8.

[139] Suto A, Nakajima H, Hirose K, et al. Interleukin 21 prevents antigen-induced IgE production by inhibiting germ line C(epsilon) transcription of IL-4-stimulated B cells. Blood 2002; 100:4565–73.

[140] Pene J, Guglielmi L, Gauchat JF, et al. IFN-gamma-mediated inhibition of human IgE synthesis by IL-21 is associated with a polymorphism in the IL-21R gene. J Immunol 2006;177:5006–13.

[141] Jin H, Malek TR. Redundant and unique regulation of activated mouse B lymphocytes by IL-4 and IL-21. J Leukoc Biol 2006;80:1416–23.

[142] Furukawa J, Hara I, Nagai H, et al. Interleukin-21 gene transfection into mouse bladder cancer cells results in tumor rejection through the cytotoxic T lymphocyte response. J Urol 2006;176:1198–203.

[143] Cappuccio A, Elishmereni M, Agur Z. Cancer immunotherapy by interleukin-21: potential treatment strategies evaluated in a mathematical model. Cancer Res 2006;66: 7293–300.

[144] He H, Wisner P, Yang G, et al. Combined IL-21 and low-dose IL-2 therapy induces anti-tumor immunity and long-term curative effects in a murine melanoma tumor model. J Transl Med 2006;4:24–40.

[145] Smyth MJ, Hayakawa Y, Cretney E, et al. IL-21 enhances tumor-specific CTL induction by anti-DR5 antibody therapy. J Immunol 2006;176:6347–55.

[146] Caven TH, Shelburne A, Sato J, et al. IL-21 dependent IgE production in human and mouse in vitro culture systems is cell density and cell division dependent and is augmented by IL-10. Cell Immunol 2005;238:123–34.

[147] Burgess SJ, Marusina AI, Pathmanathan I, et al. IL-21 down-regulates NKG2D/DAP10 expression on human NK and CD8+ T cells. J Immunol 2006;176:1490–7.

[148] Ettinger R, Sims GP, Fairhurst AM, et al. IL-21 induces differentiation of human naive and memory B cells into antibody-secreting plasma cells. J Immunol 2005;175:7867–79.

[149] Perez SA, Mahaira LG, Sotiropoulou PA, et al. Effect of IL-21 on NK cells derived from different umbilical cord blood populations. Int Immunol 2006;18:49–58.

[150] Li Y, Bleakley M, Yee C. IL-21 influences the frequency, phenotype, and affinity of the antigen-specific CD8 T cell response. J Immunol 2005;175:2261–9.

[151] Takaki R, Hayakawa Y, Nelson A, et al. IL-21 enhances tumor rejection through a NKG2D-dependent mechanism. J Immunol 2005;175:2167–73.

[152] Wood N, Bourque K, Donaldson DD, et al. IL-21 effects on human IgE production in response to IL-4 or IL-13. Cell Immunol 2004;231:133–45.

[153] Mehta DS, Wurster AL, Grusby MJ. Biology of IL-21 and the IL-21 receptor. Immunol Rev 2004;202:84–95.

[154] Moroz A, Eppolito C, Li Q, et al. IL-21 enhances and sustains CD8+ T cell responses to achieve durable tumor immunity: comparative evaluation of IL-2, IL-15, and IL-21. J Immunol 2004;173:900–9.

[155] Strengell M, Julkunen I, Matikainen S. IFN-alpha regulates IL-21 and IL-21R expression in human NK and T cells. J Leukoc Biol 2004;76:416–22.

[156] Pene J, Gauchat JF, Lecart S, et al. Cutting edge: IL-21 is a switch factor for the production of IgG1 and IgG3 by human B cells. J Immunol 2004;172:5154–7.

[157] Habib T, Nelson A, Kaushansky K. IL-21: a novel IL-2-family lymphokine that modulates B, T, and natural killer cell responses. J Allergy Clin Immunol 2003;112:1033–45.

[158] Collins M, Whitters MJ, Young DA. IL-21 and IL-21 receptor: a new cytokine pathway modulates innate and adaptive immunity. Immunol Res 2003;28:131–40.

[159] Curti BD. Immunomodulatory and antitumor effects of interleukin-21 in patients with renal cell carcinoma. Expert Rev Anticancer Ther 2006;6:905–9.

[160] Wang G, Tschoi M, Spolski R, et al. In vivo antitumor activity of interleukin 21 mediated by natural killer cells. Cancer Res 2003;63:9016–22.

[161] Kishida T, Asada H, Itokawa Y, et al. Interleukin (IL)-21 and IL-15 genetic transfer synergistically augments therapeutic antitumor immunity and promotes regression of metastatic lymphoma. Mol Ther 2003;8:552–8.

[162] Overwijk WW, de Visser KE, Tirion FH, et al. Immunological and antitumor effects of IL-23 as a cancer vaccine adjuvant. J Immunol 2006;176:5213–22.

[163] Langowski JL, Zhang X, Wu L, et al. IL-23 promotes tumour incidence and growth. Nature 2006;442:461–5.

[164] Dranoff G, Jaffee E, Lazenby A, et al. Vaccination with irradiated tumor cells engineered to secrete murine granulocyte-macrophage colony-stimulating factor stimulates potent, specific, and long-lasting anti-tumor immunity. Proc Natl Acad Sci U S A 1993;90:3539–43.

[165] Grabstein KH, Urdal DL, Tushinski RJ, et al. Induction of macrophage tumoricidal activity by granulocyte-macrophage colony-stimulating factor. Science 1986;232:506–8.

[166] Grabstein K, Mochizuki D, Kronheim S, et al. Regulation of antibody production in vitro by granulocyte-macrophage colony stimulating factor. J Mol Cell Immunol 1986;2:199–207.

[167] Leverkus M, Walczak H, McLellan A, et al. Maturation of dendritic cells leads to up-regulation of cellular FLICE-inhibitory protein and concomitant down-regulation of death ligand-mediated apoptosis. Blood 2000;96:2628–31.

[168] Hu X, Zuckerman KS. Cloning and sequencing of an alternative splicing-derived cDNA variant of the GM-CSF receptor alpha subunit, which encodes a truncated protein. Am J Hematol 1998;58:145–7.

[169] Jinushi M, Nakazaki Y, Dougan M, et al. MFG-E8-mediated uptake of apoptotic cells by APCs links the pro- and antiinflammatory activities of GM-CSF. J Clin Invest 2007;117:1902–13.

[170] Ridolfi L, Ridolfi R, Ascari-Raccagni A, et al. Intralesional granulocyte-monocyte colony-stimulating factor followed by subcutaneous interleukin-2 in metastatic melanoma: a pilot study in elderly patients. J Eur Acad Dermatol Venereol 2001;15:218–23.

[171] Dranoff G. GM-CSF-secreting melanoma vaccines. Oncogene 2003;22:3188–92.

[172] Spitler LE, Grossbard ML, Ernstoff MS, et al. Adjuvant therapy of stage III and IV malignant melanoma using granulocyte-macrophage colony-stimulating factor. J Clin Oncol 2000;18:1614–21.

[173] O'Day SJ, Boasberg PD, Piro L, et al. Maintenance biotherapy for metastatic melanoma with interleukin-2 and granulocyte macrophage-colony stimulating factor improves survival for patients responding to induction concurrent biochemotherapy. Clin Cancer Res 2002;8:2775–81.

[174] Britten CD, Kabbinavar F, Randolph Hecht J, et al. A phase I and pharmacokinetic study of sunitinib administered daily for 2 weeks, followed by a 1-week off period. Cancer Chemother Pharmacol 2007 [epub ahead of print].

[175] McKeage K, Wagstaff AJ. Sorafenib: in advanced renal cancer. Drugs 2007;67:475–83 [discussion: 484–5].

[176] Rini BI, Shaw V, Rosenberg JE, et al. Patients with metastatic renal cell carcinoma with long-term disease-free survival after treatment with sunitinib and resection of residual metastases. Clin Genitourin Cancer 2006;5:232–4.

[177] Faivre S, Delbaldo C, Vera K, et al. Safety, pharmacokinetic, and antitumor activity of SU11248, a novel oral multitarget tyrosine kinase inhibitor, in patients with cancer. J Clin Oncol 2006;24:25–35.

[178] Yang JC, Sherry RM, Steinberg SM, et al. Randomized study of high-dose and low-dose interleukin-2 in patients with metastatic renal cancer. J Clin Oncol 2003;21:3127–32.

[179] Fisher RI, Rosenberg SA, Fyfe G. Long-term survival update for high-dose recombinant interleukin-2 in patients with renal cell carcinoma. Cancer J Sci Am 2000;6(Suppl 1):S55–7.

[180] Kirkwood JM, Harris JE, Vera R, et al. A randomized study of low and high doses of leukocyte alpha-interferon in metastatic renal cell carcinoma: the American Cancer Society collaborative trial. Cancer Res 1985;45:863–71.

[181] Amato R. Modest effect of interferon alfa on metastatic renal-cell carcinoma. Lancet 1999; 353:6–7.

[182] Flanigan RC, Yonover PM. The role of radical nephrectomy in metastatic renal cell carcinoma. Semin Urol Oncol 2001;19:98–102.

[183] Flanigan RC, Salmon SE, Blumenstein BA, et al. Nephrectomy followed by interferon alfa-2b compared with interferon alfa-2b alone for metastatic renal-cell cancer. N Engl J Med 2001;345:1655–9.

[184] Atzpodien J, Schmitt E, Gertenbach U, et al. Adjuvant treatment with interleukin-2- and interferon-alpha2a-based chemoimmunotherapy in renal cell carcinoma post tumour nephrectomy: results of a prospectively randomised trial of the German Cooperative Renal Carcinoma Chemoimmunotherapy Group (DGCIN). Br J Cancer 2005;92:843–6.

[185] Atzpodien J, Korfer A, Palmer PA, et al. Treatment of metastatic renal cell cancer patients with recombinant subcutaneous human interleukin-2 and interferon-alpha. Ann Oncol 1990;1:377–8.

[186] McDermott DF, Atkins MB. Interleukin-2 therapy of metastatic renal cell carcinoma—predictors of response. Semin Oncol 2006;33:583–7.

[187] Golomb HM, Jacobs A, Fefer A, et al. Alpha-2 interferon therapy of hairy-cell leukemia: a multicenter study of 64 patients. J Clin Oncol 1986;4:900–5.

[188] Quesada JR, Gutterman JU. Alpha interferons in B-cell neoplasms. Br J Haematol 1986;64: 639–46.

[189] Golomb HM, Ratain MJ, Mick R, et al. The treatment of hairy cell leukemia: an update. Leukemia 1992;6(Suppl 2):24–7.

[190] Goodman GR, Burian C, Koziol JA, et al. Extended follow-up of patients with hairy cell leukemia after treatment with cladribine. J Clin Oncol 2003;21:891–6.

[191] Talpaz M, McCredie K, Kantarjian H, et al. Chronic myelogenous leukaemia: haematological remissions with alpha interferon. Br J Haematol 1986;64:87–95.

[192] Hehlmann R, Kister P, Willer A, et al. Therapeutic progress and comparative aspects in chronic myelogenous leukemia (CML): interferon alpha vs. hydroxyurea vs. busulfan and expression of MMTV-related endogenous retroviral sequences in CML. German CML Study Group. Leukemia 1994;8(Suppl 1):S127–32.

[193] Yasukawa M, Ohminami H, Kaneko S, et al. CD4(+) cytotoxic T-cell clones specific for bcr-abl b3a2 fusion peptide augment colony formation by chronic myelogenous leukemia cells in a b3a2-specific and HLA-DR-restricted manner. Blood 1998;92:3355–61.

[194] Foon KA, Sherwin SA, Abrams PG, et al. Treatment of advanced non-Hodgkin's lymphoma with recombinant leukocyte A interferon. N Engl J Med 1984;311:1148–52.

[195] Rohatiner AZ, Gregory WM, Peterson B, et al. Meta-analysis to evaluate the role of interferon in follicular lymphoma. J Clin Oncol 2005;23:2215–23.

[196] Schalling M, Ekman M, Kaaya EE, et al. A role for a new herpes virus (KSHV) in different forms of Kaposi's sarcoma. Nat Med 1995;1:707–8.

[197] Ezekowitz A, Mulliken J, Folkman J. Interferon alpha therapy of haemangiomas in newborns and infants. Br J Haematol 1991;79(Suppl 1):67–8.

[198] Real FX, Oettgen HF, Krown SE. Kaposi's sarcoma and the acquired immunodeficiency syndrome: treatment with high and low doses of recombinant leukocyte A interferon. J Clin Oncol 1986;4:544–51.

[199] Mauss S, Jablonowski H. Efficacy, safety, and tolerance of low-dose, long-term interferon-alpha 2b and zidovudine in early-stage AIDS-associated Kaposi's sarcoma. J Acquir Immune Defic Syndr Hum Retrovirol 1995;10:157–62.

[200] Wang HY, Wang RF. Regulatory T cells and cancer. Curr Opin Immunol 2007;19:217–23.

[201] Cesana GC, DeRaffele G, Cohen S, et al. Characterization of CD4+CD25+ regulatory T cells in patients treated with high-dose interleukin-2 for metastatic melanoma or renal cell carcinoma. J Clin Oncol 2006;24:1169–77.

[202] Ahmadzadeh M, Rosenberg SA. IL-2 administration increases CD4+CD25(hi)FoxP3+ T cells in cancer patients. Blood 2006;107:2409–14.

[203] Petrulio CA, Kaufman HL. Development of the PANVAC-VF vaccine for pancreatic cancer. Expert Rev Vaccines 2006;5:9–19.

[204] Piancatelli D, Romano P, Sebastiani P, et al. Local expression of cytokines in human colorectal carcinoma: evidence of specific interleukin-6 gene expression. J Immunother (1997) 1999;22:25–32.

[205] Nemunaitis J, Khuri F, Ganly I, et al. Phase II trial of intratumoral administration of ONYX-015, a replication-selective adenovirus, in patients with refractory head and neck cancer. J Clin Oncol 2001;19:289–98.

[206] Weber WP, Feder-Mengus C, Chiarugi A, et al. Differential effects of the tryptophan metabolite 3-hydroxyanthranilic acid on the proliferation of human CD8+ T cells induced by TCR triggering or homeostatic cytokines. Eur J Immunol 2006;36:296–304.

[207] Gaspari P, Banerjee T, Malachowski WP, et al. Structure-activity study of brassinin derivatives as indoleamine 2,3-dioxygenase inhibitors. J Med Chem 2006;49:684–92.

[208] Basu GD, Tinder TL, Bradley JM, et al. Cyclooxygenase-2 inhibitor enhances the efficacy of a breast cancer vaccine: role of IDO. J Immunol 2006;177:2391–402.

[209] Barnett B, Kryczek I, Cheng P, et al. Regulatory T cells in ovarian cancer: biology and therapeutic potential. Am J Reprod Immunol 2005;54:369–77.

[210] Dudley ME, Wunderlich JR, Yang JC, et al. Adoptive cell transfer therapy following non-myeloablative but lymphodepleting chemotherapy for the treatment of patients with refractory metastatic melanoma. J Clin Oncol 2005;23:2346–57.

[211] Dudley ME, Wunderlich JR, Yang JC, et al. A phase I study of nonmyeloablative chemotherapy and adoptive transfer of autologous tumor antigen-specific T lymphocytes in patients with metastatic melanoma. J Immunother 2002;25:243–51.

[212] Thompson RH, Allison JP, Kwon ED. Anti-cytotoxic T lymphocyte antigen-4 (CTLA-4) immunotherapy for the treatment of prostate cancer. Urol Oncol 2006;24:442–7.

[213] Hodi FS, Mihm MC, Soiffer RJ, et al. Biologic activity of cytotoxic T lymphocyte-associated antigen 4 antibody blockade in previously vaccinated metastatic melanoma and ovarian carcinoma patients. Proc Natl Acad Sci U S A 2003;100:4712–7.

[214] Egen JG, Kuhns MS, Allison JP. CTLA-4: new insights into its biological function and use in tumor immunotherapy. Nat Immun 2002;3:611–8.

[215] Ribas A, Camacho LH, Lopez-Berestein G, et al. Antitumor activity in melanoma and anti-self responses in a phase I trial with the anti-cytotoxic T lymphocyte-associated antigen 4 monoclonal antibody CP-675,206. J Clin Oncol 2005;23:8968–77.

[216] Parmiani G, Castelli C, Pilla L, et al. Opposite immune functions of GM-CSF administered as vaccine adjuvant in cancer patients. Ann Oncol 2007;18:226–32.

[217] Chakraborty M, Abrams SI, Coleman CN, et al. External beam radiation of tumors alters phenotype of tumor cells to render them susceptible to vaccine-mediated T-cell killing. Cancer Res 2004;64:4328–37.

ELSEVIER
SAUNDERS

Surg Oncol Clin N Am
16 (2007) 819–831

SURGICAL
ONCOLOGY CLINICS
OF NORTH AMERICA

Therapeutic Cancer Vaccines

Lilah F. Morris, MD[a], Antoni Ribas, MD[a,b,c],*

[a]Department of Surgery, UCLA Medical Center, 16-155 CHS.
10833 Le Conte Avenue, Los Angeles, CA 90095, USA
[b]Department of Medicine, University of California at Los Angeles,
10833 Le Conte Avenue, Los Angeles, CA 90095, USA
[c]Jonsson Comprehensive Cancer Center, University of California at Los Angeles,
10833 Le Conte Avenue, Los Angeles, CA 90095, USA

In the midst of a smallpox epidemic in 1796, English surgeon Edward Jenner extracted pus from a milkmaid's cowpox blister and injected the material into both arms of a young boy. After minor flu-like symptoms, the boy had no reaction when later injected with the more potent variola, and never contracted smallpox. The term vaccine derives from the Latin word "of a cow," "vaccinus," and references this first series of inoculations.

While significant progress was made in the development of vaccines against infectious pathogens, their use in the treatment of neoplastic disease has been very limited. In 1896, amid reports that some patients with cancer who developed bacterial infections experienced remission of their malignancies, New York surgeon William Coley locally injected streptococcal broth cultures to induce erysipelas in a patient with an inoperable neck sarcoma. Although the therapy was toxic, the patient's tumor ultimately regressed, and he lived disease-free for 8 years before succumbing to his cancer [1].

Remarkably, Coley achieved a greater than 10%, 20-year disease-free survival by injecting "Coley's toxins" into mostly inoperable sarcoma patients. During the century since Coley's first experiments, immensely more is understood about tumor immunology, enabling development of more sophisticated and far less toxic immune therapies for malignant disease.

This review will outline various cancer vaccine strategies, including tumor cell, peptide, ganglioside, DNA, viral, and dendritic cell vaccines, discussing current understanding of mechanisms and clinical progress. Finally, adoptive

This study was supported in part by University of California Los Angeles Cancer Gene Medicine Training Grant T32 CA 75,956, the Melanoma Research Foundation, and the Harry J. Lloyd Charitable Trust.

* Corresponding author. Division of Hematology-Oncology, 11-934 Factor Building, UCLA Medical Center, 10833 Le Conte Avenue, Los Angeles, CA 90095-1782.

E-mail address: aribas@mednet.ucla.edu (A. Ribas).

cell transfer, or the ex vivo expansion and manipulation of large numbers of tumor-reactive CD8+ T cells, will be discussed as an emerging and promising immunotherapeutic strategy for a variety of cancers. Although immunotherapy has been successful to some degree for hematologic malignancies [2,3], this report will focus on treatments for solid tumors.

Therapeutic cancer vaccines

Technical definitions of vaccine reference humoral immunity, or antibody production. However, the cellular arm of the immunological cascade—the recognition, proliferation, and activation of cytotoxic CD8+ T lymphocytes (CTLs)—is required for effective cancer immunotherapy. Cancer vaccines use tumor-associated antigens (TAA), protein fragments expressed on the surface of most human cancers presented by major histocompatibility complexes (MHC), to elicit a cellular immune response.

Most TAAs are nonmutated, self-antigens. Some, like the melanosomal lineage antigens MART-1, gp100, and tyrosinase, are expressed on tumor cells and on cells of the same origin, but not on other cells. Others, like the cancer-testis antigen MAGE family of antigens or NY-ESO, are expressed during embryonic life and only in immune-shielded tissues like the testis in adult life. They differ most prominently from antigens used in preventive vaccines for infectious diseases (eg, measles, chicken pox) in that they are "self," rather than "foreign" antigens. TAAs evade immune surveillance; progressive malignancies are not rejected by a normal immune system.

In order for TAAs to activate the cellular arm of the immune system, they need to be presented to the CTL by an antigen-presenting cell (APC). The most powerful professional APC is the dendritic cell (DC). Tumor antigens, produced within the cell's cytosol, and extracellular (foreign) antigens taken into the cell by phagocytosis, are both processed into peptide fragments by APCs.

The interaction between T cells and APCs occurs via the highly specific T-cell receptor (TCR) located on the T-cell's surface and the antigen presented on the APC in the context of the MHC. APCs process self-antigens and present them to CD8+ T cells via class I MHC; foreign antigens are presented to CD4+ T cells via class II MHC. (The human homolog of the MHC is the human leukocyte antigen, or HLA.)

The immune system is trained to differentiate between self and foreign antigens. Early in life, the thymus samples T cells to determine which are appropriate for release into circulation, a process known as positive and negative thymic selection. In the process of positive selection, cells survive only if they are able to interact with host's MHC. This process ensures that mature T cells will be able to recognize foreign antigens presented by self-MHC, remaining tolerant to self-antigens. In the process of negative selection, T cells that are able to recognize self-antigens are deleted. This process is responsible for so-called central tolerance, because it ensures that potentially autoreactive T cells do not go to the peripheral blood. Some autoreactive T cells escape central tolerance and are released into the periphery.

While immune therapy for the treatment of cancer holds promise, current cancer vaccines have broad limitations and few objective clinical responses. Currently, no therapeutic cancer vaccines are approved by the Food and Drug Administration (FDA) in the United States for general use. This underscores the importance of referring appropriate patients for clinical trial participation.

Challenges of cancer vaccines

Targeting tumor antigens

Unique tumor antigens were first identified in the late 1980s and include melanoma-melanocyte differentiation antigens (eg, MART-1 or gp100), cancer-testes antigens (NY-ESO-1, MAGE-1), mutated antigens (β-catenin, Caspase-8), or nonmutated shared antigens that are overexpressed on cancer cells (Her-2/neu, carcinoembryonic antigen, α-Fetoprotein) [4]. While technologies such as gene chip analysis are able to rapidly identify new antigens, few cancers have well-characterized tumor antigens. Many vaccine strategies, like peptide-based or DC vaccines, require known TAAs. Other methods, like autologous or allogeneic whole tumor cell vaccines, rely on a host of unknown TAAs to stimulate an immune response.

Vaccines can be univalent, targeting one specific TAA, or polyvalent, either employing peptides of multiple known TAAs or using tumor cell products that by nature will incorporate many TAAs.

Limitations of cancer vaccines

There are several control mechanisms that do not allow for an efficient antitumor response. As discussed above, secondary to central tolerance, T cells that are specific for a particular tumor antigen are usually extremely rare—1/100,000 in peripheral blood. By nature, because most TAAs are self-antigens, they are poorly immunogenic. Cancer cells tend to down-regulate HLA expression or fail to express HLA class I molecules, making them poor targets for CTLs. Even if a TAA is recognized by the TCR on its specific CTL, CTLs have difficulty infiltrating into tumor sites. In addition, tumors actively inhibit the immune system by secretion of signals that interfere with DC and T-cell function.

Determining success—varying definitions of treatment response

The degree of optimism associated with research into therapeutic cancer vaccines depends largely upon definitions of response to treatment. Objective complete response and partial response to cancer vaccines is measured by World Health Organization (WHO) criteria: Disappearance of all lesions versus 50% decrease in the sum of the products of perpendicular diameters of all lesions and no increase in any lesion [5]. Response Evaluation Criteria in Solid Tumors (RECIST) criteria modifies the WHO partial response criteria to allow evaluation based on unidimensional measurements only. By doing so, the definition of a partial response was set as a 30% decrease in the sum of the largest diameters of target lesions and no increase in any lesion [6]. When using these objective response evaluation criteria, the determination of efficacy of cancer vaccine clinical trials has been dramatically lowered, with objective response rates as low as 3% [7,8].

More optimistic studies use so-called "soft" criteria—"minor response," "stable disease," and so forth—to declare clinical benefit. Some trials of therapeutic cancer vaccines demonstrate immune response in nearly half of patients assessed (eg, antipeptide antibody or lymphoproliferation) after vaccination, without any change in objective clinical response [8,9]. Dim results from cancer immunotherapy must be viewed in context of the patient populations included in trials. It is obvious that response rates with cancer vaccines will be low if the enlisted patients have widely metastatic disease with failure after standard therapies [10].

The promise of immunotherapy

There are numerous reasons to continue to pursue immunotherapeutic options. First, immunotherapy for metastatic disease often offers the only hope for cure. While chemotherapy may result in higher response rates or prolonged survival, it rarely results in disappearance of disease [11]. Clearly, no "magic bullet," immunotherapy or otherwise, will conquer cancer. Immunotherapeutic strategies that use multiple modalities (eg, adoptive cell transfer combined with a small molecule immunosensitizing agent) will likely be most successful.

Cancer vaccine strategies

Whole tumor cell vaccines

Injecting inactivated tumor cells or lysates into cancer patients is one method of assisting the immune system in recognizing tumor antigens. Whole tumor cell vaccines are either autologous, requiring resection of the patient's tumor, or allogeneic, using established tumor cell lines. Tumor cell vaccines are typically delivered with an immunological adjuvant, including foreign organisms (bacilli Calmette-Guerin, or BCG) or bacterial derivatives (Detox, Corixa Corporation, Seattle, WA), which help recruit APCs to the site of vaccination. This strategy theorizes that attracted by foreign adjuvant, APCs recognize antigenic epitopes on the tumor cells, then present them to T cells, initiating a larger immune response against all cells carrying that tumor antigen.

There are several advantages to whole tumor vaccines. The tumor antigen need not be identified before vaccination. In addition, whole tumor cell vaccines are polyvalent, containing multiple common antigens [12]. Allogeneic vaccines combine several tumor cell lines. These types of vaccines do not require HLA matching because they rely on cross-presentation of TAA by host APCs. Autologous tumor cell vaccines are by definition individualized, requiring lesions that are accessible for resection. Melanoma is more likely than many other malignancies to have accessible tumor tissue for this purpose.

Melacine (Corixa Corporation, Seattle, WA) is derived from lysates of two allogeneic melanoma cell lines, administered with the immunologic adjuvant Detox [13]. Despite promising phase I/II trials, a large, randomized, phase III trial by the Southwest Oncology Group (SWOG) found no difference in 2 years of Melacine versus observation as adjuvant treatment in resected intermediate-thickness, node-negative melanoma patients (T3N0M0) [14]. Recent results from a 25-institution, randomized phase III clinical trial of Melacine in patients with resected stage III melanoma had disappointing results. This trial found no difference in overall and disease-free survival in patients treated with Melacine plus low-dose interferon alfa-2b (IFN-α-2b) versus high-dose IFN-α-2b alone [15]. (High-dose IFN-α-2b is the only FDA-approved treatment for stage III melanoma.) As is the case here, it is important to separate studies of vaccination of patients with metastatic disease versus those that examine vaccination in an adjuvant setting. In patients with metastatic disease, it is possible to evaluate response to treatment. In adjuvant treatment, the goal is to not detect cancer recurrence compared with a control group. Single-arm studies (phase II single-arm clinical trials) are mostly uninformative since they do not have a concurrent control group, and small phase II randomized clinical trials lack the statistical power to detect reasonable differences provided by the study agent. Therefore, to detect a small, statistically significant difference, adjuvant studies require a very large sample size.

Canvaxin (CancerVax Corporation, Carlsbad, California), an allogeneic whole-cell vaccine from three melanoma cell lines, was studied as adjuvant therapy in patients with stage III and IV melanoma after surgical resection. Nonrandomized phase II trials found significantly improved 5-year survival of 49% in vaccine-treated patients versus 37% in historical controls [16]. However, two phase III randomized, double-blind clinical trials in patients with stage III and IV melanoma did not support an advantage for patients receiving Canvaxin compared with placebo [17]. In fact, the study arm seemed to behave worse than the placebo arm in these clinical trials.

Autologous tumor cell vaccines for adjuvant therapy in renal cell and colon carcinoma have shown more promise. A randomized, phase III trial of an autologous renal tumor cell vaccine investigated disease progression in patients with T2-3b, N0-3, M0 renal cell carcinoma after radical nephrectomy. Patients were randomized to receive vaccine versus no adjuvant treatment. The 5-year and 70-month progression-free survival was significantly better in the treatment group (77.4% and 72%, respectively) than in the control group (67.8% and 59.3%, respectively) [18]. A randomized, phase III trial of OncoVax, an autologous tumor cell vaccine administered with BCG, significantly improved recurrence-free and overall survival in stage II, but not stage III, colon cancer after surgical resection [19]. However, neither approach has been approved for routine clinical use, in part because the results of these clinical trials are far from conclusive.

Genetically modified tumor cell vaccines

Genetically engineered tumor cell vaccines are made up of autologous or allogeneic tumor cells to which immune stimulating genes are added. Various genes have been introduced, including costimulatory molecules and cytokines [20]. Preclinical murine vaccination screening studies demonstrated that genetic modification of tumor cells to express the DC-stimulating cytokine granulocyte-macrophage colony-stimulating factor (GM-CSF) were the most powerful to generate antitumor immunity [21].

Early trials of GM-CSF–modified tumor cell vaccines, termed GVAX (Cell Genesys, Hayward, CA), used a retroviral vector, which required actively replicating tumor cell cultures before transduction. This strategy required an average of 8 weeks of ex vivo manipulation, prohibitively long for patients with aggressive disease [22]. As adenoviruses can infect nondividing cells, switching vectors was attempted. Phase I/II trials using allogeneic GVAX therapies in recurrent, hormone-refractory prostate cancer showed low side-effect profiles and favorable survival data [23]. Cell Genesys is currently conducting two phase III trials of GVAX in hormone refractory prostate cancer.

Peptide vaccines

Peptides used in cancer vaccines are tumor antigens, typically coupled with an immunogenic adjuvant (eg, incomplete Freund's adjuvant). Peptide vaccines are usually injected intradermally or subcutaneously and captured by APCs, which then migrate to regional lymph nodes. The APCs present the peptide to circulating CTLs. If the peptide is recognized by its corresponding TCR, clonal expansion of CTLs occurs. These activated, expanded CTLs then travel to the periphery, recognizing the corresponding peptide-MHC complexes on tumor cells and lysing them.

Peptide vaccines consist of 8 to 10 amino acids, presented in association with MHC class I molecules, and can be synthesized in large scale. They are easily administered to patients in an outpatient setting with few side effects. However, the frequency of peptide-specific CTLs in circulation is low. In addition, a given MHC allele is only able to bind efficiently certain peptides. For instance, common melanoma antigens MART-1 and gp100 are restricted to HLA-A2*0201.

Several peptide vaccine trials have created a polyvalent vaccine using multiple tumor antigens. Immunologic response is improved with a slight modification, which renders the peptide more immunogenic but does not change its MHC binding affinity [9]. Most peptide trials have added immunostimulatory cytokines, such as IL-2 and GM-CSF, to improve vaccination [24]. While some peptide vaccines have elicited immune responses [25], a review of a decade of peptide vaccine trials at the National Cancer Institute (NCI) revealed dismal results: an overall objective response rate of 2.9% [7].

Dendridic cell vaccines

T cells require antigen presentation to initiate an effective immune response. DCs are generated in the bone marrow from hematopoietic progenitor cells. Immature DCs residing in tissues ingest pathogenic antigens and are activated by factors secreted as part of the inflammatory response to these pathogens. Mature, or activated, DCs then migrate to draining lymph nodes to present their antigens to T cells carrying a receptor that recognizes these antigens. DCs first present their antigens to CD4+ T cells. Cross-linking of CD40 to the CD4+ T-cell CD40 ligand (CD40L) activates CD4+ T cells and DCs so that they may provide help to CD8+ T cells. DCs also secrete IL-12, which is necessary to support T-cell proliferation. Tumor antigens alone do not generate this type of response.

DC vaccines for cancer strive to harness the work of these professional APCs. Clinically, autologous DCs are harvested from patients' peripheral blood mononuclear cells (PBMCs). They are differentiated and expanded ex vivo from stem cell precursors in cytokine-containing culture (GM-CSF, IL-4). They are then "loaded" with tumor antigen and injected back into patients in an attempt to develop a more profound immune response to tumor antigen. This entire process is labor intensive and time consuming.

Most clinical trials of DCs are peptide-based, but like peptide-based vaccines, this requires HLA matching. DCs can also present known and unknown antigen if they have been exposed to tumor lysates. This polyvalent approach does not require HLA matching. DCs can also be genetically engineered with viral vectors to produce TAAs [26,27].

Clinical trials of DC vaccines have demonstrated that DCs are able to elicit a specific T-cell immune response, but have had little impact on tumor regression. A randomized phase III trial in metastatic melanoma demonstrated no difference in objective response rates between autologous peptide-pulsed DC vaccination with dacarbizine (DTIC) chemotherapy (objective response for DC vaccine 3.8% versus 5.5% for DTIC) [28].

A phase III placebo-controlled study in asymptomatic metastatic hormone-refractory prostate cancer showed more promising results. Sipuleucel-T (APC8015, or Provenge) is an autologous DC vaccine cultured with fusion protein PA2024 (prostatic acid phosphatase [PAP], a prostate TAA, linked to GM-CSF). While Sipuleucel-T did not improve time to disease progression versus placebo, an intent-to-treat analysis in patients receiving Sipuleucel-T demonstrated a statistically significant 4.5-month improvement in overall survival [29].

Ganglioside vaccines

Gangliosides are carbohydrate epitopes of TAAs that are overexpressed on cancer cells. GM2 is a ganglioside melanoma antigen and the most immunogenic ganglioside expressed on melanoma cells. A formulation of GM2 vaccine (GM2 coupled to keyhole limpet hemocyanin combined with QS-21 adjuvant), called GMK vaccine (Progenics Pharmaceuticals, Inc, Tarrytown, NJ) was tested against the only proven adjuvant for patients at high risk of recurrence—high-dose interferon alfa-2b (HDI). This prospective, randomized trial was closed early when HDI proved significantly better in terms of relapse-free survival and overall survival. However, patients with high anti-GM2 antibody titers had improved relapse-free survival and overall survival compared with nonresponders [30].

Heat shock proteins

Heat shock proteins (HSPs) are chaperones for unique, immunogenic tumor peptides. Their main function is to help, under stresses like heat, newly translated proteins fold correctly and denatured proteins to refold appropriately. They carry a peptide-binding pocket that binds antigens suited to MHC presentation. TAA-HSP complexes are presented to and taken up by APCs, then cross-presented in the context of MHC class I to elicit a CTL response. HSPs have a role in DC activation, so the activation of CTLs is achieved without CD4+ T-cell help. HSPs can bind multiple peptides, making them polyvalent vaccines.

While peptide vaccines rely on identified common tumor antigens, HSP vaccines are more personalized. Studies have demonstrated that HSPs chaperone common tumor antigens (eg, hsp70 chaperones common melanoma antigens MART-1, gp100, tyrosinase, and TRP-2), but also chaperone unique tumor antigens that have not yet been identified [31]. HSPs provide immunity against a specific tumor in a particular individual, but not of another tumor from the same cell type origin, requiring surgical resection for vaccine production [32].

For clinical trials of HSP gp96 (Oncophage, Vitespen, or HSPCC-96, Antigenics, New York, NY), resected tumor was sent for processing to Antigenics, Inc, a Lexington, Massachusetts–based central facility. HSP gp96 was purified from the tumor, and the vaccine's efficacy was derived from the unique tumor antigen contained within gp96's binding region. Tumor tissue requirements from surgical resection were stringent. However, two randomized phase III clinical trials comparing Oncophage or physician's choice of treatment in patients with stage IV metastatic melanoma or renal cell carcinoma failed to meet the primary study end point. There was a trend toward improved survival in a subset of vaccine-treated patients with the most indolent melanoma lesions (stage M1a) [33].

DNA vaccines

DNA vaccines use DNA encoding a TAA, which is cloned into a bacterial plasmid and injected intradermally or intramuscularly into a patient. The plasmid enters the nucleus of a host cell and an antigen is synthesized from the viral DNA. APCs are able to pick up and present the protein products in the appropriate MHC context with costimulatory molecules. DNA vaccines stimulate both humoral and cellular immune responses by encoding a full-length protein with several epitopes of interest, rather than a purified, recombinant peptide. This also circumvents the need for HLA matching. In addition, the bacterial vector holds immunogenic, unmethylated CpG motifs, a "built-in adjuvant" [34,35].

Despite promising preclinical data, few clinical trials of DNA cancer vaccines have been completed. Results of a phase I trial of xenogenic human tyrosinase DNA vaccines used in canines with spontaneously arising melanoma of the oral mucosa demonstrated median survival time of 389 days versus less than 150 days for historical controls [36].

Recombinant viral vaccines

Viruses have been exploited for use in cancer vaccines because of their ability to express foreign gene sequences (in this case, tumor antigen genes) in target cells. Poxviruses are able to replicate entirely within the cytoplasm of an infected cell. Poxvirus vectors are not infectious, because after transfection, the viral genome is not transcribed by cellular enzymes, and viral proteins are not made. Recombinant poxviruses that express TAAs can be used to stimulate cell-mediated immunity; the antigens are expressed intracellularly, allowing MHC class I presentation to CTLs [37]. The recombinant protein presented by poxvirus vectors is more immunogenic than the tumor antigen alone since the viral vector acts as an immunological adjuvant [38].

Costimulatory molecules, so termed because they are a second signal between the APC's surface MHC-peptide presentation and the TCR, play a vital role in prolonging and promoting the APC-TCR interaction. Initial clinical trials in prostate cancer have tested the safety of using a recombinant virus with gene sequences for both a TAA (prostate-specific antigen, or PSA) and costimulatory molecules (TRICOM, or ICAM-1, B7.1, and LFA-3) [39].

Generation of immunologic memory, a subset of circulating T cells that recognize antigen long after the initial immune response, is an important goal of vaccination. Vaccination induces a proliferation phase of antigen-specific T cells that lasts for 7 to 10 days. Numbers of these cells fall sharply, but over the next 3 months a small subset of antigen-specific T cells develop into a circulating "memory" pool that will vigorously proliferate in response to antigen restimulation. Recombinant viral vaccines use prime-boost strategies. The concept involves the priming of an immune response using one type of vector to deliver the tumor antigen, followed by boosting the induced T-cell response by immunizing with the same antigen delivered by a different vector.

In a phase II randomized trial of prostate cancer patients with biochemical progression after local therapy, a vaccinia virus was used to deliver PSA and spark the immune response, while fowlpox, unable to replicate in human cells, is administered later to boost previously initiated cellular immune response. This study compared varying vaccinia-PSA and fowlpox-PSA vaccine regimens; the prime-boost method (vaccinia followed by fowlpox) demonstrated a trend toward longer PSA progression [40]. At a mean follow up of 50 months, 80% of men receiving fowlpox-PSA or fowlpox-PSA plus vaccinia-PSA continued to be free of clinical disease progression, while 90% of men receiving vaccine-PSA followed by fowlpox-PSA prime-boost were free of disease progression [41].

Adoptive cell transfer

Adoptive transfer strategies involve the ex vivo expansion and activation of autologous tumor-reactive CTLs that are the then administered back to the patient [42]. After tumor resection, tumor-infiltrating lymphocytes (TILs) are purified, expanded, and reinjected into the patient. Early studies of this method in melanoma and renal cell carcinoma were met with some success (23% to 34% overall response rate) [43,44], while others in renal cell carcinoma showed no advantage to administration of TILs in addition to IL-2 [45]. Since those initial studies, the importance of immunodepletion before adoptive cell transfer has been elucidated [46]. Studies of adoptive transfer after immunodepletion have resulted in greater than 50% objective response rates in patients with metastatic melanoma [42,47,48].

The genes encoding the TCR specific for several TAAs have been cloned from patients who had near-complete responses to immune therapy. Recent efforts have attempted to introduce these TCRs, via a viral vector, into peripheral blood lymphocytes (PBLs) of patients with advanced cancers. A phase I clinical trial for ovarian cancer, in which a patient's T cells were genetically engineered to display a TCR for the ovarian cancer–associated antigen α-folate receptor (FR), demonstrated no antitumor response, thought to be due to poor tumor trafficking of the engineered T cells and low persistence (barely detectable at 3 weeks) [49]. A more promising study from NCI in patients with metastatic melanoma demonstrated durable (>20 months) disease regression in 2 of 17 patients whose PBLs were transduced with a retrovirus expressing the MART-1 TCR after lymphodepleting preconditioning regimens [50].

Summary

Despite seemingly slow progress in immunotherapy for aggressive diseases like metastatic melanoma, immune-based therapies are the only treatment modalities that have the potential to offer long-term survival in some patients with widely metastatic solid cancers. Some patients experience a complete response to various immunotherapeutic agents, with long-term survival and no evidence of tumor. With so many treatments in existence, if we could determine with scientific precision which patient would respond to which treatment, we could forgo the search for a catch-all treatment "magic bullet" [51,52].

Combination immunotherapies, such as DC vaccines coupled with immunostimulatory molecules, offer the best hope for vaccine-based therapy. Adoptive cell transfer has demonstrated great promise in the treatment of metastatic melanoma, and will be the future of directed immunotherapy for many cancers with known tumor antigens.

References

[1] Wiemann B, Starnes CO. Coley's toxins, tumor necrosis factor and cancer research: a historical perspective. Pharmacol Ther 1994;64:529–64.

[2] Mocellin S, Semenzato G, Mandruzzato S, et al. Part II: vaccines for haematological malignant disorders. Lancet Oncol 2004;5(12):727–37.

[3] Timmerman J. Immunotherapy for lymphomas. Int J Hematol 2003;77(5):444–55.

[4] Rosenberg SA. Progress in human tumor immunology and immunotherapy. Nature 2001; 411:380–4.

[5] Miller A, Hoogstraten B, Staquet M, et al. Reporting results of cancer treatment. Cancer 1981;47(1):207–14.

[6] Therasse P, Arbuck SG, Eisenhauer EA, et al. New guidelines to evaluate the response to treatment in solid tumors. J Natl Cancer Inst 2000;92:205–16.

[7] Rosenberg S, Yang JC, Restifo NP. Cancer immunotherapy: moving beyond current vaccines. Nat Med 2004;10(9):909–15.

[8] Nagorsen D, Thiel E. Clinical and immunologic responses to active specific cancer vaccines in human colorectal cancer. Clin Cancer Res 2006;12(10):3064–9.

[9] Rosenberg S, Yang JC, Schwartzentruber DJ, et al. Immunologic and therapeutic evaluation of a synthetic peptide vaccine for the treatment of patients with metastatic melanoma. Nat Med 1998;4(3):321–4.

[10] Mocellin S, Mandruzzato S, Bronte V, et al. Cancer vaccines: pessimism in check. Nat Med 2004;10(12):1278–80.

[11] Mocellin S, Mandruzzato S, Bronte V, et al. Part I: vaccines for solid tumors. Lancet Oncol 2004;5:681–9.

[12] Copier J, Dalgleish A. Overview of tumor cell-based vaccines. Int Rev Immunol 2006;25: 297–319.

[13] Sondak V, Sosman JA. Results of clinical trails with an allogeneic melanoma tumor cell lysate vaccine: melacine. Semin Cancer Biol 2003;13:409–15.

[14] Sondak V, Liu PY, Tuthill RJ, et al. Adjuvant immunotherapy of resected, intermediate-thickness, node-negative melanoma with an allogeneic tumor vaccine: overall results of a randomized trial of the Southwest Oncology Group. J Clin Oncol 2002;20(8): 2058–66.

[15] Mitchell M, Abrams J, Thompson JA, et al. Randomized trial of an allogeneic melanoma lysate vaccine with low-dose interferon alfa-2b compared with high-dose interferon alfa-2b for resected stage III cutaneous melanoma. J Clin Oncol 2007;25(16):2078–85.

[16] Morton D, Hsueh EC, Essner R, et al. Prolonged survival of patients receiving active immunotherapy wiht canvaxin therapeutic polyvalent vaccine after complete resection of melanoma metastatic to regional lymph nodes. Ann Surg 2002;236(4):438–49.

[17] Morton D, Mozzillo N, Thompson JF, et al. An international, randomized, phase III trial of bacillus Clamette-Guerin (BCG) plus allogenic melanoma vaccine (MCV) or placebo after complete resection of melanoma mestatic to regional or distant sites. 2007 ASCO Annual Meeting Proceedings, Part I. J Clin Oncol 2007;25(Suppl 18S):8508.

[18] Jocham D, Richter A, Hoffmann L, et al. Adjuvant autologous renal tumor cell vaccine and risk of tumor progression in patients with renal-cell carcinoma after radical nephrectomy: phase III, randomised controlled trial. Lancet 2004;363:594–9.

[19] Uyl-de Groot C, Vermorken JB, Hanna MG Jr, et al. Immunotherapy with autologous tumor cell-BCG vaccine in paitents with colon cancer: a prospective study of medical and economic benefits. Vaccine 2005;23:2379–87.

[20] Dranoff G. GM-CSF-based cancer vaccines. Immunol Rev 2002;188:147–54.

[21] Dranoff G, Jaffee E, Lazenby A, et al. Vaccination with irradiated tumor cells engineered to secrete granulocyte-macrophage colony-stimulating factor stimulates potent, specific, and long-lasting anti-tumor immunity. Proc Natl Acad Sci U S A 1993;90:3539–43.

[22] Soiffer R, Lynch T, Mihm M, et al. Vaccination with irradiated autologous melanoma cells engineered to secrete human granulocyte-macrophage colony-stimulating factor generates potent antitumor immunity in patients with metastatic melanoma. Proc Natl Acad Sci U S A 1998;95:13141–6.

[23] Hege K, Jooss K, Pardoll D. GM-CSF gene-modified cancer cell immunotherapies: of mice and men. Int Rev Immunol 2006;25:321–52.

[24] Slingluff C, Petroni GR, Yamschchikov GV, et al. Immunologic and clinical outcomes of vaccination with a multiepitope melanoma peptide vaccine plus low-dose interleukin-2 administered either concurrently or on a delayed schedule. J Clin Oncol 2004;22:4474–85.

[25] Parmiani G, Castelli C, Dalerba P, et al. Cancer immunotherapy with peptide-based vaccines: what have we achieved? Where are we going? J Natl Cancer Inst 2002;94(11): 805–18.

[26] Gilboa E. DC-based cancer vaccines. J Clin Invest 2007;117(5):1195–203.

[27] Saito H, Frleta D, Dubsky P, et al. Dendritic cell-based vaccination against cancer. Hematol Oncol Clin North Am 2006;20:689–710.

[28] Schadendorf D, Ugurel S, Schuler-Thurner B, et al. Dacarbazine (DTIC) versus vaccination with autologous peptide-pulsed dendritic cells (DC) in first-line treatament of patients with metastatic melanoma: a randomized phase III trial of the DC study group of the DeCOG. Ann Oncol 2006;17:563–70.

[29] Small E, Schellhammer PF, Higano CS, et al. Placebo-controlled phase III trial of immunologic therapy with Sipuleucel-T (APC8015) in patients with metastatic, asymptomatic hormon refractory prostate cancer. J Clin Oncol 2006;24(19):3089–94.

[30] Kirkwood J, Ibrahim JG, Sasman JA, et al. High-dose interferon alfa-2b significantly prolongs relapse-free and overall survival compared with the GM2-KLH/QS-21 vaccine patients with resected stage IIB-III melanoma: results of intergroup trial E1694/S9512/ C509801. J Clin Oncol 2001;19(9):2370–80.

[31] Castelli C, Rivoltini L, Rini F, et al. Heat shock proteins: biological functions and clinical applications as personalized vaccines for human cancer. Cancer Immunol Immunother 2004;53:227–33.

[32] Srivastava P, DeLeo AB, Old LJ. Tumor rejection antigens of chemically induced sarcomas of inbred mice. Proc Natl Acad Sci U S A 1986;83:3407–11.

[33] Richards J, Testori A, Whitman E, et al. Autologous tumor-derived HSPPC-96 vs. physician's choice (PC) in a randomized phase III trial in stage IV melanoma. J Clin Oncol 2006;24(18S):8002.

[34] Srinivasan R, Wolchok JD. Tumor antigens for cancer immunotherapy: therapeutic potential of xenogenic DNA vaccines. J Transl Med 2004;2(1):12.

[35] Stan R, Wolchok JD, Cohen AD. DNA vaccines against cancer. Hematol Oncol Clin North Am 2006;20:613–36.

[36] Bergman P, McKnight J, Novosad A, et al. Long-term survival of dogs with advanced malignant melanoma after DNA vaccination with xenogeneic human tyrosinase: a phase I trial. Clin Cancer Res 2003;9:1284–90.

[37] Moss B. Genetically engineered poxviruses for recombinant gene expression, vaccination, and safety. Proc Natl Acad Sci U S A 1996;93:11341–8.

[38] Arlen P, Dahut WL, Gulley JL. Immunotherapy for prostate cancer: what's the future? Hematol Oncol Clin North Am 2006;20:965–83.

[39] DiPaola R, Plante M, Kaufman H, et al. A phase I trial of Pox PSA vaccines (PROSTVAC-VF) with B7-1, ICAM-1, and LFA-3 co-stimulatory molecules (TRICOM) in patients with prostate cancer. J Transl Med 2006;4:1.

[40] Kaufman H, Wang W, Manola J, et al. Phase II randomized study of vaccine treatment of advanced prostate cancer (E7897): a trial of the eastern cooperative oncology group. J Clin Oncol 2004;22(11):2122–32.

[41] Kaufman H, Wang W, Manola J, et al. Phase II prime/boost vaccination using poxviruses expressing PSA in hormone dependent prostate cancer: follow-up clinical results from ECOG 7897. J Clin Oncol 2005;23(16S):4501.

[42] Gattitoni L, Powell DJ, Rosenberg SA, et al. Adoptive immunotherapy for cancer: building on success. Nat Immunol 2006;6:383–93.

[43] Kradin R, Kurnick JT, Lazarus DS, et al. Tumor-infiltrating lymphocytes and interleukin-2 in the treatment of advanced cancer. Lancet 1989;1(8638):577–80.

[44] Rosenberg S, Yannelli JR, Yang JC, et al. Treatment of patients with metastatic melanoma with autologous tumor-infiltrating lymphoctyes and interleukin 2. J Natl Cancer Inst 1994; 86(15):1159–66.

[45] Figlin R, Thompson JA, Bukowski RM, et al. Multicenter, randomized, phase III trial of CD8+ tumor-infiltrating lymphocytes in combination with recombinant interleukin-2 in metastatic renal cell carcinoma. J Clin Oncol 1999;17(8):2521–9.

[46] Dudley M, Wunderlich JR, Yang JC, et al. A phase I study of nonmyeloablative chemotherapy and adoptive transfer of autologous tumor antigen-specific T lymphocytes in patients with metastatic melanoma. J Immunother 2002;25(3):243–51.

[47] Dudley ME, Wunderlich J, Robbins PF, et al. Cancer regression and autoimmunity in patients after clonal repopulation with antitumor lymphocytes. Science 2002;298(5594): 850–4.

[48] Dudley M, Wunderlich JR, Yang JC, et al. Adoptive cell transfer therapy following non-myeloablative but lymphodepleting chemotherapy for the treatment of patients with refractory metastatic melanoma. J Clin Oncol 2005;23(10):2346–57.

[49] Kershaw M, Westwood JA, Parker LL, et al. A phase I study on adoptive immunotherapy using gene-modified T cells for ovarian cancer. Clin Cancer Res 2006;12(20): 6106–15.

[50] Morgan R, Dudley ME, Wunderlich JR, et al. Cancer regression in patients after transfer of genetically engineered lymphocytes. Science 2006;314:126–9.

[51] Itoh K, Yamada A. Personalized peptide vaccines: a new therapeutic modality for cancer. Cancer Sci 2006;97(10):970–6.

[52] Parmiani G, De Filippo A, Novellino L, et al. Unique tumor antigens: immunobiology and use in clinical trials. J Immunol 2007;178:1975–9.

ELSEVIER
SAUNDERS

Surg Oncol Clin N Am
16 (2007) 833–839

SURGICAL
ONCOLOGY CLINICS
OF NORTH AMERICA

The Surgeon's Role in Immunotherapy

Robert P. Sticca, MD, FACS[a],*,
Jonathan A. Sticca, BA[b]

[a]Department of Surgery, University of North Dakota School of Medicine and Health Sciences,
501 North Columbia Road, Grand Forks, ND 58201, USA
[b]Department of Pathology and Laboratory Medicine, Medical University of South Carolina,
Charleston, SC 29401, USA

At first glance, surgeons do not appear to have a significant role in immunotherapy for malignancy. In fact, however, surgeons play an important role in immunotherapy of solid tumors. In 1970, Morton [1], a pioneer in the field of tumor immunology, advocated the surgeon's role in immunotherapy. He stated that "the surgeon is ideally suited to use immunotherapy as a therapeutic tool and should welcome its development." In the ensuing decades, there have been many significant advances in the understanding of the molecular and clinical basis for immunotherapy. For many of these advances, surgeons were leaders or collaborators as basic scientists or clinical investigators.

Many of the leading immunotherapy programs are integrally related to surgical departments as the surgeon is often a key figure in initiating an immunotherapy protocol or treatment. Without the surgeon's assistance in obtaining tissue specimens, developing immunotherapeutic treatments, and monitoring response to treatment, it is unlikely that many successful immunotherapy trials or treatments could occur. The surgeon plays a central role in many aspects of immunotherapy treatment (Fig. 1). This article reviews the key roles that surgeons play in immunotherapy treatment and research.

Specimen procurement

During surgery to remove malignant tumors, surgeons have a unique opportunity to obtain tumor specimens for immunotherapy treatments and research protocols. Many immune-based therapies require viable autologous tumor tissue to develop and administer the treatment. The development

---

* Corresponding author.
E-mail address: rsticca@medicine.nodak.edu (R.P. Sticca).

doi:10.1016/j.soc.2007.09.001   *surgonc.theclinics.com*

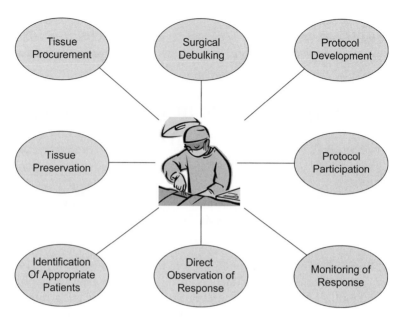

Fig. 1. The surgeon plays a central role in immunotherapy for solid tumors.

of autologous vaccines as well as the isolation of unique tumor antigens often requires timely and appropriately managed tumor specimens. To ensure highest quality specimens, tumor tissue must be procured and handled under the proper conditions. This means sterility must be maintained. In some cases, tissue must be quickly frozen. In others, precautions must be taken to ensure tissue remains fresh. Because of these requirements, the surgeon may need to obtain specimens at the time of tumor extirpation before the proteins and nucleic acids denature. The increasing emphasis on molecular characterization of tumor antigens and of key genes and proteins in the immune response necessitates timely tissue procurement and preservation.

Recent studies on tumor microenvironments have demonstrated complex interactions between the tumor and the host immune system [2,3]. The ability to accurately assess and characterize the full spectrum of the tumor interaction with the host immune system throughout the evolution of the tumor often requires serial biopsy and analysis, a situation in which surgical assistance is crucial. It is likely that in the future a primary role for surgical removal of solid tumors may be to obtain tissue for analysis of molecular tumor characteristics facilitating choice or development of treatment options, including immunotherapy.

Optimal surgical management

Optimal surgical management to enable and promote immune responses against tumors includes several aspects of surgical therapy.

Perioperative management

Many factors affect the host immune response to malignancy at the time of surgical removal of a tumor, including nutritional status, comorbidities, blood transfusions, and postoperative infectious complications. The surgeon should strive to limit immunosuppressive factors at the time of surgery for solid tumors. The immunosuppressive effect and subsequent negative impact on survival of blood transfusion during and after surgery has been reported since the 1980s [4–6]. Surgeons should make every effort to restrict blood transfusions in the perioperative period to avoid this effect.

Surgical technique

Complete removal of solid tumors with negative margins reduces residual tumor to micrometastatic disease when such disease is present. Responses to most cancer therapies improve with smaller tumor volumes. Similarly, response to immunotherapy for solid tumors improves with smaller tumor volumes [7,8]. Tumors have been shown to produce several substances (immunosuppressive cytokines, immune complex precipitates, and peptidoglycans) that interfere with normal immunologic defenses [9,10]. An increasing volume of literature indicates that immune responses to solid tumors improve with complete surgical removal. While it is still not conclusively established that immune responses improve with the removal of solid tumors, several explanations have been proposed as to why such improvement might occur. One possible explanation for this improvement is that large bulky tumors overwhelm the immune response and, once those tumors are removed, the immune response returns. Another possible explanation for this improvement is that factors in the tumor microenvironment shield tumor cells from the immune system and the removal of the tumor disrupts the microenvironment, enabling the restoration of the immune response. Yet other possible explanations relate to anatomical factors within larger tumors (altered blood flow, pH) and immunosuppressive effects of larger tumors. The removal of tumors means the removal of such anatomical factors and immunosuppressive effects, leading to restoration of the immune response. The best results with immunotherapy may be in an adjuvant setting with improved immune responses to residual micrometastatic disease.

Cytoreduction

In patients for whom complete removal of tumor is not feasible, surgical cytoreduction may be of benefit. The principle of cytoreduction (ie, the incomplete removal of large or bulky solid tumors) has been shown to be beneficial in several types of tumors (ovarian, melanoma, appendiceal, neuroendocrine) when combined with other forms of adjuvant therapy [11–14]. Cytoreduction can be attained by several methods, including surgical debulking, chemotherapy, or radiation therapy. Due to advances in surgical and critical care techniques, there has been renewed interest in surgical cytoreduction in both curative and palliative situations. The role of an experienced cancer surgeon in performing radical debulking surgery in these settings is obvious. Combining cytoreduction techniques with immunotherapy has the potential to further improve survival and quality of life. Other benefits to cytoreduction include the interruption of the metastatic cascade whereby metastases beget more metastases [8].

Monitoring of response to immunotherapy

The response to an immunotherapeutic treatment may be monitored by several methods. For some of these methods, a surgeon's involvement is indispensable. In the setting of immunotherapeutic treatments with measurable disease, evaluation of response can be monitored by radiologic techniques, physical examination, and biochemical or immunologic assays. Evaluation of tumor tissue after treatment can provide valuable information on the host immune response and host–tumor interactions. Surgical removal of tumor or host lymphoid tissue before, during, and after immunotherapeutic treatment is important to allow analysis of new or changing interactions between the host immune system and the tumor. An example of the importance of direct tissue analysis has been demonstrated in a study by Slingluff and colleagues [15], in which analysis of the immunized sentinel lymph nodes was much more accurate in documenting generation of antitumor reactions than analysis of peripheral blood.

Surgical evaluation of response to therapy for solid tumors has been used. One example of this is second-look surgery in ovarian cancer. Such surgical evaluation combines the diagnostic aspect of a surgical exploration with the therapeutic aspect of resection of residual disease if present. When immunotherapy is part of the treatment plan, opportunities such as this allow the surgeon to not only evaluate the response to therapy, but also to provide an invaluable resource of tumor tissue for study of the effects of immunotherapy on the tumor.

Protocol awareness

In many cases, the surgeon is the first oncologic specialist to diagnose the malignancy and develop a relationship with the patient. This places the surgeon in an excellent position to approach the patient about participation in immunotherapy clinical trials or recommend approved immunotherapeutic treatments. Knowledge of available research protocols and entry criteria for these studies is essential for the surgeon to encourage and promote immunotherapeutic clinical trials to their patients. It behooves the surgeon to be aware of locally and nationally available immunotherapy clinical trials for their patients who are interested. When other therapeutic options have been exhausted or when patients are interested in alternatives to standard therapies, immunotherapy clinical trials offer additional possibilities for continued treatment. Immunotherapy trials may be attractive to many patients because of lower toxicities associated with most immunotherapeutic treatments. Timely referral of patients for immunotherapy trials is important to maximize opportunity for participation in these trials. Awareness of the trial requirements before enrollment can also increase the opportunity for participation by ensuring that surgical or specimen procurement criteria are met.

Many Web sites list and categorize cancer clinical trials available in regional, national, and international forums. Some of these Web sites are listed in Table 1. These sites are useful for both patients and physicians, providing information about currently available clinical trials as well as background information on clinical trials and research methodology. In addition, local or institutional immunotherapy clinical trials may be available to interested patients and investigators. The continued advancement in immunotherapy for cancer depends on active participation of both patients and their treating physicians in immunotherapeutic clinical trials. By the nature and timing of their interactions with cancer patients, surgeons have a tremendous opportunity to promote immunotherapy clinical trials to their patients.

Protocol development

Surgical involvement in design and development of immunotherapy protocols is essential. Optimal timing of surgical excision, specimen procurement, and handling, as well as monitoring of results through timely tissue sampling or posttherapy surgical excision, requires the guidance of surgical

Table 1
Web sites related to cancer clinical trials

Web site name	Web site address	Sponsor	Sponsor funding	Location of trials
Center Watch	http://www.centerwatch.com/	Thomson Corporation	Private	International
NCI Clinical Trials	http://www.cancer.gov/clinicaltrials	National Cancer Institute	U.S. government	United States
Clinical Trials.gov	http://clinicaltrials.gov/	National Institutes of Health	U.S. government	United States
Cancer Backup	http://www.cancerbackup.org.uk/Trials/Search	Cancer Backup	Private charity	United Kingdom and Europe

members of the immunotherapy team. All surgical procedures affect the immune system and these effects should be considered when designing and implementing immune-based protocols.

Surgical personnel qualified in the design of immunotherapy protocols must evaluate the logistics and feasibility of incorporating immunotherapy in the treatment of tumors where surgery is required. Most solid tumors are initially treated with surgery as part of a multidisciplinary treatment plan. The benefits of surgical removal of the tumor with the subsequent effects on the immune response against the tumor is an integral part of the treatment plan for the patient and can be incorporated into protocols to manipulate or improve the host immune response against the tumor.

Summary

While it is unlikely that immunotherapy will replace surgical removal of most solid tumors, especially in the early stages of disease, the use of immunotherapy in the multidisciplinary care of the cancer patient will play an increasingly important role in cancer therapy for solid tumors. Strategies to optimize surgical management for an effective immune response against tumors should be acknowledged and promoted by the surgical community. Immunotherapy can serve as a beneficial adjunct to surgical excision for high-risk and recurrent tumors, with the attraction of decreased toxicity and disability over current adjuvant treatment methods. It is important that surgeons recognize immunotherapy's potential and play an active role in developing immunotherapy treatment regimens, for without surgical involvement many of these therapies may never come to fruition.

References

[1] Morton DL. Cancer immunology and the surgeon. Surgery 1970;67(2):396–8.
[2] Wang E, Marincola FM. A natural history of melanoma: serial gene expression analysis. Immunol Today 2000;21(12):619–23.
[3] Strauss L, Bergmann C, Szczepanski M, et al. A unique subset of CD4+ CD25highFoxp3+ T cells secreting interleukin-10 and transforming growth factor-beta1 mediates suppression in the tumor microenvironment. Clin Cancer Res 2007;13(15 Pt 1):4345–54.
[4] Voogt PJ, van de Velde CJH, Brand A, et al. Perioperative blood transfusion and cancer prognosis. Cancer 1987;59:836–43.
[5] Tartter PI. The association of perioperative blood transfusion with colorectal cancer recurrence. Ann Surg 1992;216:633–8.
[6] Heiss MM, Mempel W, Delanoff C, et al. Blood transfusion modulated tumor recurrence: first results of a randomized study of autologous versus allogeneic blood transfusion in colorectal cancer surgery. J Clin Oncol 1994;12:1859–67.
[7] Morton D, Ollila D, Hsueh E, et al. Cytoreductive surgery and adjuvant immunotherapy: a new management paradigm for metastatic melanoma. Ca Cancer J Clin 1999;49:101–16.
[8] McCarter M, Fong Y. Role for cytoreduction in multimodality treatments for cancer. Ann Surg Oncol 2001;8:38–43.
[9] Pollock RE, Roth JA. Cancer-induced immunosuppression: implications for therapy? Semin Surg Oncol 1989;5:414–9.

[10] Kavanaugh DY, Carbone DP. Immunologic dysfunction in cancer. Hematol Oncol Clin North Am 1996;10:927–51.

[11] Bristow RE, Montz FJ, Lagasse LD, et al. Survival impact of surgical cytoreduction in stage IV epithelial ovarian cancer. Gynecol Oncol 1999;72:278–87.

[12] Tafra L, Dale PS, Wanek LA, et al. Resection and adjuvant immunotherapy for melanoma metastatic to the lung and thorax. J Thorac Cardiovasc Surg 1995;110:119–28 [discussion: 129].

[13] Chen H, Hardacre JM, Uzar A, et al. Isolated liver metastases from neuroendocrine tumors: does resection prolong survival? J Am Coll Surg 1998;187:88–92 [discussion: 92–3].

[14] Sugarbaker PH, Chang D. Results of treatment of 385 patients with peritoneal surface spread of appendiceal malignancy. Ann Surg Oncol 1999;6:727–31.

[15] Slingluff CL Jr, Petroni GR, Yamshchikov GV, et al. Clinical and immunologic results of a randomized phase II trial of vaccination using four melanoma peptides either administered in granulocyte-macrophage colony-stimulating factor in adjuvant or pulsed on dendritic cells. J Clin Oncol 2003;21(21):4016–26.

ELSEVIER
SAUNDERS

Surg Oncol Clin N Am
16 (2007) 841–860

SURGICAL
ONCOLOGY CLINICS
OF NORTH AMERICA

Current Immunotherapeutic Strategies
in Breast Cancer

William E. Carson III, MD[a,b,*], Margaret I. Liang, BS[c]

[a]Division of Surgical Oncology, The Ohio State University School of Medicine,
N924 Doan Hall, 410 West 10th Avenue, Columbus, OH 43210-1228, USA
[b]The Ohio State University Comprehensive Cancer Center, N924 Doan Hall,
410 West 10th Avenue, Columbus, OH 43210-1228, USA
[c]The Ohio State University School of Medicine, N924 Doan Hall,
410 West 10th Avenue, Columbus, OH 43210-1228, USA

Despite significant advances in the administration of combination cytotoxic chemotherapy, the overall 5-year survival rate is about 75% for
a woman who has node-positive breast cancer and is just 20% for a patient
who has been diagnosed with metastatic disease [1]. Recent advances in our
understanding of the immune system have led to the hope that manipulation
of this organ system could be used as a cancer treatment. Initial studies have
been conducted in patients who have metastatic disease, but the ultimate
goal would be to develop treatments that could prevent the outgrowth of
micrometastatic disease in patients who have had definitive surgery for
early-stage breast cancers. Strategies that have been used in the immune
therapy of breast cancer include the administration of exogenous cytokines,
vaccines, and humanized monoclonal antibodies (mAb). Each of these
approaches is discussed in turn.

Overview of the immune system

Humans are under constant attack by rapidly dividing and highly
adaptable pathogenic organisms ranging in complexity and size from single-stranded RNA viruses to parasitic helminths. Infectious agents must
overcome or evade the sophisticated and highly integrated defense

This work was supported by Grants No. P01 CA95426-04 and U01 CA76576 from the
National Cancer Institute.
* Corresponding author. The Ohio State University School of Medicine, N924 Doan
Hall, 410 West 10th Avenue, Columbus, OH 43210-1228.
E-mail address: william.carson@osumc.edu (W.E. Carson).

mechanisms of the human immune system, which consist of an array of barriers, effector proteins, phagocytes, and lymphocytes. The cellular components of the immune response can be grouped into two distinct arms based on their phylogenetic age and their requirement for prior exposure to antigen. The effector cells of the innate immune system include polymorphonuclear neutrophils, monocytes/macrophages, natural killer (NK) cells, and eosinophils. These cells mediate a highly effective immune response to pathogens in the absence of prior antigenic sensitization and are the primary immunologic effectors in lower vertebrates. T cells and B cells compose the cellular arm of specific acquired immunity and are found exclusively within higher organisms [2]. These specialized lymphocytes cannot mount an effective immune response unless they have been previously sensitized with specific antigen, a process that is mediated through highly specialized receptors. Despite these differences, we now recognize that the innate and specific systems of immunity are highly interdependent and complementary. It is clear that monocytes and NK cells can modulate the functions of T cells and B cells by way of the production of soluble protein hormones known as cytokines, and vice versa. Importantly, NK cells and monocytes express receptors for the Fc (FcR) or "constant" region of immunoglobulin G (IgG) and can therefore recognize and destroy target cells that have become coated with the antibody products of B cells. Although the human immune system has developed as a means of resisting microbial attack, it is the hope of immunologists and clinicians alike that these highly differentiated cell types can be redirected to the task of eliminating malignant cells from the bodies of patients who have breast cancer.

Cytokine therapy of breast cancer

Clinical studies of recombinant cytokines in the mid-1980s demonstrated that these agents can exert an antitumor effect when administered at high dose to patients who have metastatic cancer. Cytokines that have shown the greatest usefulness in this regard include interleukin-2 (IL-2) and interferon-alpha (IFN-α). IFN-γ has also been the subject of multiple clinical investigations, although it has low usefulness as an anticancer treatment. Numerous other immune system cytokines (eg, tumor necrosis factor-alpha [TNF-α], IL-1) have been tested in the setting of malignant disease, but have not gained approval for clinical use because of lack of efficacy or their toxicity profile. Administration of high-dose IL-2 by way of the intravenous (IV) route stimulates immune effectors bearing the IL-2R (primarily NK cells and T cells) and produces objective antitumor responses in about 15% of patients who have metastatic melanoma or renal cell carcinoma. A subset of these patients exhibit complete and permanent disappearance of all their disease [3]. Isolated studies have reported very low response rates in the setting of metastatic breast cancer, however [4]. Similarly, IL-2 therapy had no positive effect when administered after autologous stem cell transplantation in patients who had advanced breast cancers [5]. High-dose IFN-α is used as an adjuvant in patients who have undergone resection of high-risk melanoma lesions (nodal disease or primary tumors with Breslow thickness > 4 mm). IFN-α is also used to treat individuals who have metastatic melanoma and metastatic renal cell carcinoma and produces clinical responses in 5% to 10% of patients [6]. Unfortunately, this cytokine has limited activity in patients who have metastatic breast cancer [7]. Of note, one report by Habif and colleagues [8] did show that IFNs are useful in controlling locoregional recurrences of breast cancer, even in patients who have not responded to systemic therapy. These investigators documented the ability of locally administered IFNs to elicit systemic immunologic effects in addition to their local antitumor actions. Local administration of these agents to patients who have unresectable locoregional breast cancer thus deserves further investigation.

Vaccine therapy of breast cancer

The ultimate goal of a cancer vaccine is to promote the development of antigen-specific immune effector cells with the ability to mediate an antitumor response. Generally, this has involved efforts to generate cytolytic CD8$^+$ T cells that can recognize defined tumor antigens in the context of major histocompatibility (MHC) class I molecules on antigen-presenting cells (APC). Another name for MHC is HLA, which stands for human leukocyte antigen. These terms are sometimes interchanged when describing the cell-surface antigen-presenting system. "HLA" is used in conjunction with a letter and number (eg, HLA-A2) to designate a specific gene at a given HLA location. Approximately 40% of the white population expresses the HLA-A2 gene and is therefore able to display peptides that bind to this cell surface component of the antigen-presenting machinery.

Although cytolytic CD8$^+$ T cells seem to be an important endpoint of vaccination in the setting of cancer, the need for "help" from CD4$^+$ T cells and the potential to stimulate B-cell production of immunoglobulins with tumor specificity have recently become important topics of investigation. Strategies for the delivery of antigenic peptides to patients who have advanced breast cancer include various novel approaches, such as the administration of recombinant DNA-encoding antigenic peptide sequences, mRNA transcripts and peptides collected directly from patient tumors, recombinant replication-deficient adenoviral and retroviral vectors encoding tumor antigens, synthetic peptides modified for enhanced binding to APC HLA molecules, allogeneic tumor cell lysates, peptide-loaded dendritic cells, tumor cell–dendritic cell fusion products, and irradiated autologous tumor cell preparations [9]. It is not clear thus far that any one method is superior for the generation of antigen-specific T cells, and the induction of durable clinical responses has remained an elusive goal. It may develop that multiple methods of vaccination will be used depending on the specific disease setting or the type of antigen that is being delivered. The limited activity of breast cancer vaccines is interesting given that these vaccination strategies can frequently stimulate the formation of antigenic-specific T cells. One area of research that may enhance the success of vaccination strategies is the development of improved vaccine adjuvants [10]. Below is a summary of vaccine research for three widely-expressed breast cancer antigens, namely carcinoembryonic antigen (CEA), MUC1, and HER2/neu.

Carcinoembryonic antigen

CEA is a glycoprotein of 180,000 molecular weight found in normal fetal colon. CEA is a member of the immunoglobulin superfamily and is believed to be an intercellular recognition and adhesion molecule. In the adult, CEA is overexpressed in normal colonic mucosa. In addition, CEA is overexpressed in virtually all colorectal adenocarcinomas and is present in most adenocarcinomas of the breast, lung, pancreas, and upper gastrointestinal tract. Using CEA as a target in vaccine-based therapies has two potential problems. First, CEA is expressed in normal tissues, and as such, it is likely that T-cell tolerance exists to this protein. Second, even if one were successful in eliciting an immune response to CEA, a potential side effect could be the development of autoimmune disease. The hope is that CEA vaccine therapy will produce an immune response against CEA-bearing cancer cells by stimulating the formation of cytotoxic T lymphocytes (CTL) with the capacity to lyse CEA-expressing cancer cells, while sparing the normal CEA-expressing cells in the gut. CEA is an attractive immunologic target, and several different anti-CEA vaccination strategies have been investigated in phase I and II clinical trials [11–15]. These trials have yielded promising results, and several groups have reported complete regression of metastatic disease in response to CEA vaccines [16–21].

One promising approach to CEA vaccination is the use of poxvirus-based vaccines as pioneered by Schlom and colleagues [22]. These trials have used two novel anti-CEA vaccines: recombinant (r) Vaccinia-CEA(6D)-TRICOM and rFowlpox-CEA(6D)-TRICOM. These recombinant vaccinia and fowlpox virus vector vaccines contain genes for human CEA and three costimulatory molecules that are capable of providing a critical second activating signal to antigen-specific T cells: B7.1, intercellular adhesion molecule-1 (ICAM-1), and leukocyte function-associated antigen-3 (LFA-3). The CEA gene used in these vectors has a single amino acid substitution (aspartic acid at position 6, instead of asparagine) in one nine–amino acid, HLA-A2–restricted, immunodominant epitope (designated CAP1-6D), which has been shown to induce CTL in vitro more efficiently than the native epitope. The viral vectors infect professional APCs, which in turn present peptides derived from the CEA molecule (including the CAP1-6D epitope) in the context of HLA class I and II to CD8$^+$ and CD4$^+$ T cells, respectively. Preclinical experiments and data from phase I clinical trials suggest that priming with the vaccinia vector (the parental form of which

is used as the smallpox vaccine) and boosting with the fowlpox vector significantly enhances the formation of a CEA-specific T-cell response. The vigor-
ous host response to the vaccinia virus stimulates an intense inflammatory
reaction characterized by cytokine production and T-cell proliferation that
further amplifies the immune response to the transgene antigen (in this
case, CEA). Because vaccinia actively replicates in the host, it can present
high levels of transgene antigen to the host immune system over a period of
approximately 1 week, substantially increasing the potential for immune stimulation. Granulocyte-macrophage colony-stimulating factor (GM-CSF) is
co-administered at the vaccination site because it promotes the activation,
maturation, and migration of APCs, such as dendritic cells [10].

Marshall and colleagues [23] have reported their results with the TRI-
COM vectors in patients who have advanced CEA-expressing cancers.
They treated 58 patients who had the rVaccinia-CEA(6D)-TRICOM and
the rFowlpox-CEA(6D)-TRICOM, with or without GM-CSF. The vaccine
was administered every 28 days for six doses and then once every 3 months.
No significant toxicity was observed in this phase I study. Twenty-three patients (40%) had stable disease for at least 4 months and 14 of these patients
exhibited prolonged stable disease (>6 months). Serum CEA levels decreased or remained stable in 11 patients, and 1 patient achieved a pathologic
complete response. Ten of the 13 HLA-A2–positive patients in the different
cohorts mounted CEA-specific T-cell responses that were at least twofold
greater following the vaccinations compared with baseline. The CEA-TRI-
COM vaccines can thus be safely administered in this population and can
generate a significant CEA-specific immune response. In addition, the vaccine can be of clinical benefit in some patients who have advanced cancer.

Further research with vaccinia-based vaccines will involve the use of additional vaccine adjuvants that could enhance the formation of CEA-specific
CTL and sensitize tumors to the actions of antitumor immune effectors. Our
group is currently conducting an NCI-sponsored phase I clinical trial in patients who have advanced CEA-expressing malignancies in which the rVac-
cinia-CEA(6D)-TRICOM and rFowlpox-CEA(6D)-TRICOM vectors are
given with GM-CSF and IFN-α. IFN-α enhances the expression of CEA
on cancer cells and also works in combination with GM-CSF to enhance
the formation and antigen-presenting capacity of dendritic cells [24,25]. It
is hoped that the addition of IFN-α will lead to improved antitumor
responses in vaccinated patients.

MUC1

MUC1 is a membrane-associated glycoprotein that is expressed by ductal
epithelia in the breast, lung, pancreas, and gastrointestinal tract. MUC1 is
involved in the protection of mucous membranes and has the ability to modulate the activity of the immune system. Greater than 70% of cancers overexpress aberrantly glycosylated MUC1, which is immunogenic enough to

stimulate antitumor immunity [26]. Early breast cancer patients who have a natural humoral response to MUC1 have a higher probability of freedom from distant failure and better disease-specific survival. MUC1 antibodies may control hematogenous tumor dissemination and outgrowth by aiding the destruction of circulating or seeded MUC1-expressing tumor cells [27]. In a phase I clinical trial, a 105–amino acid synthetic MUC1 peptide (containing five repeated immunodominant epitopes) was administered to 63 patients who had advanced adenocarcinomas, 9 of whom had breast cancer [28]. The vaccine was administered thrice weekly at 3-week intervals in combination with bacillus Calmette-Guerin (BCG, a bacterial vaccine adjuvant). The vaccine was well tolerated but no clinical responses were observed. Tumor biopsies showed tumor infiltration by T cells in 37 of 55 patients; however, only a minority of patients exhibited an increase in mucin-specific CTL in response to vaccination. In a subsequent trial, 16 patients who had metastatic breast carcinoma were vaccinated with a 16–amino acid MUC1 peptide conjugated to keyhole limpet hemocyanin protein in combination with DETOX adjuvant (which contains monophosphoryl lipid A and purified mycobacterial cell-wall skeleton) [29]. Only 3 patients developed an anti-MUC1 antibody response. MHC class I–restricted lysis of MUC1-expressing tumor cell lines by patient peripheral blood lymphocytes was observed in 7 of the 11 patients who were tested. Investigators have linked oxidized mannan to the MUC1 molecule to target the mannose receptor on macrophages and thereby facilitate the uptake and presentation of the MUC1 antigen. Apostolopoulos and colleagues [30] conducted a study in which 31 patients who had stage II breast cancer and no evidence of disease were randomized to subcutaneous (SC) injections of oxidized mannan-MUC1 or placebo. At 5.5 years of follow-up, there were no recurrences in the MUC1 vaccine arm, whereas 27% of patients in the placebo arm had recurrent disease ($P = .0292$). Nine of 13 patients receiving oxidized mannan-MUC1 had measurable antibodies to MUC1 and 4 of 10 had MUC-1–specific T-cell responses. In contrast, none of the placebo-treated patients exhibited an immune response to MUC1. These results suggest that MUC1 immunotherapy is beneficial in early breast cancer. Other groups, such as the one led by Dr. Olivera Finn, are currently examining the efficacy of MUC1 vaccines that use patient dendritic cells [31].

HER2/neu

The HER2/neu proto-oncogene is a cell surface glycoprotein that possesses intracellular protein tyrosine kinase activity and partners with other members of the HER family, namely HER1, HER3, and HER4. HER2 is overexpressed in about 25% of human breast cancers and represents a potential target for cancer vaccine therapy. Interestingly, patients who have HER2 overexpressing cancers exhibit increased frequencies of peripheral blood T cells recognizing HER2/neu peptides [32]. Multiple vaccination strategies have been used in the effort to develop an effective HER2/neu cancer vaccine. These include the use of immunogenic peptides, dendritic cells pulsed with HER-2/neu HLA class I and II peptides, and an HLA-A2–positive, HER2/neu-positive allogeneic breast cancer cell line genetically modified to express the costimulatory molecule CD80 (B7-1) [33–37]. Additional work will be required to determine the best method for achieving this goal, however. Led by Dr. Pravin Kaumaya, our group has developed a synthetic peptide immunogen targeting two sites in the extracellular domain of the HER2/neu oncoprotein. Our group has also examined the effectiveness of "promiscuous" nonhuman, T helper cell epitopes as a means of augmenting vaccine immunogenicity and circumventing the problem of MHC class I restriction. The end result is a novel chimeric peptide vaccine consisting of amino acids 628–647 and 316–339 of the HER2 protein (which encode two epitopes stimulatory to B cells) linked to a T-helper epitope derived from the measles virus (sequence 288–302; designated MVF). We have demonstrated that Abs elicited by the MVF-HER2 vaccine specifically bind to the HER2 protein on tumor cells and are able to reduce tumor cell proliferation both in vitro and in murine tumor models. Preclinical studies have also confirmed the ability of this construct to prevent the outgrowth of mammary tumors in HER2/neu transgenic mice [38]. Based on these studies, an NCI-sponsored phase I trial was initiated that used this multi-epitope HER2 peptide vaccine in patients who had HER2-overexpressing metastatic cancers. Twenty-seven patients have been accrued to this trial and 2 patients have experienced complete disappearance of their tumors. Analysis of serum anti-HER2 Ab titers reveal that the vaccine's effects are especially potent and long lasting. A phase II trial of this vaccine is in the planning stages.

Therapeutic monoclonal antibodies in the treatment of breast cancer

HER2/neu oncogene

About 25% of breast cancers overexpress the HER2/neu proto-oncogene. This gene encodes a cell surface glycoprotein that possesses intracellular protein tyrosine kinase activity and exhibits extensive homology to the human epidermal growth factor receptor (EGFR or HER1) [39,40]. Amplification of the HER2/neu gene has been found in multiple human malignancies, including carcinoma of the breast, ovary, uterus, stomach, and lung [41]. In breast cancer, HER2 overexpression is associated with a worse histologic grade, decreased overall survival, and altered sensitivity to chemotherapeutic regimens [41–43]. Lack of steroid receptors and the incidence of lymph node metastasis are also believed to correlate with HER2 positivity [44]. These observations suggest a correlation between HER2 content and the proliferative capacity and overall aggressiveness of a tumor. Indeed, transgenic mice bearing an activated form of the HER2 gene develop mammary adenocarcinomas in a dose-dependent manner and go on to develop metastatic disease [45–47]. Treatments that target the HER2 surface antigen thus might lead to an improved outcome in patients who have HER2-expressing breast cancer.

Development of an anti-HER2/neu monoclonal antibody

Aberrant expression of an immunogenic protein on the tumor cell surface represents an obvious target for Ab-mediated immunotherapy. Binding of a monoclonal antibody (mAb) to the extracellular domain of the HER2 protein might alter tumor cell growth by one of several different mechanisms. These include acceleration of receptor endocytosis (ie, down-regulation of HER2 expression), altered receptor phosphorylation or signaling, blockade of ligand-induced receptor activation, altered interaction of HER2 with other members of the EGFR family, complement fixation, or recruitment of immunologic effector cells with the capacity to recognize bound immunoglobulins and mediate antibody-dependent cellular cytotoxicity (ADCC) and cytokine production [43]. Carter and colleagues [48] generated a murine mAb against the extracellular domain of the HER2 receptor (mu4D5) and showed that it inhibited the proliferation of HER2-positive breast cancer cell lines in vitro. The humanized version of this Ab (recombinant anti-human HER2/neu mAb or trastuzumab) exhibited improved binding affinity to the extracellular domain of HER2 and potently inhibited the growth of HER2-overexpressing cell lines and xenografts. In addition, peripheral blood mononuclear cells (PBMCs) were able to efficiently conduct ADCC against HER2-positive tumor cells in the presence of this recombinant Ab [49–51].

Single-agent trastuzumab therapy

Promising results have been obtained in clinical trials in which trastuzumab was administered as a single agent to patients who had HER2-overexpressing breast cancers [52]. In the first phase II trial of trastuzumab, 46 patients who had HER2-overexpressing metastatic breast cancer received a loading dose of 250 mg followed by a maintenance dose of 100 mg/wk. Of the 43 evaluable patients, 12% had a complete or partial response, 37% had a minor response or stable disease, and the remaining patients (51%) had progressive disease [53]. These results were confirmed in a large multinational phase II trial that enrolled 222 women who had metastatic breast cancer and a history of having failed one or two chemotherapeutic regimens. Patients received a loading dose of 4 mg/kg trastuzumab followed by administration of 2 mg/kg on weekly basis. Using this regimen, an overall response rate of 15% was observed [54]. A role for trastuzumab as a first-line therapy in metastatic beast cancer is suggested by the results of a study conducted by Vogel and colleagues [55]. A total of 113 patients who had HER2 2+ or 3+ metastatic breast cancer and no history of prior chemotherapy for stage IV disease were randomized to receive trastuzumab at a weekly maintenance dose of 4 mg/kg or 8 mg/kg. An overall response rate of 23%

was noted (6 complete and 20 partial), all in women who had HER2 3+ tumors. These results emphasize the effectiveness of trastuzumab therapy and its apparent dependency on high-level expression of the HER2 antigen.

Administration of cytotoxic agents with trastuzumab

Early on, investigators explored the possible use of trastuzumab in combination with cytotoxic agents. In vitro experiments revealed that pretreatment of HER2-overexpressing breast cancer cells with anti-HER2 Abs led to a decreased ability to repair DNA damage induced by the cytotoxic agent cisplatin [56]. Experiments in athymic mice bearing HER2-overexpressing human breast cancer xenografts demonstrated that the combination of paclitaxel and mAb 4D5 produced a higher rate of tumor growth inhibition (93%) than either agent alone (35% growth inhibition for 4D5 or paclitaxel alone) and was able to mediate the complete regression of well-established xenografts. Importantly, paclitaxel was superior to doxorubicin in its ability to potentiate the actions of trastuzumab [57]. Proof that chemotherapy could enhance the antitumor actions of trastuzumab came in a randomized, multinational phase III trial of chemotherapy with or without trastuzumab as first-line therapy for metastatic breast cancer [58]. Patients were randomized to chemotherapy with or without trastuzumab (doxorubicin plus cyclophosphamide, or paclitaxel alone in case of prior adjuvant anthracyclines). The addition of trastuzumab to chemotherapy was associated with a longer time to disease progression (7.4 versus 4.6 months), higher response rate (50% versus 32%), longer median survival (25.1 versus 20.3 months) and a 20% reduction in the risk for death (all with $P \le .01$). Although the overall rate of adverse events was not increased by the addition of trastuzumab to these chemotherapeutic regimens, a syndrome of myocardial dysfunction was reported more commonly in patients receiving chemotherapy with trastuzumab. This finding was more pronounced for doxorubicin (28% incidence with trastuzumab, 7% without) than for paclitaxel (11% with trastuzumab, 1% without) [59].

Trastuzumab and the immune system

Clynes and colleagues [60] have reported that the antitumor effects of trastuzumab in a murine model of breast cancer required the expression of functional FcR by host immune effectors. This report suggested that FcR-dependent mechanisms contribute substantially to the actions of cytotoxic Abs directed against tumor antigens and implies that coadministration of immunomodulatory cytokines might enhance their effects. Effector cells that bear receptors for the Fc region of IgG include NK cells (FcγRIIIa or CD16), resting and activated granulocytes (FcγRII or CD32), and monocytes/macrophages (FcγRI or CD64) [61,62]. Although most immune cells coexpress activating and inhibitory FcR, NK cells are unique in that they constitutively express only an activating low-affinity FcR (FcγRIIIa) [60]. NK cells are an important source of IFN-γ and early secretion of this cytokine is critical for the optimization and coordination of the innate and specific immune responses [63]. NK cells have also been shown to be an important source of TNF-α, GM-CSF, and chemokines, such as MIP-1α/β, RANTES, and MCP-1 [64,65]. These factors are critical to the recruitment and activation of macrophages and T cells to sites of inflammation. NK cells are unique in their constitutive expression of receptors for IL-12 and IL-2 and many other cytokine receptor complexes (eg, IL-10, IL-15, IL-18). The binding of specific ligand to these receptors results in enhanced cytotoxic activity and ADCC, and increased production of immunomodulatory cytokines [64–67].

Preclinical data supporting the use of IL-12 with trastuzumab

We theorized that the immune response of FcR-bearing cells to trastuzumab-coated tumor cells might be significantly enhanced in the presence of immunomodulatory agents, such as NK cell-stimulatory agents (eg, CpG oligodeoxynucleotides [CpG ODN] see later discussion) or cytokines (eg, IL-12 and IL-2). Our initial preclinical studies involved the use of IL-12 and trastuzumab; these findings are now presented for the reader's benefit. Using a novel in vitro coculture system, in which trastuzumab-coated human breast cancer cells are cultured with purified human NK cells in the presence of IL-12, we showed that trastuzumab and IL-12 synergize to induce potent cytokine secretion [50]. The combination of IL-12 with trastuzumab-coated tumor stimulated NK cells to secrete 10-fold greater amounts of IFN-γ protein (>20 ng/mL at 48 hours) as compared with stimulation with either agent alone, a result that could not be duplicated by costimulation with IL-2, IL-10, IL-15, or IL-18. Similar results were seen with the secretion of other immunostimulatory factors, such as TNF-α, GM-CSF, and MIP-1α. Analysis by real-time reverse transcriptase polymerase chain reaction revealed an average 35-fold increase in cytokine transcript following NK cell costimulation. Inhibition of FcγRIII-mediated signaling within NK cells using a Syk/ZAP-70 inhibitor (piceatannol) or use of STAT4-deficient (ie, IL-12–resistant) NK cells resulted in abrogation of the synergistic effect on cytokine secretion, suggesting that cytokine production was critically dependent on two distinct signals emanating from the FcγRIIIa and the IL-12R. Also, coadministration of a murine anti-human HER2 mAb and IL-12 to immunocompetent mice bearing a murine adenocarcinoma transfected with the human HER2/neu gene resulted in synergistic antitumor activity that was associated with high systemic levels of IFN-γ (600 pg/mL at 24 hours). In contrast, administration of single-agent IL-12 or trastuzumab had minimal effects on tumor growth and did not induce the secretion of IFN-γ. The antitumor effects of IL-12 were completely abrogated by depletion of NK cells or Ab neutralization of IFN-γ.

Coadministration of trastuzumab and IL-12 can thus activate a potent cytokine secretion program within NK cells that has antitumor activity in vivo [50].

Phase I trial of IL-12 and trastuzumab (NCI trial T99-0032)

Based on these preclinical studies, we hypothesized that IL-12 would potentiate the antitumor actions of an anti-HER2 mAb (trastuzumab) in patients who had HER2-overexpressing malignancies. We conducted a phase I trial to determine the safety and optimal biologic dose of IL-12 when given in combination with trastuzumab [68]. Patients who had metastatic HER2-positive malignancies received trastuzumab on day 1 of each weekly cycle. Beginning in week 3, patients also received IV injections of IL-12 on days 2 and 5. The IL-12 component was dose-escalated within cohorts of 3 patients (30, 100, 300, or 500 ng/kg). Correlative assays were conducted using serum samples and peripheral blood cells obtained during the course of therapy. Fifteen patients were treated, including 12 who had HER2 2+ or 3+ breast cancer. The regimen was well tolerated with IL-12–induced grade 1 nausea and grade 2 fatigue predominating. Evaluation of dose-limiting toxicity and biologic endpoints suggested that the 300 ng/kg dose was both the maximally tolerated dose and the optimal biologic dose of IL-12 for use in combination with trastuzumab. Two patients who had HER2 3+ breast cancer within the 500 ng/kg dose level experienced grade 1 asymptomatic decreases in left ventricular ejection fraction of 12% and 19% after 3 and 10 months of therapy, respectively. There was one complete response in a patient who had HER2 3+ breast cancer metastatic to the axillary, mediastinal, and supraclavicular nodes, and 2 patients had stabilization of bone disease lasting 10 months and greater than 12 months, respectively. Correlative assays showed sustained production of IFN-γ by NK cells only in those patients exhibiting a favorable outcome (response or stabilization of disease) in response to the regimen. Elevated serum levels of MIP-1α, TNF-α, and the anti-angiogenic factors IP-10 and MIG (monokine induced by gamma) were also observed in these patients. The ability of patient peripheral blood cells to conduct ADCC against tumor targets in vitro did not correlate with clinical response or dose of IL-12. Further analyses revealed that progression-free survival following treatment with trastuzumab and IL-12 was associated with sustained production of IFN-γ and other cytokines by activated NK cells. The existence of these early indicators of clinical outcome, combined with a lack of severe toxicity, suggested that immunologically active compounds might enhance the patient immune response to therapeutic anti–breast cancer Abs [68].

Immune stimulatory effects of paclitaxel

Paclitaxel belongs to the taxane class of cytotoxic agents that mediates its effects by way of the ability to bind to beta-tubulin and stabilize the microtubule complex during mitosis and thereby inhibit cellular division. Less appreciated is that taxanes can exert immunostimulatory effects that contribute to its antineoplastic actions [69]. In vitro treatment of PBMCs with concentrations of paclitaxel that would be encountered during the course of chemotherapy does not inhibit their cytolytic activity against the NK-sensitive target K562 [70]. In fact, paclitaxel activates human macrophages in vitro and stimulates them to release cytotoxic and proinflammatory mediators, such as nitric oxide (NO), TNF-α, and IL-1 [71–73]. Pertinent to the present discussion is the observation in a murine model that paclitaxel-induced NO synthesis by IFN-γ–primed macrophages is the result of signal transduction by way of the protein kinase C (PKC) pathway [74]. Macrophage activation in response to paclitaxel might well contribute to the activity of trastuzumab regimens that contain paclitaxel [69]. These stimulatory effects may explain how paclitaxel is able to reverse tumor-induced immune suppression [75]. Interestingly, IL-12 can overcome paclitaxel-mediated suppression of T-cell proliferation [76], and this may account for the synergistic actions of IL-12 and paclitaxel in a murine model of malignant melanoma [77]. Finally, we recently reported that the administration of taxanes-based adjuvant chemotherapy to women surgically treated for regional breast cancer was associated with higher T-cell blastogenesis and NK cell lytic activity at long-term follow-up (1 year) relative to a comparison group that did not receive taxanes [78]. There is evidence to suggest that paclitaxel might be the most appropriate cytotoxic agent to administer in combination with trastuzumab.

Phase I trial of IL-12 plus trastuzumab/paclitaxel (NCI trial no. 84)

Our previous phase I trial of trastuzumab in combination with IL-12 in patients who had HER2-positive cancers showed that IFN-γ production by NK cells occurred only in patients who had a favorable response to therapy. Given that the combination of paclitaxel and trastuzumab in HER2-overexpressing breast cancers has resulted in survival benefit, we conducted a phase I clinical trial with IL-12 in combination with paclitaxel plus trastuzumab in patients who had metastatic HER2-positive cancers (NCI no. 84) [79]. Eligible patients received paclitaxel intravenously (175 mg/m^2) on day 1 every 3 weeks. Trastuzumab was given on day 1 of the weekly cycle (4 mg/kg initially and 2 mg/kg thereafter) in combination with IL-12 given intravenously on days 2 and 5 starting in week 4. The IL-2 was dose-escalated (100 and then 300 ng/kg) in cohorts of 3 patients. This trial accrued 21 patients with metastatic 2+ and 3+ HER2-positive tumors (including 7 who had breast cancer). The average age of the patients was 58 years. Sixteen of 21 patients had received at least one prior regimen of systemic chemotherapy. The IL-12 component was dose-escalated in cohorts of 3 patients, but because of dose-limiting grade 3 fatigue at the 300 ng/kg dose level, it was reduced to 200 ng/kg SC. The most common adverse event was grade 1 fevers and chills. One patient (breast cancer) had a complete response (CR),

4 patients (2 who had breast cancer, 2 who had esophageal cancer) had a partial responses (PR), and 5 patients had stable disease (SD). Ten patients (48%) had a clinical benefit (CR + PR + SD). Two patients were non-evaluable for response because of dose-limiting fatigue. All but one response occurred in patients who had HER2 3+ disease. Two SD patients (1 breast, 1 gastric) completed 1 year of therapy and went on to receive trastuzumab alone. Correlative studies showed significantly increased circulating levels of IFN-γ in patients who had clinical benefit. No Patient who had progressive disease had activation of ERK or measurable levels of IFN-γ. We concluded that IL-12 in combination with trastuzumab and paclitaxel is active in HER2-overexpressing cancers with acceptable toxicity. Secretion of IFN-γ seemed to correlate with clinical benefit. Of note, preclinical studies from our group indicate that other NK-activating cytokines, such as IL-21, can also enhance the antitumor actions of therapeutic mAbs; therefore, further studies of immune stimulatory cytokines in combination with trastuzumab and other mAbs are now in the planning stages [80].

CpG-containing oligodeoxynucleotides act through toll-like receptor 9 to enhance the natural killer cell response to antibody-coated tumor targets

Microbial pathogens express or shed factors that are recognized by the innate immune system, mainly by way of a class of receptors known as the toll-like receptors (TLR). Bacterial DNA can stimulate human innate immune cells because it contains a high frequency of unmethylated CpG motifs. In the hope of stimulating innate immune responses for the treatment of various diseases, investigators have developed synthetic oligodeoxynucleotides (ODN) that contain a high frequency of CpG dinucleotides. These CpG ODN, like intact bacterial DNA, act as agonists for TLR9, one of the key receptors for bacterial components. We have examined the ability of CpG ODN to enhance NK cell cytokine secretion in response to stimulation of the FcR by immobilized IgG or Ab-coated human breast cancer cells [81]. Purified NK cells cultured in the presence of immobilized IgG and CpG ODN were found to secrete large amounts of IFN-γ (>2000 pg/mL), whereas cells stimulated with either agent alone, or with IgG and an irrelevant control ODN, produced negligible amounts (<200 pg/mL, $P<.05$). A time-course study revealed that NK cell production of IFN-γ began within 12 hours of exposure to CpG ODN and immobilized IgG, and peaked near 72 hours. Using an in vitro system in which HER2/neu-positive human breast cancer cells were coated with a humanized anti-HER2/neu mAb (trastuzumab) and cocultured with purified human NK cells in the presence of CpG ODN, we showed that trastuzumab and CpG ODN synergize to induce potent cytokine secretion. The combination of CpG ODN with trastuzumab-coated tumor stimulated NK cells to secrete 5- to 10-fold greater amounts of IFN-γ protein as compared with stimulation with either agent alone. Similar results were observed for the secretion of an array of immune modulatory chemokines, including IL-8, macrophage-derived chemokine (MDC), and MIP-1alpha. When NK cells, T cells, B cells, and monocytes were isolated and separately cultured on IgG in the presence of CpG ODN, only NK cells responded to the costimulation with the production of IFN-γ. Furthermore, coculture of NK cells with B cells or monocytes at various ratios did not enhance NK cell production of IFN-γ, demonstrating that the effect of CpG ODN on NK cells is direct and not enhanced by APCs or their cytokine products. Interestingly, treatment of PBMC with CpG ODN significantly enhanced their lytic activity against NK cell–sensitive tumor targets (eg, K562) and Ab-coated HER2-positive breast cancer cells. As cells of the innate immune system are known to recognize and respond to CpG motifs by way of TLR9, we analyzed the expression of TLR9 on resting human NK cells by flow cytometry. Between 10% and 70% of NK cells were found to basally express TLR9 on all donors tested (mean, 35%; n = 12). Expression of TLR9 protein by NK cells was confirmed by immunoblot analysis. Furthermore, coadministration of trastuzumab-coated, HER2-positive tumor cells and CpG ODN to immune competent mice (n = 8) resulted in enhanced systemic levels of IFN-γ (215 pg/mL at 6 hours), whereas mice receiving CpG ODN or trastuzumab-coated tumor alone exhibited minimal production of this cytokine (70 pg/mL and 0 pg/mL at 6 hours, respectively). These findings suggest a potential mechanism by which concurrent administration of CpG ODN with antitumor antibodies may mediate antitumor effects during the treatment of malignancy [81].

Mechanisms by which CpG oligodeoxynucleotides could enhance the activity of trastuzumab/paclitaxel

Based on our own in vitro observations and the strong clinical and preclinical data supporting a role for trastuzumab/paclitaxel combinations in the treatment of breast cancer, we have developed a clinical trial of CpG ODN plus trastuzumab/paclitaxel in patients bearing HER2-overexpressing malignancies, including breast adenocarcinomas. We hypothesize that binding of trastuzumab to tumor cells in the presence of CpG will provide a potent costimulus to NK cells and other immune effectors that bear FcR, much as is observed for the combination of IL-12 and trastuzumab. Of prime importance is that CpG ODN can enhance NK cell cytotoxicity against Ab-coated tumor cells and NK cell cytokine production. The usefulness of an enhanced cytotoxic profile against tumor targets is obvious. The observed pattern of NK cell cytokine secretion would likely have effects on tumor cell proliferation and antigen presentation (IFN-γ) [82], T-cell activation and proliferation (MIP-1α) [83,84], and T-cell chemotaxis (MIP-1α, IL-8, MDC) [85]. Secretion of IFN-γ is of particular interest. IFN-γ is the prototypic macrophage-activating factor and markedly stimulates macrophage effector functions. Macrophage phagocytosis is greatly enhanced in the presence of IFN-γ because of up-regulation of FcRγI and other determinants of target binding [86]. Likewise, cytocidal activity of the macrophage compartment is augmented in response to IFN-γ by way of increased elaboration of reactive oxygen species and nitric oxide (a result of increased levels of key enzymes such as nitric oxide synthase) [87,88]. IFN-γ also inhibits tumor growth and promotes recognition of tumor cells by immunologic effectors. The mechanism whereby IFN-γ inhibits cellular proliferation is poorly understood; however, it is known that IFN-γ–induced activation of the JAK-STAT signaling pathway directly stimulates transcription of p21$^{\mathrm{WAF1/CIP1}}$, a potent inhibitor of cell cycle progression that is able to inactivate cyclin-dependent kinases [89]. Further, recent studies reveal that IFN-γ–mediated activation of the STAT signaling pathway can induce apoptosis in breast cancer cell lines through the induction of caspase 1 gene expression [90]. IFN-γ also up-regulates tumor expression of MHC class I molecules and multiple proteins involved in antigen presentation [63]. A randomized clinical trial of chemotherapy with or without TLR9 agonist for patients who have advanced lung cancer has recently finished accrual and additional studies are underway with other TLR agonists. Future studies of TLR9 agonists in combination with anti–breast cancer mAbs represent an exciting and innovative approach to the immunotherapy of breast cancer.

Summary

Agents used in the immunotherapy of breast cancer include exogenously administered cytokines; cancer vaccines targeting CEA, MUC1, and HER2/neu; and antitumor mAbs, such as trastuzumab, that target oncogenic cell surface proteins. Future advances in this field will likely involve the use of these agents in combination with other immunostimulatory agents with or without cytotoxic chemotherapy.

References

[1] Jatoi I, Chen BE, Anderson WF, et al. Breast cancer mortality trends in the United States according to estrogen receptor status and age at diagnosis. J Clin Oncol 2007;25(13): 1683–90.

[2] Bhardwaj N. Harnessing the immune system to treat cancer. J Clin Invest 2007;117(5): 1130–6.

[3] Eklund JW, Kuzel TM. A review of recent findings involving interleukin-2-based cancer therapy. Curr Opin Oncol 2004;16(6):542–6.

[4] Allison MA, Jones SE, McGuffey P. Phase II trial of outpatient interleukin-2 in malignant lymphoma, chronic lymphocytic leukemia, and selected solid tumors. J Clin Oncol 1989;7(1): 75–80.

[5] Gravis G, Viens P, Vey N, et al. Pilot study of immunotherapy with interleukin-2 after autologous stem cell transplantation in advanced breast cancers. Anticancer Res 2000; 20(5C):3987–91.

[6] Lens MB, Dawes M. Interferon alpha therapy for malignant melanoma: a systematic review of randomized controlled trials. J Clin Oncol 2002;20:1818–25.

[7] Padmanabhan N, Balkwill FR, Bodmer JG, et al. Recombinant DNA human interferon alpha 2 in advanced breast cancer: a phase 2 trial. Br J Cancer 1985;51(1):55–60.

[8] Habif DV, Ozzello L, De Rosa CM, et al. Regression of skin recurrences of breast carcinomas treated with intralesional injections of natural interferons alpha and gamma. Cancer Invest 1995;13(2):165–72.

[9] Acres B, Limacher JM, Bonnefoy J. Discovery and development of therapeutic cancer vaccines. Curr Opin Drug Discov Devel 2007;10(2):185–92.

[10] Carson WE. Getting melanoma cells to stimulate with frequency. J Clin Oncol 2005;23(35): 8929–31.

[11] Morse MA, Deng Y, Coleman D, et al. A phase I study of active immunotherapy with carcinoembryonic antigen peptide (CAP-1)-pulsed, autologous human cultured dendritic cells in patients with metastatic malignancies expressing carcinoembryonic antigen. Clin Cancer Res 1999;5(6):1331–8.

[12] Fong L, Hou Y, Rivas A, et al. Altered peptide ligand vaccination with Flt3 ligand expanded dendritic cells for tumor immunotherapy. Proc Natl Acad Sci U S A 2001; 98(15):8809–14.

[13] Samanci A, Yi Q, Fagerberg J, et al. Pharmacological administration of granulocyte/macrophage-colony-stimulating factor is of significant importance for the induction of a strong humoral and cellular response in patients immunized with recombinant carcinoembryonic antigen. Cancer Immunol Immunother 1998;47(3):131–42.

[14] Foon KA, John WJ, Chakraborty M, et al. Clinical and immune responses in advanced colorectal cancer patients treated with anti-idiotype monoclonal antibody vaccine that mimics the carcinoembryonic antigen. Clin Cancer Res 1997;3(8):1267–76.

[15] Foon KA, John WJ, Chakraborty M, et al. Clinical and immune responses in resected colon cancer patients treated with anti-idiotype monoclonal antibody vaccine that mimics the carcinoembryonic antigen. J Clin Oncol 1999;17(9):2889–95.

[16] Kantor J, Irvine K, Abrams S, et al. Immunogenicity and safety of a recombinant vaccinia virus vaccine expressing the carcinoembryonic antigen gene in a nonhuman primate. Cancer Res 1992;52(24):6917–25.

[17] Tsang KY, Zaremba S, Nieroda CA, et al. Generation of human cytotoxic T cells specific for human carcinoembryonic antigen epitopes from cancer patients immunized with recombinant vaccinia-CEA vaccine. J Natl Cancer Inst 1995;87(13):982–90.

[18] McAneny D, Ryan CA, Beazley RM, et al. Results of phase I trial of a recombinant vaccinia virus that expresses carcinoembryonic antigen in patients with advanced colorectal cancer. Ann Surg Oncol 1996;3(5):495–500.

[19] Tsang KY, Zhu M, Nieroda CA, et al. Phenotypic stability of a cytotoxic T-cell line directed against an immunodominant epitope of human carcinoembryonic antigen. Clin Cancer Res 1997;3(12 Pt 1):2439–49.

[20] Marshall JL, Hawkins MJ, Tsang KY, et al. Phase I study in cancer patients of a replication-defective avipox recombinant vaccine that expresses human carcinoembryonic antigen. J Clin Oncol 1999;17(1):332–7.

[21] Marshall JL, Hoyer RJ, Toomey MA, et al. Phase I study in advanced cancer patients of a diversified prime-and-boost vaccination protocol using recombinant vaccinia virus and recombinant nonreplicating avipox virus to elicit anti-carcinoembryonic antigen immune responses. J Clin Oncol 2000;18(23):3964–73.

[22] Garnett CT, Greiner JW, Tsang KY, et al. TRICOM vector based cancer vaccines. Curr Pharm Des 2006;12(3):351–61.

[23] Marshall JL, Gulley JL, Arlen PM, et al. Phase I study of sequential vaccinations with fowl-pox-CEA(6D)-TRICOM alone and sequentially with vaccinia-CEA(6D)-TRICOM, with and without granulocyte-macrophage colony-stimulating factor, in patients with carcinoembryonic antigen-expressing carcinomas. J Clin Oncol 2005;23(4):720–31.

[24] Roselli M, Guadagni F, Buonomo O, et al. Systemic administration of recombinant interferon alfa in carcinoma patients upreguates the expression of the carcinoma-associated antigens tumor-associated glycoprotein-72 and carcinoembryonic antigen. J Clin Oncol 1996; 14(7):2031–42.

[25] Santini SM, Lapenta C, Logozzi M, et al. Type I interferon as a powerful adjuvant for monocyte-derived dendritic cell development and activity in vitro and in Hu-PBL-SCID mice. J Exp Med 2000;191(10):1777–88.

[26] Yang E, Hu XF, Xing PX. Advances of MUC1 as a target for breast cancer immunotherapy. Histol Histopathol 2007;22(8):905–22.

[27] von Mensdorff-Pouilly S, Verstraeten AA, Kenemans P, et al. Survival in early breast cancer patients is favorably influenced by a natural humoral immune response to polymorphic epithelial mucin. J Clin Oncol 2000;18(3):574–83.

[28] Goydos JS, Elder E, Whiteside TL, et al. A phase I trial of a synthetic mucin peptide vaccine. Induction of specific immune reactivity in patients with adenocarcinoma. J Surg Res 1996; 63(1):298–304.

[29] Reddish M, MacLean GD, Koganty RR, et al. Anti-MUC1 class I restricted CTLs in metastatic breast cancer patients immunized with a synthetic MUC1 peptide. Int J Cancer 1998; 76(6):817–23.

[30] Apostolopoulos V, Pietersz GA, Tsibanis A, et al. Pilot phase III immunotherapy study in early-stage breast cancer patients using oxidized mannan-MUC1. Breast Cancer Res 2006; 8(3):R27.

[31] Soares MM, Mehta V, Finn OJ. Three different vaccines based on the 140-amino acid MUC1 peptide with seven tandemly repeated tumor-specific epitopes elicit distinct immune effector mechanisms in wild-type versus MUC1-transgenic mice with different potential for tumor rejection. J Immunol 2001;166(11):6555–63.

[32] Kaumaya P. HER-2/neu cancer vaccines: present status and future prospects. International Journal of Peptide Research & Therapeutics 2006;12(1):65–77.

[33] Czerniecki BJ, Koski GK, Koldovsky U, et al. Targeting HER-2/neu in early breast cancer development using dendritic cells with staged interleukin-12 burst secretion. Cancer Res 2007;67(4):1842–52.

[34] Peoples GE, Gurney JM, Hueman MT, et al. Clinical trial results of a HER2/neu (E75) vaccine to prevent recurrence in high-risk breast cancer patients. J Clin Oncol 2005;23(30): 7536–45 [Sep 12, 2005 Epub].

[35] Disis ML, Schiffman K, Guthrie K, et al. Effect of dose on immune response in patients vaccinated with an her-2/neu intracellular domain protein–based vaccine. J Clin Oncol 2004; 22(10):1916–25.

[36] Disis ML, Goodell V, Schiffman K, et al. Humoral epitope-spreading following immunization with a HER-2/neu peptide based vaccine in cancer patients. J Clin Immunol 2004;24(5): 571–8.

[37] Dols A, Smith JW 2nd, Meijer SL, et al. Vaccination of women with metastatic breast cancer, using a costimulatory gene (CD80)-modified, HLA-A2-matched, allogeneic, breast cancer cell line: clinical and immunological results. Hum Gene Ther 2003;14(11):1117–23.

[38] Dakappagari NK, Pyles J, Parihar R, et al. A chimeric multi-human epidermal growth factor receptor-2 B cell epitope peptide vaccine mediates superior antitumor responses. J Immunol 2003;170(8):4242–53.

[39] Ross JS, Fletcher JA. The HER-2/neu oncogene in breast cancer: prognostic factor, predictive factor, and target for therapy. Stem Cells 1998;16(6):413–28.

[40] Slamon DJ, Godolphin W, Jones LA, et al. Studies of the HER-2/neu proto-oncogene in human breast and ovarian cancer. Science 1989;244(4905):707–12.

[41] Revillion F, Bonneterre J, Peyrat JP. ERB-B2 oncogene in human breast cancer and its clinical significance. Eur J Cancer 1998;34(6):791–808.

[42] Tzahar E, Yarden Y. The ErbB-2/HER2 oncogenic receptor of adenocarcinomas: from orphanhood to multiple stromal ligands. Biochim Biophys Acta 1998;1377(1):M25–37.

[43] Disis ML, Cheever MA. HER-2/neu protein: a target for antigen specific immunotherapy of human cancer. Adv Cancer Res 1997;71:343–71.

[44] Baselga J, Seidman AD, Rosen PP, et al. HER2 overexpression and paclitaxel sensitivity in breast cancer: therapeutic implications. Oncology 1997;11(3 Suppl 2):43–8.

[45] Muller WJ, Sinn E, Pattengale PK, et al. Single-step induction of mammary adenocarcinoma in transgenic mice bearing the activated c-neu oncogene. Cell 1988;54(1):105–15.

[46] Bouchard L, Lamarre L, Tremblay PJ, et al. Stochastic appearance of mammary adenocarcinoma in transgenic mice bearing the activated c-neu oncogene. Cell 1989;57(6):931–6.

[47] Guy CT, Webster MA, Schaller M, et al. Expression of the neu protooncogene in the mammary epithelium of transgenic mice induces metastatic disease. Proc Natl Acad Sci U S A 1992;89(22):578–82.

[48] Carter P, Presta L, Gorman CM, et al. Humanization of an anti-p185HER2 antibody for human cancer therapy. Proc Natl Acad Sci U S A 1992;89(10):4285–9.

[49] Lewis GD, Figari I, Fendly B, et al. Differential responses of human tumor cell lines to anti-p185HER2 monoclonal antibodies. Cancer Immunol Immunother 1993;37(4):255–63.

[50] Parihar R, Dierksheide J, Hu Y, et al. IL-12 enhances the natural killer cell cytokine response to Ab-coated tumor cells. J Clin Invest 2002;110(7):983–92.

[51] Carson WE, Parihar R, Lindemann MJ, et al. Interleukin-2 enhances the natural killer cell response to Herceptin-coated Her2/neu-positive breast cancer cells. Eur J Immunol 2001; 31(10):3016–25.

[52] Baselga J. Clinical trials of single-agent trastuzumab (Herceptin). Semin Oncol 2000;27 (5 Suppl 9):20–6.

[53] Baselga J, Tripathy D, Mendelsohn J, et al. Phase II study of weekly intravenous recombinant anti-p185her2 monoclonal antibody in patients with her2/neu-overexpressing metastatic breast cancer. J Clin Oncol 1996;14(3):737–44.

[54] Cobleigh MA, Vogel CL, Tripathy D, et al. Multinational study of the efficacy and safety of humanized anti-HER2 monoclonal antibody in women who have HER2-overexpressing metastatic breast cancer that has progressed after chemotherapy for metastatic disease. J Clin Oncol 1999;17(9):2639–48.

[55] Vogel C, Cobleigh MA, Tripathy D, et al. First-line, single-agent Herceptin(trastuzumab) in metastatic breast cancer: a preliminary report. Eur J Cancer 2001;37(Suppl 1):S25–9.

[56] Pietras RJ, Fendly BM, Chazin VR, et al. Antibody to HER-2/neu receptor blocks DNA repair after cisplatin in human breast and ovarian cancer cells. Oncogene 1994;9(7): 1829–38.

[57] Baselga J, Norton L, Albanell J, et al. Recombinant humanized anti-HER2 antibody (Herceptin) enhances the antitumor activity of paclitaxel and doxorubicin against HER2/neu overexpressing human breast cancer xenografts. Cancer Res 1998;58(13):2825–31.

[58] Slamon DJ, Leyland-Jones B, Shak S, et al. Use of chemotherapy plus a monoclonal antibody against HER2 for metastatic breast cancer that overexpresses HER2. N Engl J Med 2001;344(11):783–92.

[59] Jerian S, Keegan P. Cardiotoxicity associated with paclitaxel/trastuzumab combination therapy. J Clin Oncol 1999;17(5):1647–8.

[60] Clynes RA, Towers TL, Presta LG, et al. Inhibitory Fc receptors modulate in vivo cytotoxicity against tumor targets. Nat Med 2000;6(4):443–6.

[61] Perussia B. Fc receptors on natural killer cells. Curr Top Microbiol Immunol 1998;230: 63–88.

[62] McKenzie SE, Schreiber AD. Fc gamma receptors in phagocytes. Curr Opin Hematol 1998; 5(1):16–21.

[63] Boehm U, Klamp T, Groot M, et al. Cellular responses to interferon-gamma. Annu Rev Immunol 1997;15:749–95.

[64] Carson WE, Giri JG, Lindemann MJ, et al. Interleukin-15 is a novel cytokine which activates human natural killer cells via components of the interleukin-2 receptor. J Exp Med 1994; 180(4):1395–403.

[65] Bluman E, Bartynski KJ, Avalos BR, et al. Human natural killer cells produce abundant macrophage inflammatory protein-1 alpha in response to monocyte-derived cytokines. J Clin Invest 1996;97(12):2722–7.

[66] Fehniger TA, Shah MH, Turner MJ, et al. Differential cytokine and chemokine gene expression by human NK cells following activation with IL-18 or IL-15 in combination with IL-12: implications for the innate immune response. J Immunol 1999;162(8):4511–20.

[67] Carson WE, Lindemann MJ, Baiocchi RA, et al. The functional characterization of IL-10 receptor expression on human natural killer cells. Blood 1995;85(12):3577–85.

[68] Parihar R, Nadella P, Lewis A, et al. A phase I study of interleukin 12 with trastuzumab in patients with human epidermal growth factor receptor-2-overexpressing malignancies: analysis of sustained interferon gamma production in a subset of patients. Clin Cancer Res 2004; 10(15):5027–37.

[69] Chan OT, Yang LX. The immunological effects of taxanes. Cancer Immunol Immunother 2000;49(4–5):181–5.

[70] Chen YM, Yang WK, Ting CC, et al. Depressed cytolytic activity of peripheral blood mononuclear cells in unusually high paclitaxel concentrations: reversal by IL-2 and IL-12. Zhonghua Yi Xue Za Zhi (Taipei) 1999;62(12):867–74.

[71] Manie S, Schmid-Alliana A, Kubar J, et al. Disruption of microtubule network in human monocytes induces expression of interleukin-1 but not that of interleukin-6 nor tumor necrosis factor-alpha. Involvement of protein kinase A stimulation. J Biol Chem 1993;268(18): 13675–81.

[72] Perera PY, Mayadas TN, Takeuchi O, et al. CD11b/CD18 acts in concert with CD14 and Toll-like receptor (TLR) 4 to elicit full lipopolysaccharide and Taxol-inducible gene expression. J Immunol 2001;166(1):574–81.

[73] Mullins DW, Martins RS, Burger CJ, et al. Tumor cell-derived TGF-beta and IL-10 dysregulate paclitaxel-induced macrophage activation. J Leukoc Biol 2001;69(1):129–37.

[74] Mullins DW, Walker TM, Burger CJ, et al. Taxol-mediated changes in fibrosarcoma-induced immune cell function: modulation of antitumor activities. Cancer Immunol Immunother 1997;45(1):20–8.

[75] Mullins DW, Burger CJ, Elgert KD. Paclitaxel enhances macrophage IL-12 production in tumor-bearing hosts through nitric oxide. J Immunol 1999;162(11):6811–8.

[76] Mullins DW, Koci MD, Burger CJ, et al. Interleukin-12 overcomes paclitaxel-mediated suppression of T-cell proliferation. Immunopharmacol Immunotoxicol 1998;20(4): 473–92.

[77] Zagozdzon R, Golab J, Mucha K, et al. Potentiation of antitumor effects of IL-12 in combination with paclitaxel in murine melanoma model in vivo. Int J Mol Med 1999;4(6):645–8.

[78] Carson WE, Shapiro C, Crespin TR, et al. Cellular immunity in breast cancer patients completing taxane treatment. Cellular immunity in breast cancer patients completing taxane treatment. Clin Cancer Res 2004;10(10):3401–9.

[79] Carson WE, Roda J, Parihar R, et al. 2005 ASCO Annual Meeting Proceedings. J Clin Oncol 2005;23(16S, Pt I of II):2531 [June 1 Supplement].

[80] Roda JM, Parihar R, Lehman A, et al. Interleukin-21 enhances NK cell activation in response to antibody-coated targets. J Immunol 2006;177(1):120–9.

[81] Roda JM, Parihar R, Carson WE. CpG-containing oligodeoxynucleotides act through toll-like receptor 9 to enhance the NK cell response to antibody-coated tumor targets. J Immunol 2005;175(3):1619–27.

[82] Beatty GL, Paterson Y. Regulation of tumor growth by IFN-gamma in cancer immunotherapy. Immunol Res 2001;24(2):201–10.

[83] Taub DD, Conlon K, Lloyd AR, et al. Preferential migration of activated CD4+ and CD8+ T cells in response to MIP-1 alpha and MIP-1 beta. Science 1993;260(5106):355–8.

[84] Taub DD, Turcovski-Corrales SM, Key ML, et al. Chemokines and T lymphocyte activation: I. Beta chemokines costimulate human T lymphocyte activation in vitro. J Immunol 1996;156(6):2095–103.

[85] Robertson MJ. Role of chemokines in the biology of natural killer cells. J Leukoc Biol 2002; 71(2):173–83.

[86] Allen LA, Aderem A. Mechanisms of phagocytosis. Curr Opin Immunol 1996;8(1):36–40.

[87] MacMicking J, Xie QW, Nathan C. Nitric oxide and macrophage function. Annu Rev Immunol 1997;15:323–50.

[88] Rappolee D, Werb Z. Macrophage-derived growth factors. Curr Top Microbiol Immunol 1992;181:87–140.

[89] Chin YE, Kitagawa M, Su WC, et al. Cell growth arrest and induction of cyclin-dependent kinase inhibitor p21 WAF1/CIP1 mediated by STAT1. Science 1996;272(5262):719–22.

[90] Chin YE, Kitagawa M, Kuida K, et al. Activation of the STAT signaling pathway can cause expression of caspase 1 and apoptosis. Mol Cell Biol 1997;17(9):5328–37.

ELSEVIER
SAUNDERS

Surg Oncol Clin N Am
16 (2007) 861–871

SURGICAL
ONCOLOGY CLINICS
OF NORTH AMERICA

Current Immunotherapeutic Strategies in Prostate Cancer

Joseph F. Grosso, PhD, Charles G. Drake, MD, PhD*

*Johns Hopkins Sidney Kimmel Comprehensive Cancer Center,
1650 Orleans Street, CRB 452, Baltimore, MD 21231, USA*

In 2007, more than 200,000 men will be diagnosed with prostate cancer in the United States alone [1], and most of these men will undergo primary therapy with either radical prostatectomy or radiation therapy. Although many of these patients will not have recurrent disease, approximately 27,000 men die of metastatic disease each year. For these men, the standard initial treatment is androgen ablation, which is generally efficacious [2], but which is accompanied by significant side effects [3]. Eventually most patients become resistant to androgen ablation and progress to a disease state termed "androgen-resistant" or "hormone-refractory" [4]. For men who have hormone-refractory disease, current treatment options are somewhat limited, with docetaxel the only agent showing a significant prolongation of survival [5,6].

Several groups have investigated therapeutic approaches involving stimulation of an immune response against progressive prostate cancer. Several features of prostate cancer suggest that it may be a good target for immunotherapy. First, prostate cancer is generally fairly slow growing [7], allowing the treated patient time to mount an active immune response. Second, the transcriptional profile of the prostate gland is fairly unique, suggesting the presence of a robust number of prostate-specific proteins that can serve as target antigens, including well-known gene products, such as prostate-specific antigen (PSA), prostate stem cell antigen (PSCA), and prostate-specific membrane antigen (PSMA) [8]. Finally, the prostate gland is a nonessential organ, suggesting that in patients who still have an intact gland, bystander damage to normal glandular parenchyma resulting from imperfect tumor targeting might not be expected to have serious clinical implications.

CGD is a Damon Runyon-Lilly Clinical Investigator. This work was also supported by National Institutes of Health grant CA 096948 to CGD.

* Corresponding author.

E-mail address: drakech@jhmi.edu (C.G. Drake).

doi:10.1016/j.soc.2007.07.009

As is the case for several other malignancies, however, significant barriers to successful immunotherapy exist [9]. Several groups have suggested that prostate cancer arises in the context of pre-existing inflammation, indicating that patients who have cancer have an ongoing but nonproductive immune response associated with their disease [10]. As is the case for hepatitis and gastritis, this pre-existing immune response might be a driving force for cancer development. In addition, the prostate gland of men who have cancer seems to contain a significant population of regulatory T cells, a specialized T-cell subset that inhibits a lytic CD8 T-cell response [11]. Finally, men who have advanced prostate cancer frequently have elevated levels of the cytokine TGFβ, a potent inhibitor of a protective CD8 T-cell response [12].

Overview of an antitumor immune response

To understand the various approaches to immunotherapy for prostate cancer, it is helpful to conceptually outline an antitumor immune response. Primary in such a response is the dendritic cell, a specialized cell of the innate immune system that continuously surveys its surrounding environment for signs of infection [13]. At rest, these cells are immunologically silent, and are not recognized by either T or B lymphocytes, the major cells of the adaptive immune system. When a "danger" signal is encountered, however, these dendritic cells change their phenotype dramatically, up-regulating cell surface markers necessary for cell–cell interactions, and secrete proinflammatory cytokines to attract and stimulate T cells. These activated dendritic cells display their sampled antigen on their surface in the context of HLA molecules. CD4 and CD8 T cells are attracted to activated dendritic cells; these T cells then use their unique cell surface receptors (TCRs) to scan activated dendritic cells for specific recognition. If the T cell recognizes its cognate antigen on an activated dendritic cell, the T cell itself is then activated and goes on to perform its effector function. For CD4 T cells, this involves providing help to CD8 T cells in the form of secreted cytokines. CD8 T cells, in turn, are stimulated to become activated, divide, and then traffic widely throughout the body in search of their antigenic targets. On recognition of their targets, these CD8 T cells can then kill them, either through secreted molecules that physically create open holes or pores, or through other secreted molecules that mediate programmed cell death (apoptosis). In respect to tumor cells as targets, CD8 T cells have been demonstrated to lyse even chemotherapy-resistant tumors, suggesting a potential therapeutic value for immunotherapy strategies even in chemotherapy-resistant disease. In addition, activated CD8 T cells can traffic widely, suggesting that a productive antitumor immune response may prove capable of targeting multiple sites of metastatic disease. Finally, the potential specificity of the human T cell repertoire is immense, with the capability to effectively target more than 10^8 potential peptide antigens.

A vast array of potential immunotherapeutic interventions for prostate cancer is currently under development and a comprehensive discussion of each of these is beyond the scope of this article. Instead, the authors focus on a small set of specific strategies that have advanced to either phase III or late phase II trials, because these agents are most likely to be encountered by the surgical oncologist in the near future. In addition, the immunologic principles underpinning these approaches are broadly applicable to most of the other agents currently under investigation.

Dendritic cell–based immunotherapy

Because active dendritic cells are primary players in an adaptive immune response, one approach to immunotherapy for prostate cancer might be to simply deliver activated dendritic cells, loaded with prostate-specific target antigens, to patients who have disease. To generate human dendritic cells for immunotherapy, immature monocytes from peripheral blood are isolated and cultured for 4 to 7 days in the presence of certain cytokines (typically IL-4 and GM-CSF) [14]. This process results in the production of inactive dendritic cells, which must then be activated and loaded with an appropriate target antigen. For prostate cancer, antigens targeted by dendritic cell immunotherapy approaches have included PSA, PSCA, and PSMA, among others [15]. The primary downside to such approaches is their complexity; patients must undergo a pheresis procedure to obtain the required monocytes and several days of sterile, in vitro culture are required to generate an immunotherapy product. Although several phase II trials have been reported [16,17], only one dendritic cell–based approach has advanced to multiple phase III trials in prostate cancer [18]. This product, known as sipuleucel-T (Dendreon, Seattle, Washington), is a variation on the standard dendritic cell approach. Patients must still undergo pheresis to provide a source of monocytes, but in lieu of long-term culture, these cells are cocultured for a relatively short time (approximately 36 hours) with a fusion protein that couples the major dendritic cell stimulatory factor (GM-CSF) with a prostate-targeted protein (prostatic acid phosphatase). The resulting cellular product is then infused intravenously (IV) into the patient; the procedure is repeated three times at 2-week intervals to complete a course of therapy. Phase I trials of this approach were provocative [19,20] and led to a small randomized phase III trial reported in 2006 [21]. The phase III trial showed a statistically significant increase in 3-year survival, but no difference in the primary endpoint, time to disease progression between the two arms. A second, smaller phase III trial was recently completed and based on these two data sets (and on a benign toxicity profile), Dendreon Inc. filed for a Biologics License Application, which was reviewed by the US Food and Drug Administration (FDA) in an open session on March 29, 2007 (www.fda.gov; search term "Dendreon"). Although the advisory committee voted 13 to 4 in favor of efficacy, full licensure was not granted by the agency, which requested either final or interim survival data from a larger, ongoing phase III trial involving 500 patients. These data are expected in 2008, and accrual to this important trial (IMPACT) is ongoing (Table 1).

Immunotherapy based on GM-CSF transduced, allogeneic tumor cells

A second approach to immunotherapy for prostate cancer that has advanced to phase III clinical trials involves the use of tumor cells as a vaccine. Such an approach has a long history in the realm of infectious diseases, for which heat-killed or otherwise attenuated bacteria or viruses are used in protective vaccines. Because such techniques proved to be generally ineffective in cancer treatment or prevention studies, several groups sought to increase the relative immunologic potency of tumor cells by transfecting them with genes for various cytokines. The critical experiment in this regard was published by Dranoff and colleagues [22], who showed that melanoma cells transfected to produce the cytokine GM-CSF provided nearly complete protection against tumor challenge in a poorly immunogenic murine model of melanoma. It should be noted that this result was somewhat surprising at the time, because many groups suggested that the cytokines IL-2 or perhaps interferon gamma (IFN-γ) would be most efficacious in this regard. To translate these findings to a clinical setting, initial trials used a patient's own tumor cells, transduced ex vivo with a plasmid encoding GM-CSF [23]. This trial showed that autologous cell-based immunotherapy was generally well tolerated but highlighted the variability and inherent difficulties in using patient-derived materials to produce an immunotherapy product. A solution to this obstacle came in the late 1990s, when several groups working in basic immunology described a phenomenon known as cross-priming, suggesting that immunogenic antigens from an outside source could be taken up and presented by a patient's own endogenous dendritic cells [24,25]. This finding meant that it might not be necessary to use patients' own cancer cells; perhaps allogeneic cells could function as a cell-based immunotherapy, provided they were sufficiently immunogenic. For prostate cancer, the cell lines LNCaP and PC3 were transduced with the gene for human GM-CSF and used in a phase I trial [26]. For immunotherapy, cell-based vaccines are injected intradermally, where the GM-CSF they secrete serves to attract and mature local dendritic cells. The tumor cells (which have been irradiated before injection) eventually undergo apoptosis, and this apoptotic debris is taken up by the recruited dendritic cells, thus activating specific CD4 and CD8 T cells [27]. A phase I trial showed this type of immunotherapy to be generally well tolerated, and a subsequent, recently published phase II trial showed that administration of allogeneic, GM-CSF transduced tumor cells could result in detectable immune responses in patients, as demonstrated by the induction of detectable antibodies directed at the cells that make up the product [28]. From a commercial standpoint,

Table 1
Selected immunotherapy trials in prostate cancer

Agent	Phase	Target population	No. patients	Comments
Single agent				
Sipuleucel-T (ProVenge)	III	Metastatic HRPC	500	IMPACT (Immunotherapy in Metastatic Prostate AdenoCarcinoma Treatment), 2:1 randomized, double-blinded trial comparing sipuleucel-T IV q 2 wk × 3 to empty vector. Primary endpoint is overall survival. Crossover to a second-line active treatment protocol is allowed for the control group on progression.
GVAX prostate	III	Progressive, metastatic HRPC, asymptomatic	600	VITAL-1 (Vaccine ImmunoTherapy with Allogeneic prostate cancer cell Lines), 1:1 randomized, unblinded trial comparing first-line immunotherapy (GVAX q 2 wk × 13) to standard chemotherapy (docetaxel q 3 wk × 9). Primary endpoint is overall survival. Enrollment completed 7/2007
Ipilimumab	I/II	Metastatic HRPC, no chronic narcotic pain medication, prior chemotherapy allowed	34	Open-label, multisite dose-escalation study of ipilimumab q 3 wk × 4 doses
Combinatorial				
GVAX prostate + docetaxel	III	Metastatic, symptomatic HRPC	600	VITAL-2 (Vaccine ImmunoTherapy with Allogeneic prostate cancer cell Lines), 1:1 randomized, unblinded trial comparing first line standard chemotherapy (docetaxel q 3 wk × 9) to the same regimen combined with GVAX immunotherapy. Primary endpoint is overall survival.
GVAX prostate + ipilimumab	I	Metastatic HRPC	12 + 15	Phase I dose escalation trial combining ipilimumab with GVAX prostate; 12 patients in dose-escalation phase, 15 patients at MTD
Prostvac VF + ipilimumab	I	Metastatic HRPC	24	Phase I trial combination trial based on the vaccinia-PSA-TRICOM vector, dose escalation of ipilimumab, 3–6 patients per dose.
Ipilimumab + short-term androgen ablation	II	Newly diagnosed PC, no prior chemotherapy, hormonal therapy, or radiation therapy	108	Randomized trial comparing progression-free survival in men treated either with 3 mo of androgen ablation or the same combined with a single dose of ipilimumab. Secondary endpoints include PSA response.

Current data at www.clinicaltrials.gov.
Abbreviations: HRPC, hormone refractory prostate cancer; MTD, maximum tolerated dose; PC, prostate cancer.

this approach has been developed by Cell Genesys Inc. (South San Francisco, California), which initiated two large randomized phase III trials in men who had hormone-refractory prostate cancer (see Table 1). The first of these trials (Vital-1) compares overall survival of men treated with standard-of-care docetaxel to the survival of men treated with a 6-month course of GVAX immunotherapy. This 600-patient randomized trial has recently completed accrual; an interim analysis is expected in 2008. In a second trial, the combination of GVAX immunotherapy with concurrent docetaxel chemotherapy will be compared with standard docetaxel chemotherapy, also in men who have hormone-refractory prostate cancer. This second 600-patient trial is also powered to detect a difference in overall survival, and accrual is ongoing.

Viral-based immunotherapy strategies for prostate cancer

Viral pathogens directly activate dendritic cells through several mechanisms, resulting in subsequent T cell priming and activation. Vaccinia viruses of the poxvirus family are particularly potent in this regard, resulting in a dramatic expansion of specific CD4 T cells. These viruses can be engineered to carry various specific proteins, which serve as immunologic targets in vaccination strategies [29]. For prostate cancer, an approach targeting PSA has been the subject of significant clinical development. The first phase I trial of this approach was reported by Sanda and colleagues [30], who administered a recombinant vaccinia virus encoding PSA (Prost-Vac) to men who had biochemically relapsed prostate cancer. As is the case for most of these immunotherapy approaches, the vaccines were well tolerated with only minor side effects. These data were followed soon after by dose-escalation studies of this agent, with accompanying immunologic monitoring [31,32]. One drawback to vaccinia-based vaccination is that immunogenicity is eventually limited by an antibody-mediated response against the vector itself; these concerns were borne out by clinical trial demonstrating a reduced potency of sequential doses [31]. In response to this observation, sequential addition of a second, replication-deficient pox-virus–based vector (fowlpox) targeting PSA was explored in a prime-boost strategy. A multicenter Eastern Cooperative Oncology Group (ECOG) trial optimized scheduling of vaccinia-PSA and fowlpox-PSA vectors, showing that vaccinia priming followed by fowlpox boosting resulted in the highest frequency of detectable immune responses [33]. Long-term monitoring data from this interesting trial also suggested an improvement in progression-free survival in treated patients. Further work with this approach involved the inclusion of three separate costimulatory molecules (LFA-1, ICAM, and B7-1) in an effort to further improve T cell immune responses [34]. In the case of metastatic HPRC, a randomized phase II trial has been completed, and whereas an early analysis did not show evidence of a survival benefit longer-term follow-up data are pending [35]. At the present time, a phase III trial of this approach has not yet been initiated, but current development efforts seeking to combine this agent with various other therapeutic strategies to increase potency are underway [36].

Immune checkpoint blockade

In addition to the stimulatory signals provided to T cells by activated dendritic cells, there are several signals that oppose full T-cell activation [9]. Under normal circumstances, these checkpoints most likely serve to limit the magnitude of an induced T-cell response and protect the host from developing autoimmune disease. Recent data suggest that several of these checkpoints have been co-opted by evolving tumors in an effort to escape immune recognition and destruction [37]. From a clinical standpoint, the molecule that has progressed furthest in this regard is CTLA-4. This molecule was originally described by Allison and colleagues [38] and is induced on the cell surface of CD4 and CD8 T cells during activation. Engagement of CTLA-4 during an immune response effectively dampens T cell expansion and limits expansion. Mice in which CTLA-4 has been genetically knocked out develop severe systemic autoimmunity and die before 20 weeks of age [39], demonstrating a powerful role for CTLA-4 in immunologic tolerance. A fully human monoclonal antibody directed against CTLA-4 has been developed by the Medarex Corporation (Princeton, New Jersey); this agent is known as ipilimumab, and has been the subject of several clinical trials in kidney cancer, melanoma, and prostate cancer. In general, these trials, which mostly involve treatment-refractory patients, showed a measurable response rate but also demonstrated that clinical responses are frequently associated with various autoimmune side effects, including colitis and hypophysitis [40]. The first trial of ipilimumab in prostate cancer was recently published [41], and several phase I and II trials are in progress (see Table 1).

Passive administration of antitumor antibodies

An antitumor immune response may be initiated when either dead or dying tumor cells are taken up locally by immature dendritic cells [13]. Antigen uptake and presentation is markedly enhanced when the target is coated with antibody, and this process (known as opsonization) has been implicated in the mechanism of the monoclonal antibody Rituximab (Genentech), which is widely used in lymphoma therapy [42]. In prostate cancer, several monoclonal antibodies are currently in development. In particular, a humanized anti-PSMA antibody (HuJ591, BZL Biologics, Inc.) has undergone a Phase II trial; preliminary data indicate that the antibody is well tolerated and results in PSA stabilization in some patients [43]. To enhance the cytotoxic efficacy of a monoclonal antibody, it can be conjugated to β-emitters, such as ^{90}Y and ^{111}I. From an immunologic point of view, these conjugates may operate through more complex mechanisms, including direct toxicity resulting in the liberation of tumor antigens from necrotic cancer cells. Phase I trials of ^{90}Y and lutetium^{177} conjugated anti-PSMA antibodies have been reported, with evidence of biologic activity in both studies [44,45]. Although the targeting efficiency of these PSMA-conjugated antibodies has been impressive, their clinical response rate in advanced disease has been less so. In ongoing trials, a phase II trial of a lutetium^{177} conjugated version of HuJ591 has been initiated.

Combination immunotherapy

With a few exceptions, few chemotherapy agents are used alone in the treatment of patients who have cancer. It thus seems likely that approaches combining immunotherapy with other treatment modalities, or perhaps even combining multiple immunotherapy agents, might prove useful in treating men who have prostate cancer. This concept has been studied extensively by the National Institutes of Health (NIH) group, which has tested ProstVac with radiotherapy [46], secondary androgen manipulation [47], and chemotherapy [48]. In general, these studies have been encouraging, showing improved PSA response rates and increased rates of correlative immune responses. Combination with docetaxel is particularly interesting in this regard; preclinical data from several laboratories clearly show that administration of docetaxel before immunotherapy with cell-based immunotherapy leads to improved clinical outcome, without an obvious increase in toxicity [49]. A phase III clinical trial testing this approach using the GVAX platform was initiated in 2005.

Perhaps one of the most innovative concepts involving immunotherapy for prostate cancer is the notion of combining multiple immunotherapy modalities. In this respect, Dr. Larry Fong is currently examining the combination of checkpoint blockade with anti-CTLA4 antibody (MDX-010) and GM-CSF in a phase I trial currently enrolling patients at University of California, San Francisco. From a mechanistic standpoint, it might also make sense to provide a positive stimulus to the immune system in the form of active immunotherapy, while at the same time mitigating the negative effects of co-inhibitory checkpoints. In an automotive analogy, this might correspond to applying the gas while at the same time taking the foot off the brake. Preliminary results from such an approach were presented at the American Society of Clinical Oncology (ASCO) national meeting in 2006; Gerritsen and colleagues [50] showed that men who had metastatic hormone refractory prostate cancer treated with a combination of GVAX immunotherapy for prostate cancer and ipilimumab displayed an impressively high rate of PSA and radiologic responses, along with a measurable incidence of autoimmune breakthrough events. A phase I trial currently enrolling patients at the NCI will further explore this approach by combining the ProstVac vaccine vector with MDX010 and systemic GM-CSF.

Summary

Immunotherapy for prostate cancer may be close to clinical application, as demonstrated by the recent FDA application for sipuleucel-T and by the completion of accrual to a large phase III trial of GVAX immunotherapy for prostate cancer. Earlier data for each of these agents suggest the potential for a survival benefit, which is especially impressive in light of the relatively benign toxicity profiles for each of these agents. Constant pressure by the immune system forces tumors to evolve multiple ways to escape immune assault [9], however, and it is thus unlikely that single-agent immunotherapy for prostate cancer will achieve maximal clinical benefit. Most likely, successful immunotherapy will eventually require either the combination of multiple immunologic approaches or the combination of immunologic approaches with conventional therapy.

References

[1] Jemal A, Siegel R, Ward E, et al. Cancer statistics, 2006. CA Cancer J Clin 2006;56:106–30.
[2] Denmeade SR, Isaacs JT. A history of prostate cancer treatment. Nat Rev Cancer 2002;2: 389–96.
[3] Gomella LG. Contemporary use of hormonal therapy in prostate cancer: managing complications and addressing quality-of-life issues. BJU Int 2007;99(Suppl 1):25–9.
[4] Scher HI, Heller G. Clinical states in prostate cancer: toward a dynamic model of disease progression. Urology 2000;55:323–7.
[5] Tannock IF, de Wit R, Berry WR, et al. Docetaxel plus prednisone or mitoxantrone plus prednisone for advanced prostate cancer. N Engl J Med 2004;351:1502–12.
[6] Petrylak DP, Tangen CM, Hussain MH, et al. Docetaxel and estramustine compared with mitoxantrone and prednisone for advanced refractory prostate cancer. N Engl J Med 2004;351:1513–20.
[7] Coffey DS, Isaacs JT. Prostate tumor biology and cell kinetics–theory. Urology 1981;17:40–53.
[8] Rhodes DR, Barrette TR, Rubin MA, et al. Meta-analysis of microarrays: interstudy validation of gene expression profiles reveals pathway dysregulation in prostate cancer. Cancer Res 2002;62:4427–33.
[9] Drake CG, Jaffee E, Pardoll DM. Mechanisms of immune evasion by tumors. Adv Immunol 2006;90:51–81.
[10] De Marzo AM, Platz EA, Sutcliffe S, et al. Inflammation in prostate carcinogenesis. Nat Rev Cancer 2007;7:256–69.
[11] Miller AM, Lundberg K, Ozenci V, et al. CD4+CD25high T cells are enriched in the tumor and peripheral blood of prostate cancer patients. J Immunol 2006;177:7398–405.
[12] Wahl SM, Wen J, Moutsopoulos N. TGF-beta: a mobile purveyor of immune privilege. Immunol Rev 2006;213:213–27.
[13] Steinman RM. Some interfaces of dendritic cell biology. APMIS 2003;111:675–97.
[14] Gilboa E. DC-based cancer vaccines. J Clin Invest 2007;117:1195–203.
[15] Drake CG. Basic overview of current immunotherapy approaches in urologic malignancy. Urol Oncol 2006;24:413–8.
[16] Thomas-Kaskel AK, Zeiser R, Jochim R, et al. Vaccination of advanced prostate cancer patients with PSCA and PSA peptide-loaded dendritic cells induces DTH responses that correlate with superior overall survival. Int J Cancer 2006;119:2428–34.
[17] Pandha HS, John RJ, Hutchinson J, et al. Dendritic cell immunotherapy for urological cancers using cryopreserved allogeneic tumour lysate-pulsed cells: a phase I/II study. BJU Int 2004;94:412–8.

[18] Lin AM, Hershberg RM, Small EJ. Immunotherapy for prostate cancer using prostatic acid phosphatase loaded antigen presenting cells. Urol Oncol 2006;24:434–41.

[19] Burch PA, Breen JK, Buckner JC, et al. Priming tissue-specific cellular immunity in a phase I trial of autologous dendritic cells for prostate cancer. Clin Cancer Res 2000;6:2175–82.

[20] Small EJ, Fratesi P, Reese DM, et al. Immunotherapy of hormone-refractory prostate cancer with antigen-loaded dendritic cells. J Clin Oncol 2000;18:3894–903.

[21] Small EJ, Schellhammer PF, Higano CS, et al. Placebo-controlled phase III trial of immunologic therapy with sipuleucel-T (APC8015) in patients with metastatic, asymptomatic hormone refractory prostate cancer. J Clin Oncol 2006;24:3089–94.

[22] Dranoff G, Jaffee E, Lazenby A, et al. Vaccination with irradiated tumor cells engineered to secrete murine granulocyte-macrophage colony-stimulating factor stimulates potent, specific, and long-lasting anti-tumor immunity. Proc Natl Acad Sci U S A 1993;90:3539–43.

[23] Simons JW, Mikhak B, Chang JF, et al. Induction of immunity to prostate cancer antigens: results of a clinical trial of vaccination with irradiated autologous prostate tumor cells engineered to secrete granulocyte-macrophage colony-stimulating factor using ex vivo gene transfer. Cancer Res 1999;59:5160–8.

[24] Adler AJ, Marsh DW, Yochum GS, et al. CD4+ T cell tolerance to parenchymal self-antigens requires presentation by bone marrow-derived antigen-presenting cells. J Exp Med 1998;187:1555–64.

[25] Kurts C, Kosaka H, Carbone FR, et al. Class I-restricted cross-presentation of exogenous self-antigens leads to deletion of autoreactive CD8(+) T cells. J Exp Med 1997;186: 239–45.

[26] Simons JW, Higano C, Corman J, et al. A phase I/II trial of high dose allogeneic GM-CSF gene-transduced prostate cancer cell line vaccine in patients with metastatic hormone-refractory prostate cancer [abstract]. Proc Am Soc Clin Oncol 2003;22:166.

[27] Simmons AD, Li B, Gonzalez-Edick M, et al. GM-CSF-secreting cancer immunotherapies: preclinical analysis of the mechanism of action. Cancer Immunol Immunother 2007;56(10): 1553–65.

[28] Small EJ, Sacks N, Nemunaitis J, et al. Granulocyte macrophage colony-stimulating factor–secreting allogeneic cellular immunotherapy for hormone-refractory prostate cancer. Clin Cancer Res 2007;13:3883–91.

[29] Arlen PM, Kaufman HL, DiPaola RS. Pox viral vaccine approaches. Semin Oncol 2005;32: 549–55.

[30] Sanda MG, Smith DC, Charles LG, et al. Recombinant vaccinia-PSA (PROSTVAC) can induce a prostate-specific immune response in androgen-modulated human prostate cancer. Urology 1999;53:260–6.

[31] Gulley J, Chen AP, Dahut W, et al. Phase I study of a vaccine using recombinant vaccinia virus expressing PSA (rV-PSA) in patients with metastatic androgen-independent prostate cancer. Prostate 2002;53:109–17.

[32] Eder JP, Kantoff PW, Roper K, et al. A phase I trial of a recombinant vaccinia virus expressing prostate-specific antigen in advanced prostate cancer. Clin Cancer Res 2000;6:1632–8.

[33] Kaufman HL, Wang W, Manola J, et al. Phase II randomized study of vaccine treatment of advanced prostate cancer (E7897): a trial of the Eastern Cooperative Oncology Group. J Clin Oncol 2004;22:2122–32.

[34] Dipaola R, Plante M, Kaufman H, et al. A phase I trial of pox PSA vaccines (PROST-VAC(R)-VF) with B7-1, ICAM-1, and LFA-3 co-stimulatory molecules (TRICOMtrade mark) in patients with prostate cancer. J Transl Med 2006;4:1.

[35] Schlom J, Arlen PM, Gulley JL. Cancer vaccines: moving beyond current paradigms. Clin Cancer Res 2007;13:3776–82.

[36] Gulley JL, Madan RA, Arlen PM. Enhancing efficacy of therapeutic vaccinations by combination with other modalities. Vaccine 2007 [epub ahead of print].

[37] Chen L. Co-inhibitory molecules of the B7-CD28 family in the control of T-cell immunity. Nat Rev Immunol 2004;4:336–47.

[38] Korman AJ, Peggs KS, Allison JP. Checkpoint blockade in cancer immunotherapy. Adv Immunol 2006;90:297–339.

[39] Chambers CA, Kuhns MS, Egen JG, et al. CTLA-4-mediated inhibition in regulation of T cell responses: mechanisms and manipulation in tumor immunotherapy. Annu Rev Immunol 2001;19:565–94.

[40] Blansfield JA, Beck KE, Tran K, et al. Cytotoxic T-lymphocyte-associated antigen-4 blockage can induce autoimmune hypophysitis in patients with metastatic melanoma and renal cancer. J Immunother 2005;28:593–8.

[41] Small EJ, Tchekmedyian NS, Rini BI, et al. A pilot trial of CTLA-4 blockade with human anti-CTLA-4 in patients with hormone-refractory prostate cancer. Clin Cancer Res 2007; 13:1810–5.

[42] Uchida J, Hamaguchi Y, Oliver JA, et al. The innate mononuclear phagocyte network depletes B lymphocytes through Fc receptor-dependent mechanisms during anti-CD20 antibody immunotherapy. J Exp Med 2004;199:1659–69.

[43] Nanus DM, Milowsky MI, Kostakoglu L, et al. Clinical use of monoclonal antibody HuJ591 therapy: targeting prostate specific membrane antigen. J Urol 2003;170:S84–8.

[44] Milowsky MI, Nanus DM, Kostakoglu L, et al. Phase I trial of yttrium-90-labeled anti-prostate-specific membrane antigen monoclonal antibody J591 for androgen-independent prostate cancer. J Clin Oncol 2004;22:2522–31.

[45] Bander NH, Milowsky MI, Nanus DM, et al. Phase I trial of 177lutetium-labeled J591, a monoclonal antibody to prostate-specific membrane antigen, in patients with androgen-independent prostate cancer. J Clin Oncol 2005;23:4591–601.

[46] Gulley JL, Arlen PM, Bastian A, et al. Combining a recombinant cancer vaccine with standard definitive radiotherapy in patients with localized prostate cancer. Clin Cancer Res 2005; 11:3353–62.

[47] Arlen PM, Gulley JL, Todd N, et al. Antiandrogen, vaccine and combination therapy in patients with nonmetastatic hormone refractory prostate cancer. J Urol 2005;174:539–46.

[48] Arlen PM, Gulley JL, Parker C, et al. A randomized phase II study of concurrent docetaxel plus vaccine versus vaccine alone in metastatic androgen-independent prostate cancer. Clin Cancer Res 2006;12:1260–9.

[49] Prell RA, Gearin L, Simmons A, et al. The anti-tumor efficacy of a GM-CSF-secreting tumor cell vaccine is not inhibited by docetaxel administration. Cancer Immunol Immunother 2006;55:1285–93.

[50] Gerritsen WR. 2007 ASCO Annual Meeting Proceedings, Part I. J Clin Oncol 2007;25(Suppl 18S0):5120.

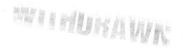

ELSEVIER
SAUNDERS

Surg Oncol Clin N Am
16 (2007) 873–900

SURGICAL
ONCOLOGY CLINICS
OF NORTH AMERICA

Current Immunotherapeutic Strategies in Colon Cancer

Michael Morse, MD[a],*, Lee Langer, BS[b],
Alexander Starodub, MD[a], Amy Hobeika, PhD[b],
Timothy Clay, PhD[b], H. Kim Lyerly, MD[b,c]

[a]*Department of Medicine, Duke University Medical Center, Box 3233, 401 MSRB,
Research Drive, Durham, NC 27710, USA*
[b]*Department of Surgery, Duke University Medical Center, 401 MSRB, Research Drive,
Durham, NC 27710, USA*
[c]*Comprehensive Cancer Center, 401 MSRB, Erwin Road, Durham, NC 27710, USA*

Immune cell infiltration into colorectal cancer

The immune surveillance theory postulates an important role for the immune system in defending against de novo carcinogenesis. Immune cells monitor normal tissues and seek out precancerous and cancerous cells and destroy them before they have a chance to propagate to a clinically significant size. This puts selective pressure on the surviving cancer cells that possess mechanisms to evade immune control. This process is summarized by the concept of immune editing [1]. Although the role of the immune system at the stage when tumors reach clinically detectable sizes has been questioned [2], evidence has been mounting that the immune system continues to play a significant role even in the later stages of tumor development [3]. For example, infiltration of immune and inflammatory cells in colorectal cancer can serve as a prognostic factor independent of Dukes' staging [4–11]. Jass and colleagues [6] observed that a peritumoral lymphocytic infiltrate was an important prognostic factor, second only to the number of lymph node metastases. In their study of 447 patients, corrected 5-year survival rates for pronounced, moderate, and little lymphocytic infiltration were 92%, 65%, and 36%, respectively. This finding was corroborated by Ali and investigators [9], who studied how the percentage of the volume of tumor infiltrated with CD4+ and CD8+ T cells correlated with the

---

* Corresponding author.
E-mail address: michael.morse@duke.edu (M. Morse).

risk of recurrence for patients with resected colon cancer. Specifically, the total percentage volume of T lymphocytes, and in particular the CD4+ T cells, was significantly lower in patients who recurred.

Pages and colleagues [10] showed that colorectal cancers (CRCs) with a high density of infiltrating memory and effector memory T cells were associated with a lower rate of dissemination to regional lymph nodes. Galon and colleagues [11] from the same group observed that colorectal cancers from patients without recurrence had higher immune cell densities (as detected by staining for CD3, CD8, Granzyme B, and CD45RO) within each "tumor region" than did colorectal cancers from patients whose tumors had recurred. They also used genomic analysis to identify a cluster of genes associated with a Th1 response, the expression of which was inversely correlated with CRC recurrence.

Infiltration of other immune cells has been linked to improved survival in CRC. Coca and colleagues [12] observed that among patients with stage III tumors, individuals with extensive natural killer cell infiltration had significantly longer 5-year survival than patients with little/moderate natural killer cell infiltration (50% versus 13%). The density of tumor eosinophils has correlated with survival, independent of staging [8,13]. An abundance of intratumoral dendritic cells (DCs), the most important of the antigen-presenting cells, is also associated with better patient outcomes for CRC [14–17].

Macrophages may possess antitumor immune effects and tumor-promoting effects. Macrophages may serve as antigen-presenting cells at the invasive margin of colon cancer [18]. Macrophages within tumor microenvironment originate from monocytes that have been recruited by a tumor cell release of monocyte chemotactic protein-1, macrophage colony stimulating factor, and vascular endothelial growth factor (VEGF). Macrophages may participate in an antibody-dependent cellular cytotoxicity through release of cytotoxic mediators such as proteinases and tumor necrosis factor-α or exhibit cytotoxicity independent of the antibodies by releasing reactive oxygen and nitrogen compounds. At the same time, these cytotoxic macrophages also can influence differentiation of naïve T-helper cells to Th1 cells, which release interferon (IFN)-γ and tumor necrosis factor-β. CRC tumors that have high levels of macrophage infiltration have significantly lower rates of lymph node and distant metastasis [19,20]. This observation is not uniform. At least in patients with metastatic liver tumors from CRC, activation of liver macrophages has been shown to be associated with a poorer prognosis.

Miyagawa and colleagues [21] found a positive relationship between liver macrophage density and microvessel density in and around tumors, which suggested the possibility that liver macrophage accumulation might be associated with angiogenesis of metastatic liver tumors. They also suggested that tumor-associated macrophages may have different properties, which have been affected by tumor cells. Tumors secrete several cytokines, including interleukin (IL)-4, IL-10, transforming growth factor-β, prostaglandin E-2, and VEGF. These factors may modulate the macrophage phenotype, changing them from cytotoxic macrophages to suppressive macrophages. Tumor-associated macrophages often do not exhibit properties attributed to activated cytotoxic macrophages described previously. They cannot effectively serve as antigen-presenting cells and have reduced cytotoxicity because of impaired production of tumor necrosis factor-α and nitric oxide [22–24].

In aggregate, the data would suggest a complex interaction of the immune system with colorectal cancers, but the presence of the innate and adaptive immune response within colorectal cancer supports the concept of augmenting this response with cancer vaccines [25].

Colorectal cancer antigens targeted by vaccines

For a cancer vaccine to be successful, the tumor must express antigens that serve as targets for recognition and destruction by immune effectors. It is generally agreed that (1) tumor-associated antigens should be expressed in the tumor and minimally or not at all in most other cells or tissues of the body, (2) they should be expressed by most of the tumor cells at the primary site and in metastases, (3) they should be expressed at the cell surface or processed and presented within major histocompatibility complex molecules, and (4) T cells should be present in the body, with T-cell receptors capable of recognizing the antigen. CRC tumor antigens recognized by T cells and antibodies are usually divided into three different groups [26]. The first group is cancer testis (CT) antigens that are normally expressed only on male germ cells but not on other normal tissues [27]. CT antigens expressed on CRC cells include MAGE 1,3,4,10, LAGE 1, SCP-1, SSX-1,2,4, CT10, NYESO-1. Their expression is likely to be regulated by methylation/demethylation of the gene promoter [28–31].

The second group includes overexpressed antigens that are expressed in normal tissues but are overexpressed in CRC cells. Examples that have been targets of cancer vaccines include (1) CEA, an intercellular adhesion glycoprotein expressed on normal colonic epithelium but overexpressed in more than 90% of CRCs [32], (2) MUC-1, a member of the family of human epithelial mucins expressed on the luminal surface of glandular epithelium that is overexpressed in more than 90% of CRCs [33], (3) Ep-Cam (EGP-2, 17-1A, GA733-2 or KSA), a glycoprotein that mediates cellular adhesion and is expressed commonly on normal epithelial cells and is overexpressed in human CRC [34], and (4) HER-2/*neu* (erbB-2, p185), a member of the epidermal growth factor receptor family that has been variously reported to be overexpressed in some CRC [35]. Overexpression of these antigens occurs through various mechanisms, such as demethylation of their promoters, decreased protein degradation, and amplification of genes.

The third group contains mutated antigens, which reflect various underlying genetic mutations and harbor new, "foreign" epitopes related to the mutation that may be important for maintaining the tumor cell. Examples include p53 [36], ras [37], and transforming growth factor-β receptor II [38]. The mismatch repair gene defects that lead to microsatellite instability in patients with hereditary nonpolyposis colon cancer also result in the expression of numerous mutant epitopes that may be targets of immune responses [39].

Approaches to immunotherapy for colorectal cancer

As has been the case for immunotherapy of other malignancies, the early strategies used for treatment of colorectal cancer were initially based on nonspecific immune stimulation with cytokines and biologic response modifiers, which had mixed results. Although IL-2 showed promising response in melanoma and renal cell carcinoma with cumulative 10% response [40], there were no responses in patients who had CRC, with results only slightly improved after combining IL-2 with injection of lymphokine-activated killers [41,42]. Several studies evaluated bacillus Calmette-Guérin (BCG) as an immune stimulant for colon cancer, but all produced negative results. The National Surgical Adjuvant Breast and Bowel Project Protocol C-01 enrolled 1166 patients with Dukes' B and C carcinoma of the colon who were randomized to one of three therapeutic categories: no further treatment after curative resection (394 patients), postoperative chemotherapy that consisted of 5-fluorouracil (5-FU), semustine, and vincristine (379 patients), or postoperative BCG (393 patients). After an average time of 77.3 months on study there was no difference in disease-free survival or adjusted overall survival between BCG and control groups [43]. Similar results were demonstrated by SWOG 7510, which showed no improvement in relapse-free survival or survival with the addition of immunotherapy to chemotherapy (methyl CCNU and 5-FU) after a median follow-up of 7 years [44].

Alfa interferon (IFN-a) also has been studied extensively in different patient cohorts with CRC. In the metastatic setting, five published randomized trials have compared 5-FU alone with the combination of 5-FU and IFN-α [45–49]. The studies revealed no improvement in the response rate, progression-free survival, or overall survival when IFN-α was added to 5-FU. In the adjuvant setting, the National Surgical Adjuvant Breast and Bowel Project performed a study that involved 2176 patients with Dukes' stage B or C colon cancer who were randomized to receive 5-FU + folinic acid (FA) or 5FU + FA + IFN-α [50]. After a follow-up period of 4 years, the addition of IFN-α did not lead to improved disease-free survival or overall survival but did increase treatment-related toxicity. In contrast to these negative studies, a positive result was obtained when polysaccharide K was administered with tegafur/uracil (UFT) as an adjuvant therapy for stage II and III colorectal cancer. Specifically, the 5-year disease-free survival rate was 73% for the group that received UFT/LV with polysaccharide K and

58.8% in the group that received UFT alone [51]. Despite these results, in general, nonspecific approaches have yielded limited results in the treatment of colorectal cancer; more specific approaches, such as active immunization against tumors or their antigens, have been studied more recently.

Active immunization

Tumor vaccines

The best results for cancer vaccines thus far have been demonstrated in clinical trials of autologous tumor combined with BCG for patients with resected stage II and III CRC (Table 1). These studies, with a total of more than 700 patients [52–54], demonstrated important lessons using the OncoVAX preparation. Benefit was confined to patients who had colon cancer (not rectal cancer, perhaps because of pelvic lymph node radiation) [52]. Benefit was greater for lower stage (stage II compared with stage III) disease [53,54]. The immune response against tumor antigen (demonstrated by the delayed-type hypersensitivity response against autologous tumor cells) correlated with an improved prognosis [53]. One limitation of this strategy is that autologous products are difficult to produce and are subject to considerable, uncontrollable variations and limitations in total amount of product available. In these studies, recurrence-free survival was significantly improved in patients vaccinated with the planned quality and dose of the vaccine, which could not be achieved in all patients [55]. Continued immunization with booster doses resulted in a better outcome, which would be limited in patients for whom inadequate vaccine could be generated from their tumor [53,54]. As a solution, allogeneic tumor or cell lines that have been well characterized and qualified may have advantages, but experience in colorectal cancer vaccine therapy is limited. A study of CancerVAX, originally designed as an allogeneic melanoma cell vaccine, did demonstrate immunogenicity and higher overall survival in patients with colorectal cancer who experienced an increase in IgM titers against antigen TA90 [56].

Modifications to tumor tissue to enhance immunogenicity seem to increase the anticancer immune response in animal models and human studies. In colorectal cancer, the limited reports regard xenogenation of tumor with Newcastle disease virus, which incites a significant inflammatory response and presumably leads to antigen release from tumors and cross-presentation of antigen by DCs. In studies of patients with various stages of colorectal cancer, immunizations with autologous tumor admixed with Newcastle disease virus resulted in longer survivals and lower rates of relapse than unvaccinated controls [57,58] and were superior to mixing tumor with BCG [59]. Survival was greater among patients who displayed a delayed-type hypersensitivity response to the vaccine [57]. Another method for modifying tumor cells to increase immunogenicity is with genes for cytokines such as granulocyte-macrophage colony stimulating factor

Table 1
Trials using autologous or allogeneic tumor cells or tumor-derived products

Clinical scenario	Study treatment	Clinical data	Immune response	Reference
Stage II, III CRC	Resection + autologous tumor + BCG versus resection	Significant improvement in OS and DFS in colon of patients who received vaccine; no improvement in rectal	DTH+ in 80%	[52]
Stage II, III colon	Resection + autologous tumor + BCG versus resection	RFS significantly longer with vaccine; trend toward improved overall survival for stage II but not stage III	DTH+ in 98%	[54]
Stage II, III colon	Resection + autologous tumor + BCG versus resection	DFS and OS trends in favor of vaccine for patients who received the "intended treatment"	DTH+ in 88%	[53]
Resected stage I–IV CRC	Resection + autologous tumor + NDV versus resection	7-year survival rates for vaccine treated patients were 56.5% versus 43.4% for resection alone, 5-year OS was 80% for those with DTH >5 mm versus 30% for those with indurations <5 mm	DTH+ in >90%	[57]
Resected stage IV CRC	Resection + autologous tumor cells incubated with NDV	Recurrence in 61% of the vaccinated patients versus 87% of a matched control group treated surgically only	DTH+ in 40%	[58]
Stage II, III CRC	Resection plus autologous tumor infected by NDV or admixed with BCG	2-year OS 98% in NDV group versus 67% in BCG group; NDV associated with mild side effects; BCG led to long-lasting ulcers	DTH+ in 68%	[59]
CRC, Resected metastasis	Allogeneic melanoma cell lines (CancerVax) +BCG	Higher overall survival in patients with IgM titers against TA90 >median	DTH+ in 89%, anti-TA90 IgG and IgM Ab detected	[56]
Colon, Resected metastasis	Autologous tumor derived HSP Gp96 (oncophage)	Responders showed significant advantage in OS and DFS over nonresponders	52% developed IFN-γ–producing T cells; within responders, CD3+, CD45RA+, and CCR7– T cells all increased	[60]

Abbreviations: DFS, disease-free survival; DTH, delayed-type hypersensitivity; HSP, heat shock protein; NDV, Newcastle disease virus; OS, overall survival.

(GM-CSF) or IL-2 that are subsequently secreted by the tumor cells after administration, although no studies for patients with colorectal cancer have been reported with this approach. Because tumors contain numerous antigens, some of which would be undesirable to activate immune responses against (if widely expressed in normal tissue) or could potentially have immune inhibitory functions, others have advocated using the most antigenic fraction of tumor cell lysates in the form of heat shock proteins. For example, vaccines based on noncovalent complexes of heat shock protein and peptides seem to derive their activity not from shared but from unique antigens that characterize each individual neoplasm. Heat shock proteins bind to DCs through a unique receptor and are internalized and their antigenic peptides processed and presented. Immune responders to a vaccine that consisted of autologous tumor-derived heat shock protein Gp96 given to patients with resected colon cancer experienced longer overall and disease-free survival compared with nonresponders [60]. The future of this approach remains uncertain because of the failure of a heat shock protein preparation to demonstrate benefit in renal cell carcinoma in a pivotal clinical trial.

Defined tumor protein vaccines

To avoid the need to use tumor cells or their products and to produce a more defined product, vaccines using proteins or immunogenic peptide epitopes known to be overexpressed or uniquely expressed in tumors have been developed. Despite the large number of known tumor antigens, most studies have focused on CEA and epithelial cell adhesion molecule (Ep-CAM; also called GA733–2E antigen, CO17-1A, EGP, KS1-4 and KSA) (Table 2). Ullenhag and colleagues [61] administered recombinant CEA with or without GM-CSF to patients with resected CRC. Immunizations were well tolerated, with only minor local side effects. The magnitude and frequency of the T-cell and IgG responses against CEA were greater in patients who received GM-CSF compared with two thirds of patients who did not receive GM-CSF. Importantly, the immune responses persisted at least 24 months after the last vaccination. Despite these results, producing CEA protein for clinical use is complicated (because CEA is heavily glycosylated and exists in a membrane-bound and secreted form), and few other clinical trials have been reported with this approach (although other forms of CEA, such as peptides and within viral vectors, have been used commonly).

Ep-CAM, which is widely expressed on epithelial malignancies, mediates $Ca2+$-independent homotypic cell-cell adhesions. Its widespread expression on malignancies has suggested it as a target for cancer immunotherapy, but its ability to disrupt the regulatory effects of cadherins leading to increased epithelial proliferation also suggests that targeting this molecule could have growth inhibitory effects. Among several clinical trials using Ep-CAM

Table 2
Trials using tumor proteins

Clinical scenario	Study treatment	Clinical data	Immune response	Reference
Stage I–III, resected CRC	CEA protein ± GM-CSF, + Alum	High, sustained IgG titers correlated with increased survival ($P<.05$)	Significant increase in DTH, proliferative T cells, and IgG in GM-CSF+ versus GM-CSF−	[61]
Resected stage II–IV CRC	Ep-CAM protein or anti-Id mimicking Ep-CAM + GM-CSF	Pts immunized with the Ep-CAM protein produced Ep-CAM-specific IgG antibodies, predominantly IgG1 and IgG3 subclasses, whereas no humoral response was induced by the anti-Id vaccine; similar rates of T-cell response by ELISPOT and proliferation	Overall, 9/13 NED with survivals 16–74+ mo	[62]
CRC, metastatic	Ep-CAM protein formulated with MPL, in liposomes and emulsified in mineral oil, with GM-CSF±	No clinical response	100% DTH+, 64% expressed proliferative T-cell response, 73% Ep-CAM antibody response	[63]
Stage I–III resected CRC, pancreas	Ep-CAM protein + Alum	Median survival (5/6) in CRC was 40 mo, with no reported cancer-related deaths at time of publication In pancreatic patients, median survival was 11 mo, with 5/6 patients dying of recurrent cancer	DTH+ in 42%, 25% demonstrated antigen-specific T-cell response; 50% showed antibody response	[64]

Abbreviations: DTH, delayed-type hypersensitivity; MPL, monophosphoryl lipid A.

protein delivered in Alum and with GM-CSF [62–64] in patients with resected colorectal cancer, encouraging disease-free and overall survivals were documented. Immune responses in the form of anti–Ep-CAM antibody were detected in 50% to 73%, delayed-type hypersensitivity responses in 42% to 100%, and T-cell responses in 25% to 64%. In one study, Ep-CAM protein was compared with anti-Id mimicking Ep-CAM; both activated similar T-cell responses, but humeral immune responses were detected in only the Ep-CAM protein group. As mentioned for CEA, the complexity of producing recombinant protein remains a complicating factor for future studies, and anti-idiotype vaccines have been a more readily developed approach for targeting this antigen (see following discussion).

Monoclonal antibodies and anti-idiotype vaccines

In addition to their more common use as signaling molecule inhibitors (eg, cetuximab) or neutralizers of promalignancy factors (eg, bevacizumab), monoclonal antibodies may be used for passive immunotherapy and as vaccines. Several different monoclonal antibodies have been studied in these roles for the treatment of CRC. The unconjugated mouse antibody 17-1A (muAb 17-1A), an IgG1a antibody that mediates antibody dependent cellular cytotoxicity directed at GA733-2 (Ep-CAM), has been used for passive immunotherapy. In a study conducted by Riethmuller and colleagues [65], 189 patients with Dukes' Stage C CRC were randomized to observation or adjuvant treatment with five injections of muAb 17-1A. A 7-year follow-up revealed that postresection MAb therapy significantly decreased distant metastasis but did not affect the rate of local relapse.

Another monoclonal antibody, MAb 33, which recognizes a 43 kDA cell surface antigen on normal human epithelium of the lower gastrointestinal tract, has been conjugated with either ^{131}I or ^{125}I radioisotopes to deliver targeted radioimmunotherapy to colon cancer cells while sparing normal tissues of intense radiation. In two phase I studies, modest antitumor effect has been observed with either conjugated MAb 33, but bone marrow toxicity was noted to be less in the study using ^{125}I [66,67].

Monoclonal antibodies also have been found to provide an immunizing effect through development of anti-idiotype and anti–anti-idiotype antibodies (and the development of T-cell responses) (Table 3). For example, mAb17-1A (being developed as IGN101) may elicit anti-idiotypic antibodies, which express epitopes that mimic Ep-CAM, and T-cell responses [62,68,69]. The induced anti-idiotypic antibodies then induce anti–anti-idiotypic responses that can recognize the tumor-expressed antigen [70]. In patients with epithelial tumors, vaccination with IGN101 induced antibodies against Ep-CAM and was associated with a significant reduction of circulating Ep-CAM positive cells in the peripheral blood. Immune responders survived significantly longer than nonresponders [71,72]. In

Table 3
Trials using anti-idiotype vaccines

Clinical scenario	Study treatment	Clinical data	Immune response	Reference
Stage II–IV resected or metastatic CRC	Polyclonal goat and rat anti-idiotypes (against CO17-1A, GA733); baculovirus expressed GA733-2E with Alum or KLH	75% of stage II patients treated with polyclonal goat Ab2 GA733 had no evidence of disease after 7–11 years of observation	Ab and T-cell response varied with stage of disease and vaccine	[68]
Stage II–IV resected CRC	Ep-CAM protein or anti-Id mimicking Ep-CAM + GM-CSF	Overall, 9/13 NED with survivals 16–74+ mo	Ep-CAM-specific IgG induced by Ep-CAM protein; no humoral response induced by the anti-Id vaccine; similar rates of T-cell response by ELISPOT	[62]
Stage II–III resected CRC	Human monoclonal anti-idiotypic Ab against mouse 17-4A Ab, mimicking Ep-CAM + Alum (± pertussis toxoid)	No clinical outcome data reported	All patients developed T-cell immunity to extracellular domain of Ep-CAM, 5/6 developed IgG response	[69]
Stage II–IV resected CRC	Anti-Id mimicking CEA (CeaVac) + Alum or QS-21	3/15 with stage II or III progressed at 19, 24, and 35 mo; 7/8 with resected stage IV remained on study from 12 to 33 mo 8/9 with unresected stage IV progressed at 6 to 31 mo	All patients developed proliferative T-cell and IgG response, 48% ADCC	[75]
Stage IV CRC	Goat IgG anti-idiotype vaccine that mimics 17-1a (Ep-CAM) (SCV 106) or unspecific goat IgG	Less disease progression with SCV 106; survival advantage of the SCV 106-treated patients who developed immune response versus controls	67% developed antibody response	[73]
Stage IV CRC	Anti-Id mimicking CD55 (105AD7) + Alum versus placebo	No significant difference in OS	Not indicated	[80]
Stage I–IV resected CRC	Anti-Id mimicking CD55 (105AD7)	65% with no evidence of disease with median follow-up 4 years	Transient CTL, CD8+ and CD4+ response; increase in natural killer activity, CD4+ and CD56+ TIL in 83%	[77–79]

Abbreviations: ADCC, antibody dependent cellular cytotoxicity; ELISPOT, enzyme-linked immunospot.

patients with metastatic CRC, a goat anti-idiotype vaccine that mimicked Ep-CAM was compared in a randomized fashion with unspecified goat IgG [73]. Fewer patients progressed on the idiotype vaccine, and immune responders experienced a longer survival than the control group.

The anti-idiotype antibody 3H1 (CeaVac), a portion of which mimics CEA [74], was studied in a phase Ib trial of 24 patients with advanced CRC. CeaVac induced anti–anti-idiotypic antibodies detectable in the sera from 17 of 23 patients, and 13 of 17 were anti-CEA responses. Although none of the patients had objective clinical responses, overall survival was 11.3 months, which was comparable to other phase II trials for patients with advanced CRC treated with conventional chemotherapy available at the time of this study. In another study, patients with surgically resected colon cancer received CeaVac with or without fluorouracil chemotherapy [75]. All patients generated IgG and T-cell proliferative responses against CEA, unaffected by the fluorouracil. Of note, 3 of 15 patients with Dukes' B and C disease progressed at 19, 24, and 35 months. Preliminary analysis of a phase III study using CeaVac showed a trend toward improved overall survival in patients with metastatic CRC receiving at least five doses of CeaVac versus placebo [76]. Unfortunately, follow-up studies have not been performed.

One other anti-idiotypic antibody, 105AD7, which mimics the tumor antigen CD55, has been tested; however, despite the ability to increase CD4 and CD8+ T-cell responses, it did not improve survival in patients with advanced CRC [77–79]. This study is complicated by the fact that only 50% of patients received the planned vaccine dose [80].

Peptide vaccines

Given the greater complexity of producing proteins compared with peptides, more studies have tested immunogenic peptide fragments of tumor antigens, although most of these studies have been phase I and involved patients with various tumor types (Table 4). Peptide targets have included muc-1 [81,82], SART3 [83], survivin [84], and beta-human chorionic gonadotropin [85]. These studies, which have generally been phase I and included several different tumor types, have demonstrated a wide variation in immune response, and clinical responses have been rare. When peptides were administered alone or as adjuvants, primarily T-cell responses were observed [81,83,84]. When the peptides were conjugated to immunogenic proteins or carbohydrate, antibody responses also were observed [82,85]. More recent clinical trials have included multiple peptide cocktails [86]. These cocktails currently contain epitopes with high HLA binding affinity and immunogenicity, and they include epitopes that are analogs that contain a single substitution that either enhanced major histocompatibility complex binding or stimulated heteroclitic T-cell activation. Helper T-cell epitopes such as PADRE are included. The main limitation in peptide vaccines (in addition to low immunogenicity without additional adjuvants) is HLA

Table 4
Trials using tumor peptides

Clinical scenario	Study treatment	Clinical data	Immune response	Reference
Stage III–IV, resected CRC	β-hCG peptide linked to diphtheria toxin (DT) + nor-MDP	Median survival of patients with ≥median β-hCG Ab titers was significantly higher (45 versus 24 wk) (P = .0002) DT Ab response showed no significant effect	73% (56/77) patients developed antibody response to β-hCG	[85]
CRC, metastatic or locally advanced	SART3 peptides (109-118) and (315-323) + IFA	1 patient showed SD after 5 mo	8% (1/12) of patients produced IgG response, 33% IgE response; 64% and 70% of patients PBCMs showed cellular immune responses to HLA-A24+ colon cancer cells and the vaccinated peptide, respectively	[83]
CRC, metastatic or locally advanced	Survivin peptide (survivin-2B80-88)	Tumor markers (CEA and CA19-9) down in (6/15), one minor responder	DTH response in 40% (6/15), Tetramer+ response in one patient	[84]
CRC breast, other, metastatic, or locally advanced	MUC-1 peptide linked to mannan (im or ip) + cyclophosphamide iv given on weeks 1 and 4	5/41 expressed SD	60% of patients had IgG1 response, with i.p. route giving highest responses, 28% of patients developed cellular response, with proliferative T cells, CTL, and CD8 T cells secreting IFN-γ and TNF-α; DTH existed as microscopic lymphocytic infiltration	[82]
Pancreas, CRC, breast, metastatic, or locally advanced	MUC-1 peptide + BCG	No clinical response	DTH+ in 5%, 80% (44/55) showed some T-cell infiltration, primarily at site of injection site, with 67% expressing intense infiltration; 32% (7/22) showed heightened mucin- specific CTLp	[81]

Abbreviations: CTLp, cytotoxic T lymphocyte precursor; DTH, delayed-type hypersensitivity; β-hCG, beta-human chorionic gonadotropin; IFA, incomplete Freund's adjuvant; TNF, tumor necrosis factor.

dependence for the class I peptides, which limits patients who may be enrolled in clinical trials.

Viral vector vaccines

Viral vectors were designed to overcome the limitations of many other vaccines. For example, they may encode full-length antigen (avoiding HLA limitations and the complexities of producing proteins), they may include additional genes to enhance the immune response (such as costimulatory molecules or "danger signals"), and they may naturally (or be engineered) to target antigen-presenting cells. Adenovirus, adeno-associated virus, and herpes simplex virus have been used for tumor antigen delivery, but the poxvectors (vaccinia, fowlpox, and ALVAC, a variant of canary poxvirus) have been studied extensively in patients with colorectal cancer (Table 5). Because these vectors do not integrate into the genome, there is no risk of insertional mutagenesis, and expression of viral products and transgenes is transient, lasting only 10 to 14 days. The development of these vectors illustrates several principles about the use of viral vectors as cancer vaccines. First, immunization with these vectors (vaccinia-CEA, ALVAC-CEA) can break tolerance to self-antigens in animal models [87] and humans [88–93] without the development of autoimmunity. To enhance the low frequency T-cell responses, costimulatory molecules have been encoded in more recent vectors. A series of recombinant ALVAC or vaccinia viruses that contain the gene that encodes for human CEA and genes for costimulatory molecules such as CD80 (B7.1) have been tested in phase I studies [94–97]. In general, there have been no serious adverse events, and CEA-specific T-cell responses have been documented in a variable number of patients.

Stability of disease and reductions in CEA levels also have been reported. An important observation in more recent studies has been that a priming stimulus with one vector encoding a tumor antigen followed by a series of boosts with a different vector, encoding the same antigen, tends to activate more potent antigen-specific T cells. For example, Marshall and colleagues [96] demonstrated a greater rate of T-cell response in patients immunized with vaccinia-CEA followed by three injections of ALVAC-CEA (VAAA) compared with three injections of ALVAC-CEA followed by vaccinia-CEA (AAAV). A further improvement in the poxvector strategy was to generate poxvectors encoding tumor antigens and a TRIad of COstimulatory Molecules (CD80 (B7.1), CD54 (ICAM-1), and CD58 (LFA-1), designated TRICOM. When used in prime-boost immunization strategies, they activate higher T-cell precursor frequencies. For example, Marshall and colleagues [97] tested the prime-boost strategy with modifications of recombinant vaccinia (rV)-CEA-TRICOM followed by a boost with recombinant fowlpox (rF)-CEA-TRICOM in patients with advanced CEA-expressing malignancies. There was minimal toxicity. One patient had a pathologic complete

Table 5
Trials using Vaccinia or ALVAC-based vectors

Clinical scenario	Study treatment	Clinical data	Immune response	Reference
CRC, other, stage IV NED, or metastatic	Vaccinia-CEA (V) versus ALVAC-CEA (A), + GM-CSF, IL-2	Higher CEA-specific TCR levels after treatment and ratios of post- and pretreatment levels were correlated with increased survival; survival was higher in VAAA versus AAAV	All patients in VAAA cohort expressed CEA-specific T cells versus 40% in AAAV; 22% (4/18) showed CEA-specific IgG response	[96]
CRC, metastatic	Dose-escalation ALVAC–p53	1 patient exhibited SD (7 wk)	Most patients exhibited T-cell and IgG response against vector component of ALVAC; 13% (2/15) showed vaccine-enhanced T-cell immunity to p53	[100,101]
CRC, stage I–III resected	ALVAC–Ep-CAM+ ± GM-CSF	75% (9/12) continued with NED (15–24 mo)	83% of patients in GM-CSF+ demonstrated T-cell response versus 33% in GM-CSF– Responses peaked 4–5 after last vaccination; 100% antibody response to vector, 0% to Ep-CAM	[102]
CRC and others, stage III–IV resected or metastatic	Vaccinia-CEA (full-length or truncated human CEA cDNAs)	Antibodies did not affect patient CEA serum levels	No observed cellular response to CEA, although prolonged in vitro culture of PBL produced CEA-specific CTL lines; 22% (7/32) of patients expressed CEA-specific IgG1 antibodies, 3 of whom also expressed IgM	[88–90]

CRC and others, locally advanced or metastatic	ALVAC–CEA B7.1 ± GM-CSF	44% (11/25) patients experienced SD in GM-CSF+ (maximum 13 mo) versus (6/22) 27% in GM-CSF− (maximum 6 mo)	T-cell responses significantly higher only in pts receiving GM-CSF− [94]
CRC other, metastatic	rF-CEA–TRICOM, rV-CEA–TRICOM, alone or sequentially, ± GM-CSF	1 CR, 40% (23/58) patients with SD, 14 with SD >6 mo; 19% (11) patients showed stable or lower serum CEA levels	77% (10/13) of class I HLA-A2 patients who received all 4 vaccines showed IFN-γ secreting T-cell response, 18% (6/33) showed increased CEA-specific IgG response [97]
CRC, stage IV	Trovax	5/22 patients with SD for 3–18 mo	16/17 showed 5T4-specific cellular responses and 14/17, antibody responses [98]

Abbreviation: PBL, peripheral blood lymphocytes.

response. Stable disease for at least 4 months occurred in 40% of the patients. CEA-specific T-cell responses were of a higher magnitude than demonstrated in their prior studies. We are currently conducting a randomized clinical trial comparing the PANVAC-VF vectors with DCs modified with these vectors in patients with resected hepatic and pulmonary metastases of colorectal cancer.

Vaccinia-based vectors have undergone other manipulations to decrease their pathogenicity, including generation of attenuated strains such as modified vaccinia Ankara. Recently, a modified vaccinia Ankara was modified to deliver the human oncofetal antigen 5T4 (TroVax), which is expressed by CRC. In a phase I study [98], patients with metastatic colorectal cancer who had responded to or stabilized on first-line chemotherapy received escalating doses of TroVax either intramuscularly or intradermally using a Bio-Jector at weeks 0, 4, and 8. Adverse events were nonserious, local reactions at the TroVax injection site. Five of 22 patients showed periods of disease stabilization ranging from 3 to 18 months. Of 17 evaluable patients, 16 showed 5T4-specific cellular responses and 14 showed antibody responses, despite the development of anti–modified vaccinia Ankara neutralizing antibodies. Time to progression was related to 5T4 antibody levels. This study illustrated several important points for further development. First, the vaccine was applied to patients with indolent disease who have the opportunity to respond to a vaccine before disease progression. An important question in immunotherapy studies in general is whether vaccine testing should be limited to patients with minimal residual disease. Second, there was no evidence that vaccination either intramuscularly or intradermally or at various doses induced a substantially stronger or long-lived immune response. This finding confirmed the notion that dose escalation studies for cancer vaccines may be irrelevant and what may be more important is finding ways to augment the immune response or limit the counterresponses that dampen the magnitude of the immune response. Third, the antibody response to the tumor antigen was associated with outcome, which could be caused by immune effects of the antibodies or possibly other inhibitory activities of the antibodies. 5T4 may be associated with tumor mobility, and an antibody against it may limit the aggressiveness of the tumor.

Trovax has been tested further in a phase II trial of vaccine administration before and after liver metastases resection [99]. Local T-cell infiltration that consisted predominantly of CD4 cells was observed in resected tumors. According to proliferation assays, 8 of 16 patients developed proliferative T-cell responses before surgery, and eventually 12 patients developed such responses. Fourteen patients have developed 5T4-specific antibody responses. The clinical benefit of this approach remains to be seen given the small patient numbers, but at a median follow up of 8.4 months, 7 of 16 patients have had disease recurrence.

In summary, viral vectors have significant versatility and may be combined with other viral vectors or peptides in prime boost strategies. The ability to clone in various antigens allows their more rapid translation form one tumor type or system to another [100–102]. Immune responses against some vectors, such as vaccinia, limit their repeat use, but others, such as fowlpox, are not affected by this limitation. The need for an additional level of regulatory review by biosafety committees and the requirement to follow patients' long-term progress does increase the complexity of studies with viral vectors. Numerous studies are underway with viral vectors encoding tumor antigens, and new viral vector platforms, such as alpha-viral particles, are being introduced into the clinic.

Dendritic cell vaccines

Because most vaccine strategies are thought to act through DC uptake and presentation of antigen, vaccines based on antigen-loaded DCs have been under intense scrutiny (Table 6). Phase I studies have generally included various tumor types and have used DCs loaded with CEA peptides [103–106], mRNA encoding CEA [107], Mage 3 peptide [108], and viral vectors encoding CEA [109]. These studies generally have demonstrated safety with few toxicities, modest clinical activity (with a few patients having minor responses or stable disease), and T-cell responses activated against the tumor antigens in as many as 50% to 70% of patients. These studies have provided for testing of other hypotheses. For example, peptide epitopes modified at certain positions to enhance the interaction with the T-cell receptor complex may enhance immune responses. In a small phase I/II clinical trial of DCs pulsed with CEA-derived altered peptide for patients who had predominantly advanced colorectal cancer, enzyme-linked immunospot analysis revealed a vaccine-induced increase in the number of CEA-derived altered peptide-specific IFN-gamma producing CD8+ T cells in five of nine γ and an increase in CD8+ T lymphocytes recognizing the native CEA peptide in three of nine patients [110]. Whether DCs improve upon antigen or viral vector alone as a delivery system is not known and is being tested in an ongoing study at our institution. The recent clinical activity of a DC vaccine in prostate cancer supports further studies with this platform for antigen delivery.

The future of colorectal cancer vaccines and challenges to further development

The availability of numerous tumor antigens, platforms for antigen delivery, and immune modulators supports the promise for development of a successful colorectal cancer vaccine. It is premature to determine which platform will be the most efficacious. A recent meta-analysis of 32 studies of active specific cancer vaccines that together enrolled 527 patients suggested that the best clinical benefit was achieved with autologous tumor vaccines (46%) followed by DC-based (17%) and peptide

Table 6
Trials using pulsed or mRNA transfected dendritic cells

Clinical scenario	Study treatment	Clinical data	Immune response	Reference
CRC, lung, metastatic, or locally advanced	CEA peptide + KLH pulsed DC	Expression of CD8+ T cells correlated significantly with clinical response, ranging from complete response to stable disease ($P = .002$)	58% (7/12) patients showed CTL response, 50% expressed tetramer+ CD8+ T cells (>0.5% staining)	[103]
CRC, metastatic	DCs pulsed with HLAA*0201- or HLA-A*2402-restricted CEA peptides, depending on patient genotype	2 patients responded with SD (12 wk), 1 of whom developed transient decrease in CEA level	70% (7/10) of patients developed CEA-specific T cells	[104]
CRC, gallbladder, metastatic	CEA (CEA652) peptide-pulsed DCs	3 patients responded with SD after vaccination (3, 4, 5 mo)	DTH+ in 12%, 33% IFN-γ–producing cells, 57% (4/7) showed CTL response after vaccination; biopsy showed infiltration at vaccine site; increase in T-cell precursors determined by tetramer assay	[105]
CRC, stomach, lung, metastatic	CEA (CEA652) peptide-pulsed DC	No definitive evidence of decrease in tumor sizes; 3/5 lung cancer patients developed prolonged or large decreases in serum CEA levels	DTH+ in 17% after 5 vaccinations, 18% developed increased CTL response after vaccination	[106]

Colon, stomach, esophagus, metastatic	MAGE-3 (HLA-A2 or A24) peptide-pulsed DC, depending on patient haplotype	Regression was seen in 3 patients, 58% (7/12) showed deceased CA19–9, SCC, or CEA levels	DTH+ in 37% after 4 vaccinations, 50% developed peptide-specific CTL response, 50% (3/6) expressed increased IFN-γ/IL-4 ratio of CD4+ cells	[108]
Stage IV metastatic or resected colon, breast, lung	CEA mRNA-transfected DC ± IL-2	In metastatic patients, 2 MR, 3SD (up to >2 y), 1CR, 8% (2/24) showed decrease in tumor markers (CEA and CA 15-3); in resection patients, 23% (3/13) have NED at >16 mo)	Most patients retained reactivity to recall antigens administered intradermally. In limited comparisons, lymphocyte infiltration and CTL activity observed	[107]
CRC and NSCLC, metastatic	rF-CEA(6D)-TRICOM infected DC	1/14 minor response; 5/14 SD through at least one cycle of immunization (3 mo)	Increase in the frequency of CEA-specific T cells in 10 patients	[109]

Abbreviation: DTH, delayed-type hypersensitivity.

vaccines (13%) [111]. Autologous tumor vaccines have complexities in manufacture that may limit their use. As new generations of vaccines are developed, several considerations will require attention.

First, because chemotherapy is standard in the treatment of colorectal cancer, it is important to demonstrate whether immunizations may be given to patients who are receiving systemic chemotherapy. Weihrauch and colleagues [112] randomized patients with metastatic colorectal cancer to receive three cycles of standard chemotherapy (irinotecan/high-dose 5-FU/ leucovorin) and vaccinations with CEA-derived CAP-1 peptide admixed with different adjuvants. Of 17 patients, 5 had complete responses, 1 had partial response, 5 had stable disease, and 6 had progressive disease, a rate of complete response higher than expected. Despite the chemotherapy, 8 patients (47%) showed elevation of CAP-1–specific CTLs.

Second, although some studies have demonstrated immune responses in patients who have metastatic colorectal carcinoma and failed standard chemotherapy (eg, after immunizations with DCs pulsed with CEA peptides), the study by Liu and colleagues [104] indicated that from a purely numeric standpoint, too many tumor cells may require immune-mediated destruction in patients with advanced disease. Many groups are studying vaccines in the adjuvant setting.

Third, it may be important to choose antigens that have functions important to the cancer cell. Researchers have argued that immunologically targeting proteins without a known protumorigenic function may ultimately fail because tumors could down-regulate these antigens without a detrimental effect to their function. Antigens derived from proteins important for maintaining the tumor may be preferred. Idenoue and colleagues [113] demonstrated that an HLA-A24–restricted antigenic peptide of the inhibitor of apoptosis, survivin-2B80-88 (AYACNTSTL), could be used to activate specific CD8(+) CTL in six of seven (83%) patients with colorectal cancers, but no data were available on whether tumors down-regulated their survivin expression; such data will be important to collect in future studies.

Fourth, the best adjuvant is not well established and may depend on the type of immune response desired. Ullenhag and colleagues [61] immunized 24 patients who had resected CRC without macroscopic disease with recombinant CEA with and without GM-CSF. Patients who received GM-CSF had a 100% rate of immune response (T cell and antibody) against CEA compared with 66% to 75% in the protein alone group. Studies with viral vectors also have suggested a benefit for adding GM-CSF in terms of increases in CEA-specific T-cell precursors compared with no GM-CSF [97]. Weihrauch and colleagues [112] did not note a difference, however, among the ability of GM-CSF/IL2, IL-2 alone, or a CpG-containing DNA molecule to elicite CAP-1–specific immune responses. We are currently conducting a clinical trial comparing DCs infected with poxvectors encoding muc-1 and CEA with the vectors administered with GM-CSF in patients with resected metastases of colorectal cancer.

Fifth, the immune system is "programmed" to down-regulate immune responses once they have become activated to avoid the development of autoimmune disease. Activated T cells experience a negative feedback from tumor-associated regulatory T cells [114]. Multiple types of Treg recently have been discovered. There are CD4+ and CD8+ Treg lymphocytes. The former are subdivided into naturally occurring CD4+/CD25+ cells, Tr1 cells secreting IFN-γ and IL-10, and Th3 cells secreting high levels of transforming growth factor-β, IL-4, and IL-10 [115–117]. They are generated or induced only after antigen priming, which suggests that they can be important mediators of tumor anergy. Several preclinical studies conducted using murine model of colon cancer demonstrated enhanced vaccine-induced antitumor immune responses after depletion of Treg [118,119] using monoclonal antibody against CD25. There has been an intriguing report from a rat colon cancer model that injection of a single dose of cyclophosphamide produced profound depletion of Treg (CD4+/CD25+) [120]. When this was followed by injection of autologous cells mixed with BCG, all animals were cured from the cancer. Depletion of regulatory T cells by cyclophosphamide has been observed in human studies [121]. Other approaches to targeting Tregs that are currently in clinical trials include the immunotoxin denileukin diftitox, which binds to CD25 expressed by Treg. Although there is some debate as to whether Tregs are depleted with denileukin diftitox [122], others have identified an enhanced immune response when it has been combined with a vaccine [123]. We are currently performing a phase I clinical trial of denileukin diftitox followed by DCs modified with a recombinant fowlpox vaccine encoding CEA.

Because CTLA-4 engagement by B7 on antigen-presenting cells decreases T-cell responses to maintain T-cell homeostasis, it has been hypothesized that inhibiting CTLA-4 after immunization would enhance cancer vaccine efficacy. Antitumor vaccination combined with CTLA-4 blockade protects animals against tumor progression [124]. Recently, 11 patients with progressive advanced malignancy after administration of a cancer vaccine (including 3 with colorectal cancer) received the human anti–CTLA-4 monoclonal antibody (ipilimumab) [125]. Two of the patients who had colorectal cancers maintained stable disease and 1 patient experienced progressive disease. The mechanism of activity of the ipilimumab was not clear, however, because there was no increase in vaccine-specific T-cell and CD4$^+$CD25$^+$CD62L$^+$. Tregs, although initially observed to decline, rebounded to levels at or above baseline values at the time of a subsequent infusion. Also, autoimmunity has been observed in animal and human studies after anti–CTLA-4 blockade.

References

[1] Smyth MJ, Dunn GP, Schreiber RD. Cancer immunosurveillance and immunoediting: the roles of immunity in suppressing tumor development and shaping tumor immunogenicity. Adv Immunol 2006;90:1–5.

[2] Gajewski TF, Meng Y, Blank C, et al. Immune resistance orchestrated by the tumor microenvironment. Immunol Rev 2006;213:131–45.

[3] Schreiber RD. Cancer vaccines 2004 opening address. The molecular and cellular basis of cancer immunosurveillance and immunoediting. Cancer Immun 2005;5(Suppl 1):1.

[4] Watt AG, House AK. Colonic carcinoma: a quantitative assessment of lymphocyte infiltration of the periphery of colonic tumors related to prognosis. Cancer 1978;41:279–82.

[5] Jass JR. Lymphocytic infiltration and survival in rectal cancer. J Clin Pathol 1986;39:585–9.

[6] Jass JR, Love SB, Northover JMA. A new prognostic classification of rectal cancer. Lancet 1987;6:1303–6.

[7] Di Giorgio A, Botti C, Tocchi A, et al. The influence of tumor lymphocytic infiltration on long term survival of surgically treated colorectal cancer patients. Int Surg 1992;77:256–60.

[8] Nielsen HJ, Hansen U, Christensen IJ, et al. Independent prognostic value of eosinophil and mast cell infiltration in colorectal cancer tissue. J Pathol 1999;189:487–95.

[9] Ali AA, McMillan DC, Matalka II, et al. Tumour T-lymphocyte subset infiltration and tumour recurrence following curative resection for colorectal cancer. Eur J Surg Oncol 2004;30:292–5.

[10] Pages F, Berger A, Camus M, et al. Effector memory T cells, early metastasis, and survival in colorectal cancer. N Engl J Med 2005;353:2654–66.

[11] Galon J, Costes A, Sanchez-Cabo F, et al. Type, density, and location of immune cells within human colorectal tumors predict clinical outcome. Science 2006;313(5795):1960–4.

[12] Coca S, Perez-Piqueras J, Martinez D, et al. The prognostic significance of intratumoral natural killer cells in patients with colorectal carcinoma. Cancer 1997;79:2320–8.

[13] Fernandez-Acenero MJ, Galindo-Gallego M, Sanz J, et al. Prognostic influence of tumor-associated eosinophilic infiltrate in colorectal carcinoma. Cancer 2000;88:1544–8.

[14] Schwaab T, Weiss JE, Schned AR, et al. Dendritic cell infiltration in colon cancer. J Immunother 2001;24:130–7.

[15] van den Broeke LT, Daschbach E, Thomas EK, et al. Dendritic cell-induced activation of adaptive and innate antitumor immunity. J Immunol 2003;171(11):5842–52.

[16] Suzuki A, Masuda A, Nagata H, et al. Mature dendritic cells make clusters with T cells in the invasive margin of colorectal carcinoma. J Pathol 2002;196:37–43.

[17] Miyagawa S, Soeda J, Takagi S, et al. Prognostic significance of mature dendritic cells and factors associated with their accumulation in metastatic liver tumors from colorectal cancer. Hum Pathol 2004;35:1392–6.

[18] Klimp AH, de Vries EG, Scherphof GL, et al. A potential role of macrophage activation in the treatment of cancer. Crit Rev Oncol Hematol 2002;44(2):143–61.

[19] Ichim CV. Revisiting immunosurveillance and immunostimulation: implications for cancer immunotherapy. J Transl Med 2005;3(1):8.

[20] Shunyakov L, Ryan CK, Sahasrabudhe DM, et al. The influence of host response on colorectal cancer prognosis. Clin Colorectal Cancer 2004;4(1):38–45.

[21] Miyagawa S, Miwa S, Soeda J, et al. Morphometric analysis of liver macrophages in patients with colorectal liver metastasis. Clin Exp Metastasis 2002;19(2):119–25.

[22] Denis M, Ghadirian E. Human monocyte tumouristatic ability: modulation by cytokines and tumour cell products. Int J Immunopharmacol 1990;12(5):509–13.

[23] Kambayashi T, Alexander HR, Fong M, et al. Potential involvement of IL-10 in suppressing tumor-associated macrophages: colon-26-derived prostaglandin E2 inhibits TNF-alpha release via a mechanism involving IL-10. J Immunol 1995;154(7):3383–90.

[24] Maeda H, Kuwahara H, Ichimura Y, et al. TGF-beta enhances macrophage ability to produce IL-10 in normal and tumor-bearing mice. J Immunol 1995;155(10):4926–32.

[25] Reddy GK. The role of immunotherapy in the treatment of colorectal cancer. Clin Colorectal Cancer 2006;5(5):324–6.

[26] Novellino L, Castelli C, Parmiani G. A listing of human tumor antigens recognized by T cells: March 2004 update. Cancer Immunol Immunother 2005;54(3):187–207.

[27] Scanlan MJ, Simpson AJ, Old LJ. The cancer/testis genes: review, standardization, and commentary. Cancer Immun 2004;4:1.

[28] Gnjatic S, Nishikawa H, Jungbluth AA, et al. NY-ESO-1: review of an immunogenic tumor antigen. Adv Cancer Res 2006;95:1–30.

[29] Monte M, Simonatto M, Peche LY, et al. MAGE-A tumor antigens target p53 transactivation function through histone deacetylase recruitment and confer resistance to chemotherapeutic agents. Proc Natl Acad Sci U S A 2006;103(30):11160–5.

[30] Wischnewski F, Pantel K, Schwarzenbach H. Promoter demethylation and histone acetylation mediate gene expression of MAGE-A1, -A2, -A3, and -A12 in human cancer cells. Mol Cancer Res 2006;4(5):339–49.

[31] Tureci O, Chen YT, Sahin U, et al. Expression of SSX genes in human tumors. Int J Cancer 1998;77(1):19–23.

[32] Wagener C, Petzold P, Kohler W, et al. Binding of five monoclonal anti-CEA antibodies with different epitope specificities to various carcinoma tissues. Int J Cancer 1984;33: 469–75.

[33] Finn OJ, Jerome KR, Henderson RA, et al. MUC-1 epithelial tumor mucin-based immunity and cancer vaccines. Immunol Rev 1995;145:61–89.

[34] Mosolits S, Harmenberg U, Ruden U, et al. Autoantibodies against the tumour-associated antigen GA733-2 in patients with colorectal carcinoma. Cancer Immunol Immunother 1999;47:315–20.

[35] Midgley R, Kerr D. Colorectal cancer. Lancet 1999;353:391–9.

[36] Nasif WA, El-Emshaty HM, Tabll A, et al. Immunoreactivity evaluation of mutant p53 gene product with DNA ploidy pattern in colorectal carcinoma. Hepatogastroenterology 2004;51(58):1001–6.

[37] Liang JT, Huang KC, Jeng YM, et al. Microvessel density, cyclo-oxygenase 2 expression, K-ras mutation and p53 overexpression in colonic cancer. Br J Surg 2004;91(3):355–61.

[38] Iacopetta BJ, Welch J, Soong R, et al. Mutation of the transforming growth factor-beta type II receptor gene in right-sided colorectal cancer: relationship to clinicopathological features and genetic alterations. J Pathol 1998;184(4):390–5.

[39] Schwitalle Y, Linnebacher M, Ripberger E, et al. Immunogenic peptides generated by frameshift mutations in DNA mismatch repair-deficient cancer cells. Cancer Immun 2004;4:14.

[40] Rosenberg SA, Yang JC, White DE, et al. Durability of complete responses in patients with metastatic cancer treated with high-dose interleukin-2: identification of the antigens mediating response. Ann Surg 1998;228(3):307–19.

[41] Hawkins MJ, Atkins MB, Dutcher JP, et al. A phase II clinical trial of interleukin-2 and lymphokine-activated killer cells in advanced colorectal carcinoma. J Immunother 1994; 15:74–8.

[42] Dillman RO, Oldham RK, Tauer KW, et al. Continuous interleukin-2 and lymphokine-activated killer cells for advanced cancer: a National Biotherapy Study Group trial. J Clin Oncol 1991;9:1233–40.

[43] Smith RE, Colangelo L, Wieand HS, et al. Randomized trial of adjuvant therapy in colon carcinoma: 10-year results of NSABP protocol C-01. J Natl Cancer Inst 2004;96(15): 1128–32.

[44] Panettiere FJ, Goodman PJ, Costanzi JJ, et al. Adjuvant therapy in large bowel adenocarcinoma: long-term results of a Southwest Oncology Group Study. J Clin Oncol 1988;6(6): 947–54.

[45] Hill M, Norman A, Cunningham D, et al. Impact of protracted venous infusion fluorouracil with or without interferon alfa-2b on tumor response, survival, and quality of life in advanced colorectal cancer. J Clin Oncol 1995;13:2317–23.

[46] Hill M, Norman A, Cunningham D, et al. Royal Marsden phase III trial of fluorouracil with or without interferon alfa-2b in advanced colorectal cancer. J Clin Oncol 1995;13: 1297–302.

[47] Dufour P, Husseini F, Dreyfus B, et al. 5-Fluorouracil versus 5-fluorouracil plus alpha-interferon as treatment of metastatic colorectal carcinoma: a randomized study. Ann Oncol 1996;7:575–9.

[48] Greco FA, Figlin R, York M, et al. Phase III randomized study to compare interferon alfa-2a in combination with fluorouracil versus fluorouracil alone in patients with advanced colorectal cancer. J Clin Oncol 1996;14:2674–81.

[49] Palmeri S, Meli M, Danova M, et al. 5-Fluorouracil plus interferon alpha-2a compared to 5-fluorouracil alone in the treatment of advanced colon carcinoma: a multicentric randomized study. J Cancer Res Clin Oncol 1998;124:191–8.

[50] Wolmark N, Bryant J, Smith R, et al. Adjuvant 5-fluorouracil and leucovorin with or without interferon alfa-2a in colon carcinoma: National Surgical Adjuvant Breast and Bowel Project protocol C-05. J Natl Cancer Inst 1998;90:1810–6.

[51] Ohwada S, Ikeya T, Yokomori T, et al. Adjuvant immunochemotherapy with oral Tegafur/Uracil plus PSK in patients with stage II or III colorectal cancer: a randomised controlled study. Br J Cancer 2004;90:1003–10.

[52] Hoover HC Jr, Brandhorst JS, Peters LC, et al. Adjuvant active specific immunotherapy for human colorectal cancer: 6.5 year median follow-up of a phase III prospectively randomized trial. J Clin Oncol 1993;11:390–9.

[53] Harris JE, Ryan L, Hoover HC Jr, et al. Adjuvant active specific immunotherapy for stage II and III colon cancer with an autologous tumor cell vaccine: Eastern Cooperative Oncology Group Study E5283. J Clin Oncol 2000;18:148–57.

[54] Vermorken JB, Claessen AM, van Tinteren H, et al. Active specific immunotherapy for stage II and stage III human colon cancer: a randomized trial. Lancet 1999;353:345–50.

[55] Hanna MG Jr, Hoover HC Jr, Vermorken JB, et al. Adjuvant active specific immunotherapy of stage II and stage III colon cancer with an autologous tumor cell vaccine: first randomized phase III trials show promise. Vaccine 2001;19:2576–82.

[56] Habal N, Gupta RK, Bilchik AJ, et al. CancerVax, an allogeneic tumor cell vaccine, induces specific humoral and cellular immune responses in advanced colon cancer. Ann Surg Oncol 2001;8:389–401.

[57] Liang W, Wang H, Sun TM, et al. Application of autologous tumor cell vaccine and NDV vaccine in treatment of tumors of digestive tract. World J Gastroenterol 2003;9:495–8.

[58] Schlag P, Manasterski M, Gerneth T, et al. Active specific immunotherapy with Newcastle-disease-virus-modified autologous tumor cells following resection of liver metastases in colorectal cancer: first evaluation of clinical response of a phase II trial. Cancer Immunol Immunother 1992;35:325–30.

[59] Ockert D, Schirrmacher V, Beck N, et al. Newcastle disease virus-infected intact autologous tumor cell vaccine for adjuvant active specific immunotherapy of resected colorectal carcinoma. Clin Cancer Res 1996;2:21–8.

[60] Mazzaferro V, Coppa J, Carrabba MG, et al. Vaccination with autologous tumor-derived heat-shock protein gp96 after liver resection for metastatic colorectal cancer. Clin Cancer Res 2003;9:3235–45.

[61] Ullenhag GJ, Frodin JE, Jeddi-Tehrani M, et al. Durable carcinoembryonic antigen (CEA)-specific humoral and cellular immune responses in colorectal carcinoma patients vaccinated with recombinant CEA and granulocyte/macrophage colony-stimulating factor. Clin Cancer Res 2004;10:3273–81.

[62] Mosolits S, Markovic K, Frodin JE, et al. Vaccination with Ep-CAM protein or anti-idiotypic antibody induces Th1-biased response against MHC Class I- and II-restricted Ep-CAM epitopes in colorectal carcinoma patients. Clin Cancer Res 2004;10:5391–402.

[63] Neidhart J, Allen KO, Barlow DL, et al. Immunization of colorectal cancer patients with recombinant baculovirus-derived KSA (Ep-CAM) formulated with monophosphoryl lipid A in liposomal emulsion, with and without granulocyte-macrophage colony-stimulating factor. Vaccine 2004;22:773–80.

[64] Staib L, Birebent B, Somasundaram R, et al. Immunogenicity of recombinant GA733–2E antigen (CO17-1A, EGP, KS1-4, KSA, Ep-CAM) in gastrointestinal carcinoma patients. Int J Cancer 2001;92:79–87.

[65] Riethmuller G, Holz E, Schlimok G, et al. Monoclonal antibody therapy for resected Dukes' C colorectal cancer: seven-year outcome of a multicenter randomized trial. J Clin Oncol 1998;16(5):1788–94.

[66] Welt S, Scott AM, Divgi CR, et al. Phase I/II study of iodine 125-labeled monoclonal antibody A33 in patients with advanced colon cancer. J Clin Oncol 1996;14(6):1787–97.

[67] Welt S, Divgi CR, Kemeny N, et al. Phase I/II study of iodine 131-labeled monoclonal antibody A33 in patients with advanced colon cancer. J Clin Oncol 1994;12(8):1561–71.

[68] Basak S, Eck S, Gutzmer R, et al. Colorectal cancer vaccines: anti-idiotypic antibody, recombinant protein, and viral vector. Ann N Y Acad Sci 2000;910:252–3 [discussion: 252–3].

[69] Fagerberg J, Steinitz M, Wigzell H, et al. Human anti-idiotypic antibodies induced a humoral and cellular immune response against a colorectal carcinoma-associated antigen in patients. Proc Natl Acad Sci U S A 1995;92:4773–7.

[70] Fagerberg J, Hjelm AL, Ragnhammar P, et al. Tumor regression in monoclonal antibody-treated patients correlates with the presence of anti-idiotype-reactive T lymphocytes. Cancer Res 1995;55:1824–7.

[71] Himmler G, Schuster M, Janzek E, et al. Murine monoclonal antibody 17–1A used as vaccine antigen (IGN101): direct induction of anti-EpCAM antibodies by vaccination of cancer patients. Proceedings of the American Society of Oncology 2003;22:183.

[72] Loibner H, Eller N, Groiss F, et al. A randomized placebo-controlled phase II study with the cancer vaccine IGN101 in patients with epithelial solid organ tumors (IGN101/2–01). Proceedings of the American Society of Oncology 2004;22(14S):2619.

[73] Samonigg H, Wilders-Truschnig M, Kuss I, et al. A double-blind randomized phase II trial comparing immunization with anti-idiotype goat antibody vaccine SCV 106 versus unspecific goat antibodies in patients with metastatic colorectal cancer. J Immunother 1999;22: 481–8.

[74] Foon KA, John WJ, Chakraborty M, et al. Clinical and immune responses in advanced colorectal cancer patients treated with anti-idiotype monoclonal antibody vaccine that mimics the carcinoembryonic antigen. Clin Cancer Res 1997;3:1267–76.

[75] Foon KA, John WJ, Chakraborty M, et al. Clinical and immune responses in resected colon cancer patients treated with anti-idiotype monoclonal antibody vaccine that mimics the carcinoembryonic antigen. J Clin Oncol 1999;17:2889–95.

[76] Titan Pharmaceuticals. Available at: http://www.titanpharm.com/press/CeaVac_PhaseIII_Results.html. Accessed June 4, 2007.

[77] Durrant LG, Buckley DJ, Robins RA, et al. 105Ad7 cancer vaccine stimulates anti-tumour helper and cytotoxic T-cell responses in colorectal cancer patients but repeated immunisations are required to maintain these responses. Int J Cancer 2000;85:87–92.

[78] Durrant LG, Maxwell-Armstrong C, Buckley D, et al. A neoadjuvant clinical trial in colorectal cancer patients of the human anti-idiotypic antibody 105AD7, which mimics CD55. Clin Cancer Res 2000;6:422–30.

[79] Amin S, Robins RA, Maxwell-Armstrong CA, et al. Vaccine-induced apoptosis: a novel clinical trial end point? Cancer Res 2000;60:3132–6.

[80] Maxwell-Armstrong CA, Durrant LG, Buckley TJ, et al. Randomized double-blind phase II survival study comparing immunization with the anti-idiotypic monoclonal antibody 105AD7 against placebo in advanced colorectal cancer. Br J Cancer 2001;84:1443–6.

[81] Goydos JS, Elder E, Whiteside TL, et al. A phase I trial of a synthetic mucin peptide vaccine: induction of specific immune reactivity in patients with adenocarcinoma. J Surg Res 1996;63:298–304.

[82] Karanikas V, Thynne G, Mitchell P, et al. Mannan mucin-1 peptide immunization: influence of cyclophosphamide and the route of injection. J Immunother 2001;24:172–83.

[83] Miyagi Y, Imai N, Sasatomi T, et al. Induction of cellular immune responses to tumor cells and peptides in colorectal cancer patients by vaccination with SART3 peptides. Clin Cancer Res 2001;7:3950–62.

[84] Tsuruma T, Hata F, Torigoe T, et al. Phase I clinical study of antiapoptosis protein, survivin-derived peptide vaccine therapy for patients with advanced or recurrent colorectal cancer. J Transl Med 2004;2:19.

[85] Moulton HM, Yoshihara PH, Mason DH, et al. Active specific immunotherapy with a beta-human chorionic gonadotropin peptide vaccine in patients with metastatic colorectal cancer: antibody response is associated with improved survival. Clin Cancer Res 2002;8: 2044–51.

[86] Ishioka GY, Disis ML, Morse MA, et al. A phase I trial of a multi-epitope cancer vaccine (EP-2101) in non-small cell lung (NSCLC) and colon cancer patients. J Clin Oncol 2004 ASCO annual meeting proceedings. 2004;22(14S):2525.

[87] Kass E, Schlom J, Thompson J, et al. Induction of protective host immunity to carcinoembryonic antigen (CEA) a self-antigen in CEA transgenic mice, by immunizing with a recombinant vaccinia-CEA virus. Cancer Res 1999;59:676–83.

[88] Tsang KY, Zaremba S, Nieroda CA, et al. Generation of human cytotoxic T cells specific for human carcinoembryonic antigen epitopes from patients immunized with recombinant vaccinia-CEA vaccine. J Natl Cancer Inst 1995;87:982–90.

[89] Conry RM, Allen KO, Lee S, et al. Human autoantibodies to carcinoembryonic antigen (CEA) induced by a vaccinia-CEA vaccine. Clin Cancer Res 2000;6:34–41.

[90] Conry RM, Khazaeli MB, Saleh MN, et al. Phase I trial of a recombinant vaccinia virus encoding carcinoembryonic antigen in metastatic adenocarcinoma: comparison of intradermal versus subcutaneous administration. Clin Cancer Res 1999;5:2330–7.

[91] Marshall J, Hawkins MJ, Tsang KY, et al. Phase I study in cancer patients of a replication-defective avipox recombinant vaccine that expresses human carcinoembryonic antigen. J Clin Oncol 1999;17:332–7.

[92] Zhu MZ, Marshall J, Cole D, et al. Specific cytolytic T-cell responses to human CEA from patients immunized with recombinant avipox-CEA vaccine. Clin Cancer Res 2000; 6:24–33.

[93] von Mehren M, Arlen P, Tsang KY, et al. Pilot study of a dual gene recombinant avipox vaccine containing both carcinoembryonic antigen (CEA) and B7.1 transgenes in patients with recurrent CEA-expressing adenocarcinomas. Clin Cancer Res 2000;6: 2219–28.

[94] von Mehren M, Arlen P, Gulley J, et al. The influence of granulocyte macrophage colony-stimulating factor and prior chemotherapy on the immunological response to a vaccine (ALVAC-CEA B7.1) in patients with metastatic carcinoma. Clin Cancer Res 2001;7: 1181–91.

[95] Horig H, Leeds DS, Conkright W, et al. Phase I clinical trial of a recombinant canarypox-virus (ALVAC) vaccine expressing human carcinoembryonic antigen and the B7.1 co-stimulatory molecule. Cancer Immunol Immunother 2000;49:504–14.

[96] Marshall J, Hoyer RJ, Toomey MA, et al. Phase I study in advanced cancer patients of a diversified prime-and-boost vaccination protocol using recombinant vaccinia virus and recombinant nonreplicating avipox virus to elicit anti-carcinoembryonic antigen immune responses. J Clin Oncol 2000;18:3964–74.

[97] Marshall JL, Gulley JL, Arlen PM, et al. Phase I study of sequential vaccinations with fowl-pox-CEA(6D)-TRICOM alone and sequentially with vaccinia-CEA(6D)-TRICOM, with and without granulocyte-macrophage colony-stimulating factor, in patients with carcinoembryonic antigen-expressing carcinomas. J Clin Oncol 2005;23:720–31.

[98] Harrop R, Connolly N, Redchenko I, et al. Vaccination of colorectal cancer patients with modified vaccinia Ankara delivering the tumor antigen 5T4 (TroVax) induces immune responses which correlate with disease control: a phase I/II trial. Clin Cancer Res 2006; 12:3416–24.

[99] Dangoor A, Burt D, Harrop R, et al. A vaccinia-based vaccine (TroVax) targeting the on-cofetal antigen 5T4 administered before and after surgical resection of colorectal cancer liver metastases: phase II trial. J Clin Oncol 2006 ASCO annual meeting proceedings part I. 2006;24(18S):2574.

[100] Menon AG, Kuppen PJ, van der Burg SH, et al. Safety of intravenous administration of a canarypox virus encoding the human wild-type p53 gene in colorectal cancer patients. Cancer Gene Ther 2003;10:509–17.

[101] van der Burg SH, Menon AG, Redeker A, et al. Induction of p53-specific immune responses in colorectal cancer patients receiving a recombinant ALVAC-p53 candidate vaccine. Clin Cancer Res 2002;8:1019–27.

[102] Ullenhag GJ, Frodin JE, Mosolits S, et al. Immunization of colorectal carcinoma patients with a recombinant canarypox virus expressing the tumor antigen Ep-CAM/KSA (ALVAC-KSA) and granulocyte macrophage colony-stimulating factor induced a tumor-specific cellular immune response. Clin Cancer Res 2003;9:2447–56.

[103] Fong L, Hou Y, Rivas A, et al. Altered peptide ligand vaccination with Flt3 ligand ex-panded dendritic cells for tumor immunotherapy. Proc Natl Acad Sci U S A 2001;98:8809–14.

[104] Liu KJ, Wang CC, Chen LT, et al. Generation of carcinoembryonic antigen (CEA)-specific T-cell responses in HLA-A*0201 and HLAA*2402 late-stage colorectal cancer patients after vaccination with dendritic cells loaded with CEA peptides. Clin Cancer Res 2004;10:2645–51.

[105] Matsuda K, Tsunoda T, Tanaka H, et al. Enhancement of cytotoxic T-lymphocyte re-sponses in patients with gastrointestinal malignancies following vaccination with CEA pep-tide-pulsed dendritic cells. Cancer Immunol Immunother 2004;53:609–16.

[106] Morse MA, Nair SK, Mosca PJ, et al. Immunotherapy with autologous, human dendritic cells transfected with carcinoembryonic antigen mRNA. Cancer Invest 2003;21:341–9.

[107] Ueda Y, Itoh T, Nukaya I, et al. Dendritic cell-based immunotherapy of cancer with carci-noembryonic antigen-derived, HLA-A24-restricted CTL epitope: clinical outcomes of 18 patients with metastatic gastrointestinal or lung adenocarcinomas. Int J Oncol 2004;24:909–17.

[108] Sadanaga N, Nagashima H, Mashino K, et al. Dendritic cell vaccination with MAGE pep-tide is a novel therapeutic approach for gastrointestinal carcinomas. Clin Cancer Res 2001;7:2277–84.

[109] Morse MA, Clay TM, Hobeika AC, et al. Phase I study of immunization with dendritic cells modified with fowlpox encoding carcinoembryonic antigen and costimulatory molecules. Clin Cancer Res 2005;11:3017–24.

[110] Babatz J, Rollig C, Lobel B, et al. Induction of cellular immune responses against carci-noembryonic antigen in patients with metastatic tumors after vaccination with altered pep-tide ligand-loaded dendritic cells. Cancer Immunol Immunother 2006;55:268–76.

[111] Nagorsen D, Thiel E. Clinical and immunologic responses to active specific cancer vaccines in human colorectal cancer. Clin Cancer Res 2006;12(10):3064–9.

[112] Weihrauch MR, Ansen S, Jurkiewicz E, et al. Phase I/II combined chemoimmunotherapy with carcinoembryonic antigen-derived HLA-A2-restricted CAP-1 peptide and irinotecan, 5-fluorouracil, and leucovorin in patients with primary metastatic colorectal cancer. Clin Cancer Res 2005;11:5993–6001.

[113] Idenoue S, Hirohashi Y, Torigoe T, et al. A potent immunogenic general cancer vaccine that targets survivin, an inhibitor of apoptosis proteins. Clin Cancer Res 2005;11:1474–82.

[114] Wang RF. Regulatory T cells and innate immune regulation in tumor immunity. Springer Semin Immunopathol 2006;28(1):17–23.

[115] Roncarolo MG, Levings MK. The role of different subsets of T regulatory cells in control-ling autoimmunity. Curr Opin Immunol 2000;12:676–83.

[116] Francois Bach J. Regulatory T cells under scrutiny. Nat Rev Immunol 2003;3:189–98.

[117] Weiner HL. Induction and mechanism of action of transforming growth factor-beta-secreting Th3 regulatory cells. Immunol Rev 2001;182:207–14.

[118] Shimizu J, Yamazaki S, Sakaguchi S. Induction of tumor immunity by removing CD25+CD4+ T cells: a common basis between tumor immunity and autoimmunity. J Immunol 1999;163:5211–8.

[119] Onizuka S, Tawara I, Shimizu J, et al. Tumor rejection by in vivo administration of anti-CD25 (interleukin-2 receptor alpha) monoclonal antibody. Cancer Res 1999;59: 3128–33.

[120] Ghiringhelli F, Larmonier N, Schmitt E, et al. CD4+CD25+ regulatory T cells suppress tumor immunity but are sensitive to cyclophosphamide which allows immunotherapy of established tumors to be curative. Eur J Immunol 2004;34(2):336–44.

[121] Ghiringhelli F, Menard C, Puig PE, et al. Metronomic cyclophosphamide regimen selectively depletes CD4(+)CD25 (+) regulatory T cells and restores T and NK effector functions in end stage cancer patients. Cancer Immunol Immunother 2007;56:641–8.

[122] Attia P, Maker AV, Haworth LR, et al. Inability of a fusion protein of IL-2 and diphtheria toxin (Denileukin Diftitox, DAB389IL-2, ONTAK) to eliminate regulatory T lymphocytes in patients with melanoma. J Immunother 2005;28:582–92.

[123] Dannull J, Su Z, Rizzieri D, et al. Enhancement of vaccine-mediated antitumor immunity in cancer patients after depletion of regulatory T cells. J Clin Invest 2005;115:3623–33.

[124] Kwon ED, Hurwitz AA, Foster BA, et al. Manipulation of T cell costimulatory and inhibitory signals for immunotherapy of prostate cancer. Proc Natl Acad Sci U S A 1997;94: 8099–103.

[125] O'Mahony D, Morris JC, Quinn C, et al. A pilot study of CTLA-4 blockade after cancer vaccine failure in patients with advanced malignancy. Clin Cancer Res 2007;13:958–64.

ELSEVIER
SAUNDERS

Surg Oncol Clin N Am
16 (2007) 901–918

SURGICAL
ONCOLOGY CLINICS
OF NORTH AMERICA

Current Immunotherapeutic Strategies in Lung Cancer

Dominik Rüttinger, MD[a,*],
Rudolf A. Hatz, MD, PhD[a],
Karl-Walter Jauch, MD, PhD[a],
Bernard A. Fox, PhD[b,c,d,e]

[a]Department of Surgery, Laboratory of Clinical and Experimental Tumor Immunology,
Grosshadern Medical Center, Ludwig-Maximilians-University Munich,
Marchioninistrasse 15, 81377 Munich, Germany
[b]Laboratory of Molecular and Tumor Immunology, Robert W. Franz Cancer Research Center,
Earle A. Chiles Research Institute, Providence Portland Medical Center,
4805 NE Glisan Street, Portland, OR 97213, USA
[c]Department of Environmental and Biomolecular Systems, Oregon Health and Science
University, Portland, OR 97239, USA
[d]Department of Molecular Microbiology and Immunology, Oregon Health and Science
University, Portland, OR 97239, USA
[e]OHSU Cancer Institute, Oregon Health and Science University, Portland, OR 97239, USA

Lung cancer is the deadliest cancer in the world. In 2005 in the United States, there were an estimated 163,510 deaths in patients suffering from lung cancer, including 15,000 to 20,000 lifelong nonsmokers [1]. These numbers clearly demonstrate that despite progress in the treatment of this disease over the past two decades, there are still few long-term survivors: only about 10% of all patients will ever be cured of this devastating disease [2].

Only few patients present with resectable tumors, and even these "early stage" patients often relapse, develop metastases, and eventually die of disease. As a consequence, next to surgery and radiation therapy, systemic

This work was supported by the Chiles Foundation, Portland, Oregon, USA, NIH grants CA 80964, CA 119123, and DAMD PC020094, the FöFoLe-program of the Ludwig-Maximilians-University, Munich, Germany, and the Walter-Schulz Foundation, Munich, Germany.

D.Rüttinger was a Chiles Foundation Visiting Fellow. The authors represent the Munich NSCLC vaccine study group.

* Corresponding author.

E-mail address: dominik.ruettinger@med.uni-muenchen.de (D. Rüttinger).

treatment modalities have become a standard component of today's lung cancer management. However, the optimal chemotherapy regimens available (platinum-based regimens consisting of paclitaxel, docetaxel, gemcitabine, or vinorelbine) have demonstrated only limited activity, with median survival rates of less than 11 months and 1-year survival rates of 31% to 36%. Large randomized trials assessing systemic chemotherapy for lung cancer included patients with metastatic disease, who represent the majority of non-small-cell lung cancer (NSCLC) patients [3–5]. Given the modest effect and considerable toxicity of chemotherapy in the adjuvant setting, systemic chemotherapy for lung cancer of all stages is given with limited effect on survival and palliative intent in metastatic disease. Based on these facts, a wide variety of immunotherapeutic agents are currently being tested in lung cancer. However, any categorization of immunotherapeutic approaches is difficult because of frequent overlaps in mechanisms of action.

This article reviews strategies based on the humeral and cellular immune system that are already in clinical use or well progressed in early clinical trials. Because non-small-cell lung cancer accounts for approximately 80% of all lung cancers, the focus is mainly set on immunotherapy of NSCLC.

Antibody-based immunotherapy

For a long time, only a single monoclonal antibody (mAB), muromonab-CD3 (Orthoclone, OKT3) was licensed by the US Food and Drug Administration (FDA). The general reasons for the low therapeutic efficacy of mABs in the fight against cancer were: their immunogenicity in humans because of their murine origin, their short in vivo survival, and the failure to kill target cells efficiently because they failed to fix human complement or elicit antibody-dependent cellular cytotoxicity with human mononuclear cells. In addition, many mABs were not directed against cell-surface structures, such as growth factor receptors. With the development of human or humanized antibodies, and the discovery of antigenic cell-surface targets, these problems have been mostly overcome. Today, at least 12 mABs have received FDA approval and over 400 others are being tested in clinical trials [6]. In lung cancer, a primary focus was put on mABs targeting the epidermal growth factor receptor (EGFR) and the vascular endothelial growth factor (VEGF) (reviewed in Ref. [7]). The most advanced mABs in development are the anti-EGFR mAB cetuximab (Erbitux) and the anti-VEGF mAB bevacizumab (Avastin).

Antibodies targeting growth factors

To block growth factors and their receptors seems an obvious strategy in fighting cancer, because they are known to augment tumor cell proliferation and invasion, and have been shown to be overexpressed in many solid malignancies where the overexpression has been associated with a more aggressive course of disease and poor survival [8]. C-erb B-1 and c-erb B-2 are the two growth receptor families that have been studied most extensively. C-erb B-1 is better known under the name HER1 or epithelial growth factor receptor. HER2 is the more common name for c-erb B-2.

Anti-EGFR (anti-c-erb B-1) monoclonal antibodies

Cetuximab (Erbitux), a chimeric human:murine form of the original mAB 225, has demonstrated safety and was well tolerated in early phase clinical trials, but low patient numbers currently do not allow for final assessment of its therapeutic efficacy in lung cancer. Cetuximab has a 28% partial response rate, and 17% of patients with stable disease were observed in a Phase II trial with combination of cetuximab and docetaxel, which exceeds response rates usually seen with docetaxel alone [9]. In another phase II trial, patients with recurrent or progressive NSCLC were treated with cetuximab after receiving at least one prior chemotherapy regimen [10]. The response rate for all patients (n = 66) was 4.5% and the stable disease rate was 30.3%. The median time to progression for all patients was 2.3 months and median survival time was 8.9 months. The investigators of this study concluded that, although the response rate with single-agent cetuximab in this heavily pretreated patient population with advanced NSCLC was only 4.5%, the disease control rates and overall survival seemed comparable to that of pemetrexed, docetaxel, and erlotinib in similar groups of patients. More Phase I and II clinical trials have been conducted on the use of cetuximab in combination with systemic chemotherapy and radiation therapy, confirming the low toxicity but also the low clinical response rates [11,12]. Grade 3 toxicities associated with the use of cetuximab were fatigue, infections, and papulopustular rash. Development of the rash, usually located on the face and upper torso, has been related to a clinical response and has been suggested to potentially serve as a surrogate marker for cetuximab activity [13].

Other anti-EGFR mABs currently in development include panitumumab (ABX-EGF), matuzumab (EMD 72,000), pertuzumab (2C4), and MDX214 (reviewed in Ref. [14]). Early phase clinical trials with these agents in patients with lung cancer are currently ongoing, with results pending.

Anti-HER2 (anti-c-erb B-2) monoclonal antibodies

Trastuzumab (Herceptin), a humanized monoclonal antibody that targets the HER2 receptor, has been approved for metastatic breast cancer. However, to date, it has failed to demonstrate clinical efficacy in patients suffering from lung cancer [15,16]. Only few investigators suggest further investigation of trastuzumab in HER2-positive lung cancer [17]. In contrast, pertuzumab (2C4), a mAB designed to inhibit the dimerization of HER2 with EGFR and other HER tyrosine kinases, and therefore being independent of HER2 overexpression, is currently under evaluation in NSCLC in early phase clinical trials [14].

Monoclonal antibodies against other growth factors

Other factors relevant for tumor cell proliferation, such as the intercellular adhesion molecule-1 (ICAM-1) [18], have been identified as targets for mABs. Of these, bevacizumab (Avastin), which targets the VEGF, recently gained approval for the treatment of colorectal cancer. A phase II clinical trial using bevacizumab alone, or in combination with chemotherapy, in patients with metastatic NSCLC revealed promising results [19]. Other studies investigated the use of bevacizumab, in combination with the EGFR-tyrosine kinase inhibitor erlotinib (Tarceva) or as combination therapy with paclitaxel and carboplatin in the neoadjuvant setting [20,21]. In the largest trial evaluating bevacizumab, 878 subjects with recurrent or advanced NSCLC (stages IIIB and IV), were included [22]. The median survival was 12.3 months in the group assigned to chemotherapy plus bevacizumab, as compared with 10.3 months in the chemotherapy-alone group. The median progression-free survival in the two groups was 6.2 and 4.5 months, respectively, with corresponding response rates of 35% and 15%. Rates of clinically significant bleeding were 4.4% and 0.7%, respectively.

Active immunization with monoclonal antibodies

In small cell lung cancer (SCLC), an anti-idiotype vaccine targeting the ganglioside GD3 (BEC2) has been evaluated (reviewed in Ref. [23]). A pilot study of BEC2 plus BCG was performed in 15 subjects with both limited and extensive SCLC, following demonstration of a substantial response to chemotherapy. Compared with historical data the median survival was encouraging [24]. The European Organization for Research and Treatment of Cancer recently published data from a phase III trial using BEC2 in combination with induction chemoradiotherapy in limited stage SCLC [25]. A total of 515 subjects were randomly assigned to receive five vaccinations of BEC2 (2.5 mg)/BCG vaccine or follow-up. The primary toxicities of vaccination were transient skin ulcerations and mild flu-like symptoms. There was no improvement in survival, progression-free survival, or quality of life in the vaccination arm. Among vaccinated patients, a trend toward prolonged survival was observed in those who developed a humeral response. The investigators concluded that vaccination with BEC2/BCG has no impact on outcome of patients with limited-disease SCLC responding to combined-modality treatment.

Antibodies linked to cytotoxic agents

To increase their cytocidal potency, mABs are also being linked to cytocidal agents, such as toxins, chemotherapeutic drugs, or radionuclides. Approved for clinical use are drugs such as gemtuzumab ozogamicin (Mylotarg), which links the toxin calicheamicin to a CD33-specific antibody for use in the treatment of myelogenous leukemia, and ibritumomab tiuxetan (Zevalin), which links ^{90}Y to a CD20-specific mAB. To date, the available data on comparable antibodies for the treatment of lung cancer is very limited.

A phase I study investigating the immunotoxin SS1(dsFv)-PE38 is currently ongoing in patients with advanced mesothelin-expressing malignancies. Other Phase I trials evaluated the murine monoclonal antibody KS1/4 linked to methotrexate in patients with NSCLC stages IIIB and IV [26]. In this study, six subjects received KS1/4 alone and five patients received KS1/4-methotrexate conjugate. Mild to moderate side effects in both groups included fever, chills, anorexia, nausea, diarrhea, anemia, and brief transaminasemia. One patient who received antibody alone had an apparent acute immune complex-mediated reaction. Ten of 11 patients had a human antimouse response. Posttreatment carcinoma biopsies revealed binding of monoclonal antibody KS1/4 and deposition of C3d and C4c complement fragments. There was one possible clinical response. Twenty-one subjects (18 relapsed, three primary refractory) with SCLC were entered onto another phase I study investigating the murine mAB N901 that binds to the neural cell adhesion molecule (NCAM, CD56), also found on SCLC cells [27]. Specific binding of the immunotoxin to tumor cells in bone marrow, liver, and lung was observed. No patient developed clinically significant neuropathy. One patient with refractory SCLC achieved a partial response.

Ross and colleagues [28] conducted a phase II study with 59 recurrent or metastatic NSCLC subjects, evaluating survival, safety, efficacy, and quality of life (QOL) of treatment with SGN-15, an antibody-drug conjugate consisting of a chimeric murine monoclonal antibody recognizing the Lewis Y (Le(y)) antigen, conjugated to doxorubicin. SGN-15 plus docetaxel (compared with docetaxel alone) was well tolerated and showed some superiority in survival and QOL analyses. Other strategies consist of radioimmunoconjugates, such as the iodine-131-labeled chimeric tumor necrosis treatment, which has demonstrated some clinical efficacy in advanced NSCLC when given systemically or intratumorally [29].

Other immunoconjugate-based approaches, such as the antibody-directed enzyme prodrug therapy or bispecific antibodies, are currently under investigation and have not found their way into clinical application in patients with lung cancer. Another very interesting strategy for the surgical oncologist may be the technique of radioimmuno-guided surgery, where radio-labelled mABs are used for determination of tumor-free margins [30].

This section has only touched upon the extensive body of data that is available on antibody-based immunotherapy for lung cancer.

Tyrosine kinase receptor inhibitors

Even though, strictly speaking, tyrosine kinase (TK) inhibitors are not components of the humeral or cellular immune system, they should be mentioned in this article because some have progressed in clinical development and are part of anti-EGFR and anti-VEGFR strategies. The most advanced in development are the EGFR-TK inhibitors gefitinib (Iressa) and erlotinib (Tarceva). Gefitinib, a small molecule competing with adenosine triphosphate for binding to the intracellular catalytic domain of tyrosine kinase, is commercially available. Gefitinib was given conditional approval by the US FDA in 2003 for treatment of advanced, chemorefractory NSCLC, but was relabelled for restricted use for patients that were already receiving and benefiting from it, after the negative result of the phase III Iressa Survival Evaluation in Advanced Lung Cancer (ISEL) trial [31]. By contrast, erlotinib, another EGFR tyrosine kinase inhibitor, showed an overall survival benefit compared with placebo and best supportive care in the National Cancer Institute of Canada's BR.21 trial [32], and now has full FDA approval for treatment of patients with NSCLC who have progressed after treatment with chemotherapy. Although the ISEL trial result was negative overall, preplanned subgroup analyses showed a significant overall survival benefit for gefitinib treatment in lifelong nonsmokers and in patients of Asian origin.

Although the currently available EGFR inhibitors represent important advances, the overall magnitude of this benefit has been modest, and most of the time resistance emerges. New agents are currently being tested in Phase I and II studies. These include lapatinib (GW572016), canertinib (CI-1033), EKB-569, HKI272, and with additional anti-VEGFR activity, ZD6474 and AEE788 (reviewed in Ref. [14]).

Table 1 lists antibodies and tyrosine kinase inhibitors currently under clinical investigation for lung cancer.

Therapeutic lung cancer vaccines

In contrast to the prophylactic vaccination against infectious disease or cancers associated with viral infection (cervical cancer, hepatocellular carcinoma), for cancer patients the only relevant vaccination strategy must be therapeutic. Generally speaking, cancer vaccines incorporate a source of tumor antigens combined with some type of adjuvant to make these tumor antigens visible to the immune system. Sources of tumor-associated antigens include whole autologous or allogeneic tumor cells, defined proteins, or specific peptide epitopes (Fig. 1). Most likely because of the heterogeneous histology of lung cancers, the relevant immunologically dominant antigens remain unknown. Therefore, the use of autologous tumor cells might be especially suitable for vaccination strategies in lung cancer, because no prior knowledge of specific tumor antigens is necessary and the induced immunity may not be confined to a single, specific antigen that could be down-regulated by the tumor. Fig. 2 illustrates the mechanisms of action of therapeutic lung cancer vaccines on the cellular level.

Table 1
Monoclonal antibodies and tyrosine kinase inhibitors in clinical development for lung cancer

Agent	Target	Stage of development
Monoclonal antibodies		
Cetuximab (Erbitux)	EGFR	III
Panitumumab (ABX-EGF)	EGFR	II
Matuzumab (EMD 72,000)	EGFR	II
Pertuzumab (2C4)	EGFR-ErbB2 heterodimerization	II
MDX214	EGFR	II
Trastuzumab	HER2 (ErbB2)	I/II
Bevacizumab (Avastin)	VEGF	III
KS1/4-methotrexate	Epithelial-cell derived carcinoma antigen	I
N901-blocked ricin	NCAM (CD56)	I
SGN-15 (-doxorubicin)	Lewis Y antigen	II
Tyrosine kinase inhibitors (TKI)		
Erlotinib (Tarceva)	EGFR-TK	III
Gefitinib (Iressa)	EGFR-TK	III
Lapatinib (GW572016)	EGFR/ErbB2-TK	II
Canertinib (CI-1033)	EGFR/ErbB2/ErbB3-TK	II
HKI272	EGFR/ErbB2-TK	I
ZD6474	EGFR/VEGFR-2-TK	II
AEE788	EGFR/VEGFR-2-TK	II

Nonspecific vaccine approaches

The most advanced nonspecific vaccine approach for NSCLC uses a preparation of killed *Mycobacterium vaccae* in combination with systemic chemotherapy. With this strategy, the nonspecific immune stimulation is supposed to enhance recognition of tumor antigens that are released by chemotherapy-induced tumor destruction. After a small phase II study with 20 previously untreated NSCLC subjects had produced promising results [33], a phase III randomized trial was initiated. With almost 200 advanced NSCLC subjects in the vaccination cohort, this trial failed to demonstrate a survival improvement when compared with combination chemotherapy (mitomycin-C, vinblastine, and cisplatin or carboplatin) alone [34]. Improved quality of life was found in patients randomized to vaccine plus chemotherapy.

Granulocyte-macrophage colony-stimulating factor-secreting, autologous tumor cells

The genetic modification of autologous tumor cells to secrete immunomodulatory cytokines has been shown to induce antitumor immunity in a number of preclinical models. Of these cytokines, Granulocyte-macrophage colony-stimulating factor (GM-CSF) has demonstrated the greatest induction of antitumor immunity [35]. Two early phase clinical trials using GM-CSF-secreting, autologous tumor cells (GVAX) in patients with NSCLC have revealed encouraging preliminary results. Salgia and

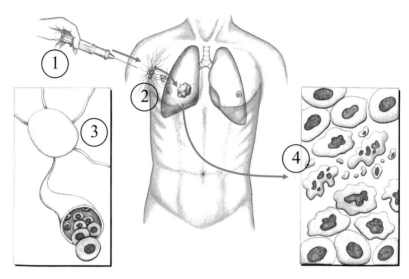

Fig. 1. Therapeutic vaccination in lung cancer. Patients are vaccinated with formulations of tumor antigens (whole tumor cells, proteins, peptides, etc.), mostly subcutaneously or intradermally (1). Antigens are then taken up by antigen-presenting cells (eg, dendritic cells), transported to the draining lymph nodes and presented to the immune system (2). Antigen (tumor)-specific T lymphocytes traffic to the tumor site (3) and elicit their anti-tumor activity (4).

colleagues [36] reported on safety and feasibility of this approach in 33 advanced NSCLC patients, with the most common toxicities being local injection site reactions and flu-like symptoms. A mixed response in one patient and long recurrence-free intervals in two other patients, following isolated metasectomy, were observed. In another phase I and II trial involving patients with early-stage (n = 10) and advanced-stage (n = 33) NSCLC, using the GVAX platform, autologous tumor cells were transduced with GM-CSF through an adenoviral vector (Ad-GM) and administered as a vaccine [37]. Seventy-eight percent of patients developed antibody reactivity against allogeneic NSCLC cell lines. Three durable complete responses were observed. Two of these responses were seen in patients with bronchoalveolar carcinoma. Subset analyses in this trial demonstrated a correlation between the amount of GM-CSF secreted by the vaccine and survival.

In an effort to have high GM-CSF secretion at a constant level, autologous NSCLC cells were mixed with an allogeneic GM-CSF-secreting cell line (K562 cells) ("bystander" GVAX). The Phase I and II trial of this vaccine failed, however, to produce objective tumor responses despite significant increased GM-CSF secretion with 49 subjects vaccinated [38]. While the reason for the failure remains unknown, the significant increase in GM-CSF secretion by the "bystander" GVAX (25-fold higher than the autologous vaccine) may have had a negative effect. In this context, Serafini and colleagues [39] have reported that tumor vaccines that secrete high levels

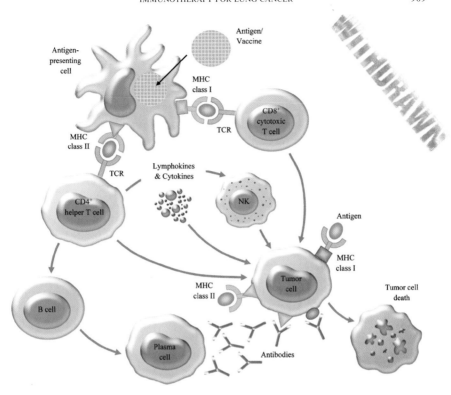

Fig. 2. Induction of an immune response by antigen vaccination. Active immunization occurs following administration of tumor antigens, which are processed by antigen-presenting cells, resulting in activation of immune effector cells, such as T lymphocytes and B lymphocytes. Effector cells fight the tumor through several different effector pathways, such as antibodies, cytokines, or direct cellular interaction. Ideally, this results in immunologic memory with long-lasting immunity against the tumor. MHC, major histocompatibility complex; TCR, T cell receptor.

of GM-CSF induce myeloid suppressor cells that, in turn, inhibit anti-tumor immunity.

Mucin-1 vaccines

Mucin-1 (MUC1) is expressed on the cell surface of many common adenocarcinomas, including lung cancer. Because of its involvement in cell-cell interaction between malignant and endothelial cells, anti-MUC1 strategies may be useful in preventing metastatic spread of tumor cells in addition to their direct anti-tumor effect. A phase I study using a modified vaccinia virus (Ankara) expressing human MUC1, which also contains a coding sequence for human interleukin-2 (IL-2) (TG4010), revealed a safe toxicity profile and some clinical activity [40]. The phase II trial is currently underway as a multicenter study.

MUC1 has also been targeted in another trial of subjects with NSCLC, using the vaccine L-BLP25 (Stimuvax). A multicenter phase IIB study investigating the vaccine in NSCLC subjects with stages IIIB and IV has recently been updated, with promising results for safety and clinical effectiveness in the first publication [41,42]. All subjects had shown stable disease or a clinical response following standard first-line chemotherapy, and were then vaccinated with Stimuvax or received best supportive care alone. Although the overall survival did not reach statistical significance, the survival in patients with stage IIIB (locoregional disease) was improved at 3 years, as compared with stage IIIB patients with malignant pleural effusion and stage IV patients, with 48.6% and 26.7%, respectively. An international, randomized, multicenter phase III trial for unresectable stage III NSCLC subjects with stable disease or better, following first-line chemoradiation, has been initiated, and the first subject has entered the trial in the United States.

Melanoma-associated antigen E-3 protein vaccine

Another protein vaccination strategy aims at the melanoma-associated antigen E-3 (MAGE-3), which is expressed in about 30% to 50% of lung cancers, depending on stage and histologica subtype and may be associated with poor prognosis [43]. First results reporting the successful induction of humeral and cellular immune responses in patients with NSCLC, following vaccination with MAGE-3 with and without adjuvant chemotherapy, have been published in 2004 [44]. Seventeen patients were enrolled following surgical resection with no evidence of disease. Nine patients received 300µg of the MAGE-3 protein alone, whereas 8 patients were treated with MAGE-3 combined with the adjuvant AS02B. In the first cohort (no adjuvant), only one patient showed a $CD4^+$ T cell response. In contrast, 4 patients out of the second cohort (MAGE-3 plus adjuvant) developed $CD4^+$ T cell responses against the MAGE-3 DP4-peptide. Based on these results, a multinational phase II trial investigating the therapeutic efficacy of the MAGE-3 vaccine in subjects with resected MAGE-3-positive stage IB/II NSCLC was initiated and recently completed. In this placebo-controlled study, 122 early-stage subjects (MAGE-3-positive NSCLC) were vaccinated five times at 3-week intervals. Preliminary analyses presented at the 2006 American Society of Clinical Oncology meeting [45] revealed a 33% disease-free survival improvement for the resected and vaccinated subjects. No significant toxicities were observed. A large multicenter phase III study is currently being initiated based on these results.

Non-small cell lung cancer dendritic cell vaccines

For the NSCLC dendritic cell vaccine approach, dendritic cells (DC) as antigen-presenting cells are pulsed with different antigens and administered subcutaneously or intradermally. In a phase I and II clinical trial, 16 subjects with NSCLC stages IB to IIIB were enrolled, after previously being treated with surgery, chemoradiation, or multimodality therapy [46]. Six of these patients showed an antigen-specific response following vaccination (DC loaded with apoptotic bodies of an allogeneic NSCLC cell line overexpressing HER2/neu, MAGE-2, and others); however, the clinical outcome also failed to show a clear correlation with the induced immune responses.

Another DC-based vaccination approach used subcutaneous or intradermal injections of ex vivo generated dendritic cells modified with a recombinant fowlpox vector encoding carcinoembryonic antigen (CEA), and a triad of costimulatory molecules (rF-CEA(6D)-TRICOM) [47]. Only very few lung cancer patients have been treated with this vaccine; however, potent anti-CEA immune responses were observed. Further studies using DC-based vaccines in NSCLC are currently underway.

B7.1 vaccine

To induce a polyvalent immune response, Raez and colleagues [48] are using an allogeneic whole cell-based vaccine expressing the costimulatory molecule B7.1 (CD80). To test this hypothesis, a phase I trial for NSCLC with advanced stages (IIIB/IV) was initiated. Eighteen patients were vaccinated intradermally once every 2 weeks for three cycles, which was repeated three times. All but one patient had a measurable $CD8^+$ T cell response following the third vaccination. One patient showed a partial response, and five patients had stable disease. As of March 2006 (data updated in Ref. [49]), three of five patients who achieved stable disease, and the patient with a partial response, were still alive, with survival ranging from 36 to 63 or more months. This study demonstrated unexpectedly long survival for some patients, which may suggest clinical efficacy of the vaccine, but further investigation is needed (phase II trials are being initiated at the University of Miami).

Other vaccination strategies

More lung cancer vaccines are currently being tested (most recently reviewed in Refs. [49,50]), but review of all strategies in clinical development would go beyond the scope of this article. However, the authors believe some approaches should be mentioned in brief because of their promising early clinical results:

- Belagenpumatucel (Lucanix), a nonviral gene-based allogeneic vaccine that incorporates the TGF-β2 antisense gene into a cocktail of four different NSCLC cell lines [51]
- EP2101 vaccine, a multi-peptide vaccine containing 10 lung cancer epitopes (p53, CEA, HER2/neu, MAGE-2/3) [50]
- Epidermal growth factor vaccine, consisting of human recombinant EGF linked to a recombinant carrier protein from Neisseria meningitides [52,53]

- α(1,3)-Galactosyltransferase (agal), a vaccine made out of three irradiated lung cancer cell lines, gene-modified to express xenotransplantation antigens by retroviral transduction with the murine α-gal gene [54]

Other strategies aim at manipulating the host before vaccination (reviewed in Ref. [55]). The combination of immunotherapy and chemotherapy has been shown to augment the immune response in both preclinical and human trials. Recent preclinical studies suggest an even higher therapeutic efficacy of cancer vaccines if the system had been made lymphopenic and reconstituted with autologous peripheral blood mononuclear cells (PBMC) [55]. Dudley and colleagues [56] combined the adoptive transfer of both $CD4^+$ and $CD8^+$ tumor infiltrating lymphocytes in patients with metastatic melanoma with a nonmyeloablative chemotherapy regimen, and observed impressive clinical response rates. A recent update has 16 of 32 patients experiencing an objective clinical response. Currently, clinical trials are being initiated that transfer parts of this strategy to the treatment of other solid tumors, such as lung cancer, combining preparative chemotherapy with adoptive transfer of peripheral blood T cells and vaccination. A phase I study in patients with NSCLC stages IB-IIIA is currently ongoing in the

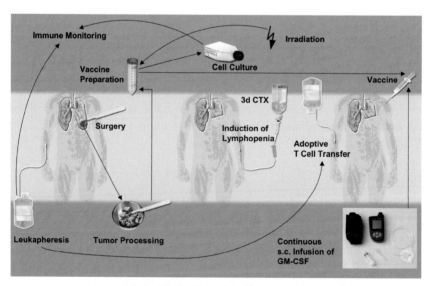

Fig. 3. Clinical trial protocol of combination therapy using preparative chemotherapy, adoptive T cell transfer, and vaccination. Non-small-cell lung cancer patients stages IB-IIIA undergo curative surgery to prepare an autologous vaccine. Immediately following the intradermal vaccination (biweekly, total of up to five vaccinations) GM-CSF is infused subcutaneously for 6 days at a rate of 50 μg per 24-hour period. Before vaccination plus GM-CSF administration, lymphopenia is induced by a 3-day combination chemotherapy (cyclophosphamide 350 mg/m^2 and fludarabine 20 mg/m^2) followed by reconstitution with autologous peripheral blood mononuclear cells. Two additional leukaphereses are harvested pre- and postvaccination for immune-monitoring purposes. CTX, chemotherapy.

Table 2
Therapeutic lung cancer vaccines in clinical development

Phase	Vaccine	No. of patients[a]	Best response[b]	Reference
Autologous/Allogeneic tumor cells				
I	GVAX	34	SD in 5 patients	Salgia et al. [36]
I	GVAX	43	CR in 3 patients	Nemunaitis et al. [37]
I	B7.1 (CD80)	19	PR in 1, SD in 5 patients	Raez et al. [48]
I	α(1,3)-galactosyl-transferase	7	SD in 4 patients	Morris et al. [54]
I	CTX + GM-CSF	4	Under evaluation	Rüttinger et al. [57]
II	Belagenpumatucel-L	75	PR in 15% of patients with stage IIIB/IV disease	Nemunaitis et al. [51]
Protein/Peptide				
I IIB	MUC1	17	SD in 4 patients	Palmer et al. [41]
(Phase III ongoing)	MUC1	88	Sign. advantage for stage IIIB (locoregional)	Butts et al. [42]
I/II	ALVAC-CEA/B7.1	3	No clinical response in phase I	Horig et al. [58]
I	WT1	10	Decreased tumor markers in 3 patient	Oka et al. [59]
I	HER-2/neu	1	No response reported	Salazar et al. [60]
I/II	Telomerase (GV1001/ HR2822)	26	CR in 1 patient, Immunol. response in 13 patients	Brunsvig et al. [61]
II	MAGE-3	17	No response reported	Atanackovic et al. [44]
II (Phase III ongoing)	MAGE-A3	122	Advantage for stage II (adjuvant)	Halmos et al. [45]
II	EGF	40	Seroconversion in 90% of patients, SD in 12 patients	Gonzalez et al. [53]
Dendritic cells				
I	DC rF-CEA(6D)-TRICOM	3	Increase in CEA-specific T cells	Morse et al. [47]
II	DC	16	Antigen-spec. response in 6 patients	Hirschowitz et al. [46]

Abbreviations: CR, complete response; PR, partial response; SD, stable disease.
[a] Number of lung cancer patients on trial.
[b] Clinical or immunological responses.

authors' clinic (Grosshadern Medical Center, Ludwig-Maximilians-University Munich, Germany). These patients receive immunomodulatory doses of cyclophosphamide and fludarabine, and a reinfusion of autologous peripheral blood mononuclear cells (PBMCs), before therapeutic vaccination with irradiated autologous tumor cells in combination with the continuous infusion of GM-CSF at the vaccination site (Fig. 3) [57]. Table 2 [58–61] summarizes therapeutic lung cancer vaccines currently under clinical evaluation.

Summary

For a long time, lung cancer was not considered an immune-sensitive malignancy. Because of this, and because of the insufficient knowledge of relevant tumor antigens, lung cancer immunotherapy lags behind similar efforts in melanoma, renal cell, and prostate cancer. However, there is increasing evidence that NSCLC and SCLC can evoke specific humeral and cellular antitumor immune responses. With increasing knowledge about the link between the induced immune response and a resulting objective clinical response, targeted agents may hold great promise in sequence with other (adjuvant) anti-tumor therapeutics. Obviously, not all of the immunotherapeutic approaches in the treatment of lung cancer can be mentioned in this review. For example, adoptive cell transfer, (immuno)-gene therapy, inducers of apoptosis, certain signal transduction inhibitors, and others (reviewed in Refs. [62–65]) have either not found their way into later clinical development—and therefore, weren't included in the focus of this review—or are in clinical development for small subgroups of lung cancer patients only. Currently active immunotherapy trials for NSCLC and SCLC are published in the National Cancer Institute's Physician Data Query database of cancer clinical trials (http://www.cancer.gov/search/clinicaltrials).

Acknowledgments

The authors wish to thank E. Hanesch and A. Steeger for technical assistance.

References

[1] Thun MJ, Henley J, Burns D, et al. Lung cancer death rates in lifelong nonsmokers. J Natl Cancer Inst 2006;98:691–9.
[2] Krasna MJ, Reed CE, Nugent WC, et al. Lung cancer staging and treatment in multidisciplinary trials: Cancer and Leukemia Group B cooperative group approach. Thoracic surgeons of CALGB. Ann Thorac Surg 1999;68:201–7.
[3] Scagliotti GV, De Marinis F, Rinaldi M, et al. Phase III randomized trial comparing three platinum-based doublets in advanced non-small-cell lung cancer. J Clin Oncol 2002;20: 4285–91.
[4] Schiller JH, Harrington D, Belani CP, et al. Comparison of four chemotherapy regimens for advanced non-small-cell lung cancer. N Engl J Med 2002;346:92–8.
[5] Fossella F, Pereira JR, von Pawel J, et al. Randomized, multinational, phase III study of docetaxel plus platinum combinations versus vinorelbine plus cisplatin for advanced non-small-cell lung cancer: the TAX 326 study group. J Clin Oncol 2003;21:3016–24.
[6] Gura T. Magic bullets hit the target. Nature 2002;417:584–6.

[7] Egri G, Takats A. Monoclonal antibodies in the treatment of lung cancer. Eur J Surg Oncol 2006;32:385–94.

[8] Reissmann PT, Koga H, Figlin RA, et al. Amplification and overexpression of the cyclin D1 and epidermal growth factor receptor genes in non-small cell lung cancer. Lung Cancer Study Group. J Cancer Res Clin Oncol 1999;125:61–70.

[9] Kim ES, Mauer AM, Tran HT, et al. A phase II study of cetuximab, an epidermal growth factor receptor (EGFR) blocking antibody, in combination with docetaxel in chemotherapy refractory/resistant patients with advanced non-small cell lung cancer: final report. Proc Am Soc Clin Oncol 2003;22:642a.

[10] Hanna N, Lilenbaum R, Ansari R, et al. Phase II trial of cetuximab in patients with previously treated non-small-cell lung cancer. J Clin Oncol 2006;24:5253–8.

[11] Robert F, Blumenschein G, Herbst RS, et al. Phase I/IIa study of cetuximab with gemcitabine plus carboplatin in patients with chemotherapy-naïve advanced non-small-cell lung cancer. J Clin Oncol 2005;23:9089–96.

[12] Jensen AD, Munter MW, Bischoff H, et al. Treatment of non-small cell lung cancer with intensity-modulated radiation therapy in combination with cetuximab: the NEAR protocol (NCT00115518). BMC Cancer 2006;6:122.

[13] Perez-Soler R, Saltz L. Cutaneous adverse effects with HER1/EGFR-targeted agents: is there a silver lining? J Clin Oncol 2005;23:5235–46.

[14] Heymach JV, Nilsson M, Blumenschein G, et al. Epidermal growth factor receptor inhibitors in development for the treatment on non-small cell lung cancer. Clin Cancer Res 2006;12:4441s–5s.

[15] Gatzemeier U, Groth G, Butts C, et al. Randomized phase II trial of gemcitabine-cisplatin with or without trastuzumab in HER2-positive non-small cell lung cancer. Ann Oncol 2004; 15:19–27.

[16] Clamon G, Herndon J, Kern J, et al. Lack of trastuzumab activity in non-small cell lung carcinoma with overexpression of erb-B2: 39810: a phase II trial of Cancer and Leukemia Group B. Cancer 2005;103:1670–5.

[17] Langer CJ, Stephenson P, Thor A, et al. Eastern Cooperative Oncology Group Study 2598: trastuzumab in the treatment of advanced non-small-cell lung cancer: is there a role? Focus on Eastern Cooperative Oncology Group Study 2598. J Clin Oncol 2004;22:1180–7.

[18] Finzel AH, Reininger AJ, Bode PA, et al. ICAM-1 supports adhesion of human small cell lung carcinoma to endothelial cells. Clin Exp Metastasis 2004;21:185–9.

[19] Johnson DH, Fehrenbacher L, Novotny WF, et al. Randomized phase II trial comparing bevacizumab plus carboplatin and paclitaxel with carboplatin and paclitaxel alone in previously untreated locally advanced or metastatic non-small-cell lung cancer. J Clin Oncol 2004; 22:2184–91.

[20] Sandler AB, Johnson DH, Herbst RS. Anti-vascular endothelial growth factor monoclonals in non-small cell lung cancer. Clin Cancer Res 2004;10:4258s–62s.

[21] Herbst RS, Johnson DH, Mininberg E, et al. Phase I/II trial evaluating the anti-vascular endothelial growth factor monoclonal antibody bevacizumab in combination with the HER-1/epidermal growth factor receptor tyrosine kinase inhibitor erlotinib for patients with recurrent non-small-cell lung cancer. J Clin Oncol 2005;23:2544–55.

[22] Sandler A, Gray R, Perry MC, et al. Paclitaxel-carboplatin alone or with bevacizumab for non-small-cell lung cancer. N Engl J Med 2006;355:2542–50.

[23] Krug LM. Vaccine therapy for small cell lung cancer. Semin Oncol 2004;31:112–6.

[24] Grant SC, Kris MG, Houghton AN, et al. Long survival of patients with small cell lung cancer after adjuvant treatment with the anti-idiotypic antibody BEC2 plus Bacillus Calmette-Guerin. Clin Cancer Res 1999;5:1319–23.

[25] Giaccone G, Debruyne C, Felip E, et al. Phase III study of adjuvant vaccination with Bec2/bacille Calmette-Guerin in responding patients with limited-disease small-cell lung cancer (European Organisation for Research and Treatment of Cancer 08971-08971B;Silva Study). J Clin Oncol 2005;23:6854–64.

[26] Elias DJ, Hirschowitz L, Kline LE, et al. Phase I clinical comparative study of monoclonal antibody KS1/4 and KS1/4-methotrexate immunoconjugate in patients with non-small cell lung carcinoma. Cancer Res 1990;50:4154–9.

[27] Lynch TJ Jr, Lambert JM, Coral F, et al. Immunotoxin therapy of small-cell lung cancer: a phase I study of N901-blocked ricin. J Clin Oncol 1997;15:723–34.

[28] Ross HJ, Hart LL, Swanson PM, et al. A randomized, multicenter study to determine the safety and efficacy of the immunoconjugate SGN-15 plus docetaxel for the treatment of non-small cell lung carcinoma. Lung Cancer 2006;54:69–77.

[29] Chen S, Yu L, Jiang C, et al. Pivotal study of iodine-131-labeled chimeric tumor necrosis treatment radioimmunotherapy in patients with advanced lung cancer. J Clin Oncol 2005; 23:1538–47.

[30] Bakalakos EA, Burak WE Jr. The radioimmunoguided surgery (RIGS) system as a diagnostic tool. Surg Oncol Clin N Am 1999;8:129–44.

[31] Thatcher N, Chang A, Parikh P, et al. Gefitinib plus best supportive care in previously treated patients with refractory advanced non-small-cell lung cancer: results from a randomized, placebo-controlled, multicentre study (Iressa Survival Evaluation in Lung Cancer). Lancet 2005;366:1527–37.

[32] Bezjak A, Tu D, Seymour L, et al. Symptom improvement in lung cancer patients treated with erlotinib: quality of life analysis of the National Institute of Canada Clinical Trials Group Study BR.21. J Clin Oncol 2006;24:3831–7.

[33] O'Brien ME, Saini A, Smith IE, et al. A randomized phase II study of SRL172 (Mycobacterium vaccae) combined with chemotherapy in patients with advanced inoperable non-small-cell lung cancer and mesothelioma. Br J Cancer 2000;83:853–7.

[34] O'Brien ME, Anderson H, Kaukel E, et al. SRL172 (killed Mycobacterium vaccae) in addition to standard chemotherapy improves quality of life without affecting survival, in patients with advanced non-small-cell lung cancer: phase III results. Ann Oncol 2004;15: 906–14.

[35] Dranoff G, Jaffee E, Lazenbay A. Vaccination with irradiated tumor cells engineered to secrete murine granulocyte-macrophage colony-stimulating factor stimulates potent, specific, and long-lasting anti-tumor immunity. Proc Natl Acad Sci U S A 1993;90:3539–43.

[36] Salgia R, Lynch T, Skarin A, et al. Vaccination with irradiated autologous tumor cells engineered to secrete Granulocyte-Macrophage Colony Stimulating Factor augments anti-tumor immunity in patients with metastatic non-small cell lung carcinoma. J Clin Oncol 2003;21:624–30.

[37] Nemunaitis J, Sterman D, Jablons D, et al. Granulocyte-macrophage colony-stimulating factor gene-modified autologous tumor vaccines in non-small-cell lung cancer. J Natl Cancer Inst 2004;96:326–31.

[38] Nemunaitis J, Jahan T, Ross H, et al. Phase I/II trial of autologous tumour mixed with an allogeneic GVAX vaccine in advanced-stage non-small-cell lung cancer. Cancer Gene Ther 2006;13:555–62.

[39] Serafini P, Carbley R, Noonan KA, et al. High-dose granulocyte-macrophage colony-stimulating factor-producing vaccines impair the immune response through the recruitment of myeloid suppressor cells. Cancer Res 2004;64:6337–43.

[40] Rochlitz C, Figlin R, Squiban P, et al. Phase I immunotherapy with a modified vaccinia virus (MVA) expressing human MUC1 as antigen-specific immunotherapy in patients with MUC1-positive advanced cancer. J Gene Med 2003;5:690–9.

[41] Palmer M, Parker J, Modi S, et al. Phase I study of the BLP25 (MUC1 Peptide) liposomale vaccine for active specific immunotherapy in stage IIIB/IV non-small-cell lung cancer. Clin Lung Cancer 2001;3:49–57.

[42] Butts C, Murray N, Maksymiuk A, et al. Randomized Phase IIB trial of BLP25 liposome vaccine in stage IIIB and IV non-small-cell lung cancer. J Clin Oncol 2005;23: 6674–81.

[43] Gure AO, Chua R, Williamson B, et al. Cancer-testis genes are coordinately expressed and are markers of poor outcome in non-small cell lung cancer. Clin Cancer Res 2005;11: 8055–62.

[44] Atanackovic D, Altorki NK, Stockert E, et al. Vaccine-induced CD4 + T cell responses to MAGE-3 protein in lung cancer patients. J Immunol 2004;172:3289–96.

[45] Halmos BH. Lung cancer II. Presented at the ASCO Annual Meeting Summaries. Atlanta (GA), June 2–6, 2006.

[46] Hirschowitz EA, Foody T, Kryscio R, et al. Autologous dendritic cell vaccines for non-small cell lung cancer. J Clin Oncol 2004;22:2808–15.

[47] Morse MA, Clay TM, Hobeika AC, et al. Phase I study of immunization with dendritic cells modified with fowlpox encoding carcinoembryonic antigen and costimulatory molecules. Clin Cancer Res 2005;11:3017–24.

[48] Raez LE, Cassileth PA, Schlesselmann JJ, et al. Allogeneic vaccination with a B7.1 HLA-A gene-modified adenocarcinoma cell line in patients with advanced non-small-cell lung cancer. J Clin Oncol 2004;22:2800–7.

[49] Raez LE, Rosenblatt JD, Podack ER. Present and future of lung cancer vaccines. Expert Opin Emerg Drugs 2006;11:445–59.

[50] Nemunaitis J, Nemunaitis J. A review of vaccine clinical trials for non-small cell lung cancer. Expert Opin Biol Ther 2007;7:89–102.

[51] Nemunaitis J, Dillman RO, Schwarzenberger PO, et al. Phase II study of LucanixTM (bela-genpumatucel) a transforming growth factor 2 (TGF-beta 2) antisense gene modified alloge-neic tumour cell vaccine in non small cell lung cancer (NSCLC). J Clin Oncol 2006;24: 4721–30.

[52] Ramos TC, Vinageras E, Ferrer MC, et al. Treatment of NSCLC patients with an EGF-based cancer vaccine: report of a Phase I trial. Cancer Biol Ther 2006;5:145–9.

[53] Gonzalez G, Crombet T, Catala M, et al. A novel cancer vaccine composed of human-recombinant epidermal growth factor linked to a carrier protein: report of a pilot clinical trial. Ann Oncol 1998;9:431–5.

[54] Morris JC, Vahanian N, Janik JE, et al. Phase I study of an antitumor vaccination using α-(1,3) galactosyltransferase expressing allogeneic tumor cells in patients with refractory or recurrent non-small cell lung cancer (NSCLC). J Clin Oncol 2005;23(16S):187s [abstract 2586].

[55] Ma J, Poehlein CH, Jensen S, et al. Manipulating the host response to autologous tumor vac-cines. Dev Biol (Basel) 2004;116:93–107.

[56] Dudley ME, Wunderlich JR, Robbins PF, et al. Cancer regression and autoimmunity in patients after clonal repopulation with antitumor lymphocytes. Science 2002;298:850–4.

[57] Rüttinger D, Winter H, van den Engel NK, et al. Preliminary results of a Pilot-Phase I clin-ical trial for lung cancer patients using an autologous tumor cell vaccine following prepara-tive chemotherapy and reconstitution with autologous PBMC. J Immunother 2006;29:655 [abstract].

[58] Horig H, Lee DS, Conkright W, et al. Phase I clinical trial of a recombinant canarypoxvirus (ALVAC) vaccine expressing human carcinoembryonic antigen and the B7.1 co-stimulatory molecule. Cancer Immunol Immunother 2000;49:504–14.

[59] Oka Y, Tsuboi A, Taguchi T, et al. Induction of WT1 (Wilm's tumor gene)-specific cytotoxic T lymphocytes by WT1 peptide vaccine and the resultant cancer regression. Proc Natl Acad Sci USA 2004;101:13885–90.

[60] Salazar LG, Fikes J, Southwood S, et al. Immunization of cancer patients with Her-2/neu-derived peptides demonstrating high-affinity binding to multiple class II alleles. Clin Cancer Res 2003;9:5559–65.

[61] Brunsvig PF, Aamdal S, Gjertsen MK, et al. Telomerase peptide vaccination: a phase I/II study in patients with non-small cell lung cancer. Cancer Immunol Immunother 2006;55: 1553–64.

[62] Hege KM, Carbone DP. Lung cancer vaccines and gene therapy. Lung Cancer 2003;41: S103–13.

[63] Maione P, Rossi A, Airoma G, et al. The role of targeted therapy in non-small cell lung cancer. Crit Rev Oncol Hematol 2004;51:29–44.

[64] Rossi A, Maione P, Colantuoni G, et al. The role of new targeted therapies in small-cell lung cancer. Crit Rev Oncol Hematol 2004;51:45–53.

[65] Rüttinger D, Winter H, van den Engel NK, et al. Immunotherapy of lung cancer: an update. Onkologie 2006;29:33–8.

ELSEVIER
SAUNDERS

Surg Oncol Clin N Am
16 (2007) 919–943

SURGICAL
ONCOLOGY CLINICS
OF NORTH AMERICA

Current Immunotherapeutic Strategies in Pancreatic Cancer

Janet M.D. Plate, PhD

Division of Oncology and Hematology, Department of Immunology/Microbiology,
Rush University Medical Center, 1653 West Congress Parkway,
Chicago, IL 60612, USA

Evidence for immune cell activation by pancreatic tumor cells has accumulated over the past 30 years (reviewed in [1]). Both antibody and cellular responses in patients with pancreatic cancer have demonstrated an immunity specifically directed against antigens expressed on pancreatic tumor cells (Table 1) [2–16]. As early as 1977, studies described active cellular immunity in the majority of patients with pancreatic cancer under study. Studies also demonstrated a specific immunity in patients with pancreatic cancer that was not present in patients with chronic pancreatitis or hepatocellular carcinomas [17–23]. The characterization of the targets of such immunity, tumor-specific antigenic epitopes, was largely accomplished with antibodies, both as a result of immunity induced in patients with pancreatic cancer and by the production of monoclonal antibodies in mice immunized with human pancreatic tumor cell extracts. Antibodies detected in the sera of patients with pancreatic cancer have defined a number of antigenic epitopes that are recognized because they are either overexpressed, underglycosylated, mutated, or inappropriately expressed in their pancreatic tumor cells (Table 2) [24–28]. Inappropriately expressed molecules are often proteins expressed during ontogeny that are turned off in differentiated tissues, then become expressed once again in tumor cells, due to a process of dedifferentiation observed particularly with tumors of epithelial cell origin. This process has come to be characterized as epithelial-to-mesenchymal transition (EMT). Specific immunity to tumors in cancer patients led investigators to postulate that by enhancing preexisting immunity, or by activating broader immune responses to pancreatic tumor antigens, the patients' immune systems might arrest tumor growth or even eradicate the tumors. As antigens expressed by pancreatic tumors were

This work was supported in part by the Wadsworth Foundation.

E-mail address: jplate@rush.edu

1055-3207/07/$ - see front matter © 2007 Elsevier Inc. All rights reserved.
doi:10.1016/j.soc.2007.07.012

Table 1
Immune responses to pancreatic cancer-associated antigens

Type of immunity	Sources of antigen	Antigen identified	Assay	References
Cellular-mediated	Pancreatic tumor extracts, purified GI antigens	Pancreatic tumor-specific sialo-peptide	Leucocyte adherence inhibition (LAI)	[17–22]
Antibody	Pancreatic tumor and cell line extracts	Mucin 1 (MUC1)[a]	Immunohistochemistry	[3–9,39]
Antibody	Ascetic fluid from pancreatic tumor	Span-1	Immunoradiometric	[10–12]
T cell	Synthetic peptides	Mucin 1 (MUC1)[a]	Cell-mediated cytotoxicity	[6,13,14]
T cell	Synthetic peptides	Her2/neu peptides	Cell-mediated cytotoxicity	[15]
T cell	Synthetic peptides	Mutated Ras	Thymidine incorporation	[16]
T cell	Allogeneic, GM-CSF transfected tumor cells	Mesothelin	Epitope binding, Elispot	[2]
T cell	mRNA from pancreatic tumor cells	Unknown, and MHC-associated	Elispot	[94]

[a] Alternatively identified as DF3-reactive antigen CA-15.3, and DU-PAN 2. Commonly referred to as MUC1.

defined, vaccines were developed to boost the patients' immune responses. Many of these vaccines are currently in clinical trials for patients with pancreatic cancer (Table 3) [29–32]. Some of the early phase II trials have shown promise, encouraging further development of vaccines against tumor antigens for clinical trials [33,34].

Table 2
Other antigenic markers associated with pancreatic cancer

Detection agent	Source of antigen	Antigen identified	Assay	References
mAb	Patient serum	SPan-1	Immunoradiometric	[9–11]
mAb	Ascitic fluid from pancreatic tumor	Du-Pan2	Competitive immunoradiometric	[6]
mAb	Tumor cell line	Ca-19.9	Radioimmunoassay	[24]
mAb	Ascitic fluid from pancreatic tumor	MUSE11	Immunohistochemistry	[25,26]
mAb	Membrane-enriched tumor extract	Tag-72	Radioimmunoassay	[27]
mAb	Patient sera	PAO[a]	Immunodiffusion	[28]

[a] Pancreatic oncofetal antigen.

Table 3
Immunotherapy in clinical trials for pancreatic cancer

Type of immune modulator	Agent	Carrier	Phase	Status	References[a]
Vaccines					
Vaccine	MUC1 peptides	SB-AS2	I	Closed	NCT00008099[b]
Vaccine with cytokine	MUC1 peptide-linked to GM-CSF	[c]	II	Not yet accruing	NCT00162500
Vaccine with cytokine	Mutated ras peptide plus GM-CSF			Closed	[54]
Vaccine with cytokine	Pancreatic tumor cells transfected with GM-CSF	Irradiated allogeneic transfected tumor cells	II	Active	NCT00389610
Vaccine with cytokine + mAb	Pancreatic tumor cells transfected with GM-CSF, mAb	Irradiated allogeneic transfected tumor cells + anti-EGFR[d] + chemotherapy	II	Active	NCT00305760
Vaccine	Mutated ras peptides	Saccharomyces Cerevisiae	II	Active	NCT00300950
Vaccine	Alpha (1,3) galactosyl-epitopes	Allogeneic pancreatic tumor cells transfected with α-gal 1,3 transferase	I, II	Active	NCT00255827
Vaccine + cytokine	telomerase peptide GV1001 + GM-CSF (TELOVAC)	[e]Administered in combination with gemcitabine with[f] or without[g] capecitabine	III	Active	NCT00425360 NCT00358566
Vaccine + cytokine	CEA[h] peptide + GM-CSF	Modified peptide CAP1-6D [29] in adjuvant, montanide	II	Active	NCT00203892
Vaccine	CEA + MUC1 + GM-CSF	Recombinant poxvirus[i]	III	Closed	[30]
Cytokines					
Cytokine	GM-CSF	Modified HSV I (OncoVEX)	I	Active	NCT00402025
Cytokine	TNF-α	Replication deficient adenovirus[j] [31]	III	Active	NCT00051467

(continued on next page)

Table 3 (continued)

Type of immune modulator	Agent	Carrier	Phase	Status	References[a]
Monoclonal Antibodies					
mAb	Anti-VEGF[k]	Antibody ± chemotherapy[l,m,n,o,p,q,r,s,t,u,v] Antibody + chemotherapy + radiation therapy[w,x]	II	Active	NCT00366457 NCT00066677 NCT00417976 NCT00307723 NCT00429858 NCT00260364 NCT00410774 NCT00365144 NCT00100815 NCT00126633 NCT00460174 NCT00428324
mAb	Anti-EGFR[y]	Antibody + chemoradiation[z,aa]	II	Active	NCT00338039 NCT00408564
mAb	Anti-EGFR	Antibody + chemotherapy[bb,cc]		Active	NCT00044838 NCT00395252
mAbs	Anti-EGFR and anti-VEGF	Antibody ± chemotherapy[dd]	II	Active	NCT00326911
mAb	Anti-α5β1 integrin[ee]	Antibody+ chemotherapy[ff]	II	Not active	NCT00401570
mAb	Anti-mesothelin[gg]	Antibody	I	Active	NCT00325494
Radio-immunotherapy	Anti-muc1[hh]	Antibody + yttrium Y^{90}	I	Active	NCT00303680
		Antibody + indium I^{111}		Active	NCT00364364
mAb	Anti-CTLA-4[ii]	Antibody	II	Active	NCT00112580

a www.clinicaltrials.gov.

b If reader is online, depress Ctrl key and left-click anywhere in blue highlighted reference to be directed immediately to the clinical trial Web site summary. Otherwise, highlight and copy the reference number, go to www.clinicaltrials.gov, then search; paste reference number in search box and press Enter to reach the online summary of the respective clinical trial.

c Unknown.

d Erbitux (cetuximab) and cyclophosphamide.

[e] Proprietary formulation of vaccine.

[f] NCT00425360.

[g] NCT00358566.

[h] Carcinoembryonic antigen.

[i] PANVAC-VF +TRICOM™. A triad of costimulatory molecules.

[j] TNFerade. Combined with 5-FU and radiation; radiation required as TNF expression is under regulation by a promoter induced by radiation [31].

[k] Bevacizumab.

[l] NCT00366457 combines gemcitabine and erlotinib with bevacizumab.

[m] NCT00066677 tests bevacizumab with or without docetaxel.

[n] NCT00417976 combines infusional 5-FU and gemcitabine with bevacizumab.

[o] NCT00425360 combines gemcitabine with bevacizumab.

[p] NCT00307723 combines 5-FU, oxaliplatin and radiation with bevacizumab, followed by gemcitabine and bevacizumab.

[q] NCT00429858 adds bevacizumab to gemcitabine to evaluate changes in gene expression.

[r] NCT00260364 combines erlotinib and gemcitabine plus capecitabine with bevacizumab.

[s] NCT00410774 combines gemcitabine with bevacizumab after surgical resection.

[t] NCT00365144 combines erlotinib with bevacizumab in patients with metastatic tumors who failed gemcitabine.

[u] NCT00100815 combines gemcitabine and capecitabine with bevacizumab in patients with metastatic or unresectable tumors.

[v] NCT00126633 combines gemcitabine and cisplatin with bevacizumab for patients who have metastatic cancer.

[w] NCT00460174 combines gemcitabine with bevacizumab and radiation for patients who have localized tumor.

[x] NCT00428324 combines gemcitabine with fractionation radiotherapy preoperatively in patients with resectable tumors.

[y] Cetuximab.

[z] NCT00338039 combines gemcitabine and oxaliplatin with cetuximab, followed by chemoradiation.

[aa] NCT00408564 combines gemcitabine and oxaliplatin with cetuximab, followed by surgery or radiation.

[bb] NCT00448838 combines gemcitabine, and oxaliplatin with cetuximab.

[cc] NCT00395252 combines gemcitabine with cetuximab as adjuvant therapy in patients who have resected tumors.

[dd] NCT00326911 combines cetuximab and bevacizumab with or without gemcitabine.

[ee] Volociximab (M200).

[ff] NCT00401570 combined volociximab with gemcitabine.

[gg] MORAb-009.

[hh] DOTA hPAM4.

[ii] Ipilimumab, MDX-010.

Immunotherapy is clearly a rational approach to the treatment of pancreatic cancer, based on the following established findings. The fact that immunity to autologous pancreatic tumors and allogeneic pancreatic tumor cell lines is detected in patients with pancreatic cancer supports the evidence for tumor-associated antigens in pancreatic tumors. Further, these findings support the rationale that the immune systems of pancreatic tumor patients are capable of responding to such tumor antigens. In many cases, not only are lymphocytes from patients with pancreatic cancer capable of recognizing pancreatic tumor antigens, but they are also capable of lysing pancreatic tumor cell targets [1]. Finally, there is evidence for activated but down-regulated T cells within pancreatic tumors, suggesting that pancreatic tumors have evolved immune escape mechanisms (Table 4) [35–38]. These down-regulatory mechanisms must be overcome for immunotherapeutic treatments to be effective in eradicating pancreatic tumors.

Immunotherapy in clinical trials for pancreatic cancer

Vaccines

One of the first antigenic moieties to be defined as expressed in pancreatic cancer cells and not detectable in the healthy pancreas is the mucin

Table 4
Tumor-associated mechanisms of escape from immune surveillance

Pathways triggered to escape from immune attack	Immune activation or immune effector function	Tumor escape mechanism
Decreased MHC expression	Both affected	
Decreased APC function	Immune activation	Soluble MUC1, VEGF
Induction of T-cell anergy, tolerance and/or suppressed functionally	Both affected	TGF-α, TGF-β, IL-10, VEGF, IDO[a]
Induction of regulatory CD4+, CD25+, FOXP3+ T cells [35,36]	Both affected	Prostaglandin E$_2$, TGF-β, IL-10 [37]
Inhibition of T- and NK-cell activity	Immune effector cells	Soluble MICA/B
Decreased CD3 ζ-Chain signaling	Immune effector cells	ROS, IDO [38]
PD-1 signaling	Immune effector cells	Soluble PD-1 ligand
Fas-triggered apoptosis	Immune effector cells	Fas-ligand
Trail-triggered apoptosis	Immune effector cells	Trail ligand
Activated T-cell apoptosis	Immune effector cells	Galectins

[a] Indoleamine 2,3-dioxygenase [32].

Data from Plate JM, Harris JE. Immunobiotherapy directed against mutated and aberrantly expressed gene products in pancreas cancer. J Cell Biochem 2005;94:1069–77; and Rabinovich GA, Gabrilovich D, Sotomayor EM. Immunosuppressive strategies that are mediated by tumor cells. Ann Rev Immunol 2007;25:267–96.

molecule, mucin 1 (MUC1). The MUC1 molecule is normally expressed on the apical surface of healthy epithelial cells and is highly glycosylated. Thus, the protein backbone of this glycoprotein is unexposed to the immune system. During transformation of epithelial cells to cancer cells, MUC1 becomes overexpressed over the entire cell surface with many of the MUC1 molecules becoming underglycosylated, such that its protein backbone becomes revealed [39]. The immune system, which had not been previously tolerized against this self protein, recognizes it as a foreign antigen and develops specifically targeted cytolytic T cells that are detectable in both epithelial-type tumors and the peripheral blood of patients with pancreatic cancer [40]. MUC1 overexpression and underglycosylation is not specific to pancreatic tumors but is observed in many epithelial tumor types. Since immune responses to antigenic epitopes of the MUC1 protein backbone had been detected in patients with pancreatic cancer, a vaccine trial to stimulate enhanced immune responses to MUC1 held great promise [40,41].

The protein backbone of MUC1 contains tandem repeats of 20 amino acids, wherein lies the antigenic epitope recognized by cytotoxic T lymphocytes [42]. A MUC1 vaccine was designed with five of these, linked as tandem repeats, and admixed with SB-AS2 adjuvant to present the 100-mer peptide to boost MUC1-specific immune responses. Clinical trials of this synthetic MUC1 peptide, however, revealed little initial success [43,44]. Although the vaccine plus adjuvant was found to be a safe therapy in a phase I clinical trial, and some changes in immune activities were observed in the vaccinated subjects, the immune activity did not lead to significant changes in survival of these patients as compared with historical survival data. After realizing the importance of presenting a vaccine with an agent that both induces uptake of antigen by dendritic cells and then induces their maturation into effective antigen presenting cells, other investigators directly linked the MUC1 antigenic moiety to an inducing cytokine such as granulocyte macrophage colony-stimulating factor (GM-CSF) (Table 3, NCT00162500). GM-CSF is a myeloid-lineage, specific growth factor that induces maturation of dendritic cells [45]. The current clinical trial using this vaccine is focusing on multiple myeloma patients and is not yet available for patients with pancreatic cancer.

The rationale for the development of most vaccines is grounded in an understanding of the immune system, and how antigens are processed and presented to T cells. The use of ex vivo irradiated, allogeneic tumor cells that are transfected with GM-CSF, for example, is based on the fact that this vaccine triggers a chemokine cascade resulting in the chemotaxis of monocytes, including immature dendritic cells, into the vaccination site to engulf the transfected tumor cells of the vaccine (Table 3, NCT00389610) [46,47]. GM-CSF expressed in the transfected tumor cells then induces maturation of the dendritic cells that are processing the proteins expressed by the phagocytized tumor cells. During the breakdown of the tumor cell proteins in the phagocytes or dendritic cells, cleaved peptides become associated with the subjects' own major histocompatibility complex (MHC), HLA antigens. The HLA-peptide complexes are then transported to the surface membranes of the antigen presenting cells, where they are presented as novel antigens to antigen receptors on T cells and activate specific T-cell immune responses [48,49]. MHC incompatibility with the irradiated, and transfected, allogeneic tumor cells therefore is a non-issue with respect to the ability of tumor antigens to be presented to the recipients, T-cell receptors.

The main assumption of this vaccine is that unknown tumor-specific antigens will be common and shared between in the tumors of unrelated patients. Although this may often be true for pancreatic tumors in which there appears to be a more consistent phenotype between tumors of different patients, the diversity of tumors arising in other tissue types, such as in lung cancer, does not yet lend itself to allogeneic sources as promising for vaccines. Until tumors of other tissue types are grouped into subsets — based on gene expression microarrays, genomic chromosome hybridization arrays, or proteomics — such vaccines would depend upon using the patients' own autochthonous tumor cells. Personalized, autochthonous tumor vaccines are unlikely to be accessible to the general public because of limited availability of tissue and sheer cost of construction of the vaccine. Information gained from genomic expression microarrays has already resulted in the ability to subdivide several tumor types, within a generalized categorization of tumors of a specific tissue or organ, into distinct subtypes, such as in breast cancer and chronic lymphocytic leukemia [50,51]. The reclassification of tumors based on a more similar array of genes expressed defines tumor subtypes that are more like each other and have a greater chance of sharing tumor-specific markers. Thus, allogeneic vaccines created within defined tumor subsets that would benefit each specific subset could eventually be developed.

A mutated ras vaccine, on the other hand, makes no assumptions about the potential that pancreatic tumors express true tumor-specific antigenic epitopes that are not present in the recipients' normal cells, hence would be applicable to all patients whose tumors had specific ras mutations. Greater than 90% of tumors from patients with pancreatic cancer, for example, express a mutated ras gene, most in codon #12, although the nucleotide substitutions may not be identical [52,53]. Clinical trials with mutated ras vaccines require that the patients' tumors be genotyped with respect to the specific mutation site and nucleotide substitution. The use of ras peptides that include the patients' own mutated epitope as a vaccine is a sound approach. In fact, initial clinical trials using a K-ras mutant peptide-based vaccine in combination with GM-CSF showed promise. K-ras peptide-vaccinated patients whose T cells demonstrated antigen-specific responses survived longer than those who did not experience immune responses to K-ras [54].

One criticism of such an approach is that the cytokine, or adjuvant, is merely mixed with peptide and not directly linked to it. Hence, there is no assurance that the activating factor (cytokine or adjuvant) will be available to induce dendritic cell maturation once the patient has ingested the peptide. For an effective and prolonged immune response, peptides must be directly linked to an adjuvant so that they can function within the same antigen-presenting cells. A variety of adjuvants have been used in vaccines for many years. Specific, innate immune cell stimulators or dendritic maturation agents such as GM-CSF, however, have definite advantages over an agent such as alum which is often used in vaccines developed to immunize against childhood diseases. A ras vaccine in current clinical trials, for example, uses yeast expression of the ras mutant protein as an *intrinsic* adjuvant (Table 3, NCT00300950) [55]. Yeast are engulfed quickly by phagocytic cells and also function to induce the maturation of dendritic cells into effective antigen-presenting cells [56]. The probability of inducing tumor-specific responses to the patients' tumors in this trial is increased by the fact that the protocol requires matching of the specific K-ras gene mutation in the tumor with the mutation exhibited in the yeast vaccine administered. The requirement for matching the tumor K-ras mutation with the vaccine, however, may hinder the possibility that these vaccinations will become the treatment of choice in hospitals where genotyping of tumor samples is not yet available. Also, patients whose tumors are not resectable are currently excluded from the clinical trial, as the trial is meant to determine whether the vaccine is effective in limiting the growth of minimal residual disease, and whether it can induce long-term immunity that would destroy newly emerging tumor cells either from tumor stem cells or newly mutated cells. If, in fact, these vaccines are effective in ablating minimal residual disease and providing long-term survival, then extension of the study to determine the value of these vaccines to patients with nonresectable or metastatic disease may be possible. The unfortunate reality, however, is that large tumor masses provide hostile environments for the effective functioning of immune cells and enable tumor escape from immune surveillance [57,58]. Potential ways to circumvent tumor escape from immune surveillance are discussed later in this review (Table 4).

Another approach to attracting dendritic cells and enhancing antigen presentation uses a glycosyl-transferase to modify host tumor cells (Table 3, NCT00255827). The idea here is that anti-species, specific, natural antibodies will induce opsonization of modified tumor cells or cell fragments and serve as an adjuvant to boost immune responses [59]. These natural antibodies comprise 1% of circulating IgG in all humans and are developed in response to α-gal epitopes (Galα1-3Galβ1-4GlcNAc-R) from environmental exposure. The effect of α-gal antibodies is most notably recorded in xenotransplantation as virtually all other nonprimammalian species (excluding apes and old world monkeys) have an α-gal linked to a variety of their proteins including blood group antigens. The natural anti-α-gal antibodies bind to α-gal epitopes expressed on transplanted xeno-grafted tissues like pig, for example, and initiate immediate rejection [60]. Harnessing the power of this xenograft response for protective immunity to tumor cells is the goal of this vaccine. The addition of α-gal epitopes onto tumor cells will target them via antibody-mediated opsonization for uptake and processing by phagocytic cells, including dendritic cells. During processing by phagocytic cells, the tumor proteins, including those containing the α-gal substitutions, are cleaved into peptides. The peptides combine with host MHC, enabling them to be presented as antigens to T cells. Antigen-presenting cells (APC) express both classes of HLA antigens, hence can present antigen to CD4$^+$ helper T cells via MHC-class II and to CD8$^+$ effector T cells via MHC-class I. The interactions of the helper CD4$^+$ T cells with CD8$^+$ effector T cells contribute signals secondary to activation of the T-cell receptor (which is triggered by interaction with the antigen presented by APCs) and assure that these T cells will mature into antigen-specific helper and cytotoxic cells directed against the tumors. Peptides from proteins that are specifically expressed on tumor cells as a result of their transformation from normal cells to cancer cells will then be recognized as foreign, or tumor-specific antigens.

This approach does not require that tumor-specific antigens be defined for a given tumor before preparation of the vaccine. Thus, it overcomes the lack of information regarding tumor-specific antigens expressed on any given tumor. It does, however, require that the patient's tumor be available for α-gal substitution before the vaccine can be prepared and administered. Membrane fragments of the tumor are prepared and, following removal of terminal sialic acid residues with neuraminidase (disialicylation), incubated with a source of galactose and the recombinant enzyme α1,2 galactosyltransferase, so that galactose can be added to available sugar backbones as side chains on proteins and lipids expressed on the tumor cell membranes. Preclinical and animal studies have demonstrated proof of the principle of this approach [59]. Although clinical trials using this approach have been initiated in patients with pancreatic cancer, no data are yet available to verify its validity as a vaccine in these patients.

Proteins that are only expressed during ontogeny and not in adult tissues, but become re-expressed in tumor cells, can be recognized by the immune system and might serve as effective targets for immunotherapy. Earlier, the 20-mer repetitive peptide of the MUC1 protein was discussed as an example of an antigen that the immune system can recognize but does not because it is normally shielded from recognition with extensive carbohydrate side chains. Two other proteins that are frequently overexpressed in cancer cells are the carcinoembryonic antigen (CEA) and the enzyme telomerase. CEA is associated with gastrointestinal tumors and is not specific to pancreatic tumors. A particular epitope from CEA was demonstrated to target activation of CD8$^+$ effector T cells [61]. The amino acid sequence of the CTL epitope was identified and synthesized for use as a vaccine. A clinical trial using this CEA peptide that was modified to enhance immune responses is currently enrolling patients with pancreatic cancer (Table 3,

NCT00203892). Telomerase is expressed in normal hematopoietic cells and telomerase activity is often elevated in a variety of solid tumor cells [62]. A phase I/II trial of a telomerase peptide vaccine, GV1001, demonstrated favorable induction of immune activity, with median survival data indicating a significant survival effect of the vaccine [63]. A phase III trial of telomerase peptide plus GM-CSF as a vaccine, TELOVAC, is currently recruiting patients with pancreatic cancer for administration of the vaccine in combination with chemotherapy (NCT00425360). The discouraging fact about pancreatic cancer, however, is that the statistical significance demonstrated by a particular therapy still does not approach a cure or stabilization of disease progression.

It may seem illogical to combine chemotherapy with a vaccine trial, as chemotherapeutic drugs often inhibit lymphocyte proliferation and are immunosuppressive. Our studies of patients with pancreatic cancer receiving chemotherapy with gemcitabine, however, indicated that there is a window of opportunity during which immune activity may be accelerated [64]. A marker for a CD1a subset of myeloid dendritic cells indicated that gemcitabine had an immediate impact on their circulation in the blood with a significant depression of circulating $BDCA-1^+$ monocytes which rebounded quickly with significant increases in the percentage of $BDCA-1^+$ cells observed after the second and third injections of gemcitabine. The yield of adherent cells obtained by culturing mononuclear cells from the blood of these patients also increased with continued therapy (data not presented). It was apparent in these studies that immune cell activities increased during gemcitabine therapy, with the abilities of unstimulated lymphocytes to produce gamma-interferon in control-cell cultures also increasing (cultures where dendritic cells had not been cultured with tumor-cell RNA). In our data, the increases in background gamma-interferon-producing control-cell responses of cells cultured from blood draws taken following continued therapy were subtracted from the experimental cell cultures, causing it to appear that specific responses as calculated and presented were decreased. In fact, nonspecific hyperactivity with respect to cytokine production resulted from the Gemzar® therapy (data not presented). Augmentation of peptide-specific cytotoxic T-lymphocyte responses against pancreatic cancer cells with vaccines in combination with gemcitabine therapy has also been recently reported [65]. Whether other chemotherapeutic drugs such as capecitabine will have detrimental or supportive effects on responses to vaccines is yet to be determined.

It is our conclusion that by carefully selecting the chemotherapeutic agents or local, targeted, radiation for adjuvant therapy of pancreatic cancer, a combination therapy with immunologic reagents such as vaccines and/or antibody therapies may lead to an effective therapy. One advantage of localized irradiation is that radiation often kills cells by inducing them to undergo programmed cell death via an apoptotic pathway [66]. Apoptotic cells are cleared from the body by phagocytic cells which can then present processed antigen. Apoptosis, however, is a noninflammatory response. This could be a disadvantage for generating immune responses unless local radiation damage results in some level of inflammation. Inflammatory cytokines would then induce phagocytic cells to process molecules from the apoptotic bodies and mature into antigen-presenting cells to induce and/or enhance immune responses to the tumor.

Cytokines

The rationale behind using cytokines for therapy of pancreatic cancer is that cytokines can modify immune responses. While some cytokines such as IL-4, IL-10, or TGF-β can suppress ongoing immune responses and may be useful in treatment of autoimmune diseases, other cytokines can boost various phases of immune responses, such as antigen presentation and induction of responses, expansion of activated T cells, and maturation of effector T cells. The latter types of cytokines have found some effectiveness in cancer therapy. IL-2, for example, affects the growth and expansion of activated T cells. IL-2 is currently being used as an effective immunotherapeutic agent for renal cell cancer but early trials in pancreatic cancer revealed that IL-2 monotherapy was insufficient to accomplish effective responses. Currently, cytokines are being tested in patients with pancreatic cancer largely to aid in the inductive phase of immune responses, or to directly kill tumor cells, rather than in attempts to boost ongoing immune responses in these patients.

The OncoVEX GM-CSF trial uses a conditionally replicative herpes simplex virus (HSV) constructed to express GM-CSF in the local environment (Table 3, NCT00402025). The theory behind the use of OncoVEX GM-CSF is that the HSV will infect and kill tumor cells. During the infective phase, the cotransduced GM-CSF gene will be expressed in the infected cells before they are killed by the virus. It is expected that the dead tumor cells will be phagocytized and the expressed GM-CSF will then induce phagocytic cells to mature to effectively process tumor cell antigens, then present peptides from those tumor cells to T cells to induce the development of immunity specific to the tumor cells. The current clinical trial is for patients who have surgically unresectable pancreatic tumors and requires that the vaccine be injected directly into the tumor by endoscopic ultrasound (EUS)-guided fine needle injection.

The TNFerade trial uses a replication defective adenovirus construct carrying the TNF gene to infect tumor cells (Table 3, NCT00051467). The viral constructs are injected directly into tumors by EUS-guided fine needles. The expression of the TNF gene in these viral constructs is regulated by a chemoradiation-inducible gene promoter. TNF expression therefore only occurs in virally-infected cells after the tumor site has been irradiated. The TNF expressed by the adenoviral constructs is expected to directly kill infected tumor cells. Although TNF has been demonstrated to directly kill tumor cells that express p75, type 2 TNF receptors, TNF cannot be administered systemically as other cells also express either or both p55, type 1 and p75, type 2 TNF receptors, and significant adverse events would result. The endoscopically-guided administration of this therapeutic agent, followed by irradiation focused on the tumor, makes it likely that the expressed TNF will be localized to the tumor site and effect its cytotoxic activity there. As stated above, these clinical trials are limited to patients whose pancreatic tumors are locally advanced and nonresectable.

Antibodies

Although immunotherapy with humanized (or fully human) monoclonal antibodies largely effects passive immunity and does not directly activate the recipient's adaptive immunity to tumor-specific antigens, it has had significant beneficial effects in a variety of tumors, such as with the use of Herceptin in breast cancer, Rituxan in non-Hodgkins' lymphoma, and Erbitux in colon cancer. The effectiveness of some of these monoclonal antibody therapies is dependent upon innate immune cells such as those that are involved in antibody-dependent cell-mediated cytotoxicity (ADCC), while other antibody therapies directly induce death of tumor cells. The induction of adaptive immunity from these therapies depends on the immediate environmental signals with phagocytic cells ingesting and processing killed tumor cells, then maturing into effective APCs to present processed peptides to T cells. Clinical trials with monoclonal antibody therapy in patients with pancreatic cancer are in early phases relative to their use in other cancers (Table 3). Also, unlike treatment for tumors of other tissue types, monoclonal antibodies in most trials for pancreatic cancer are being tested in combination with chemotherapy lutic drugs and/or radiation.

Initial trials of bevacizumab, a recombinant, humanized, monoclonal antibody directed against the vascular endothelial growth factor (VEGF), although initially full of promise because patients had partial responses to this therapy, failed to demonstrate significant prolonged survival of patients with pancreatic cancer [67]. There is now a plethora of clinical trials combining anti-VEGF therapy with chemotherapy with or without radiation and potential surgery (Table 3). VEGF is a pro-angiogenesis growth factor that stimulates blood vessel formation and endothelial cell growth, as evidenced in the neovascularization of a variety of solid tumors [68,69]. Inhibiting VEGF and its ability to induce neovascularization of solid tumors has met with some success in colorectal tumors. The sheer size of pancreatic tumors at diagnosis and the manner in which pancreatic tumor cells grow may indicate that they are less dependent upon vascularization for sustenance. Alternatively, other angiogenesis factors may be more predominant growth factors for vascularization of pancreatic tumors. Current trials with inhibitors of VEGF in pancreatic cancer, therefore, include gemcitabine and/or other chemotherapeutic agents in a variety of combinations (Table 3, NCT00366457, NCT00066677, NCT00417976, NCT00307723, NCT00429858) [70]. There is some evidence that part of gemcitabine function, which is the standard-of-care prescribed drug in pancreatic cancer, may serve to inhibit angiogenesis [71,72]. Three trials, NCT00366457, NCT00260364 and NCT00326911, exemplify the recent trend toward directing therapy at combinations of defined signal transduction pathways either in the same cell or in multiple cell types within a tumor. Bevacizumab, by virtue of its ability to bind to VEGF so that it blocks VEGF from binding to its receptor, prevents the transduction of VEGFR-triggered downstream signals, thereby preventing continued neovascularization and capillary growth in the tumors.

Erlotinib is the combination drug of choice in the NCT00366457 and NCT00365144 trials. Erlotinib is a small-molecule tyrosine kinase inhibitor that blocks the kinase domain of the epidermal growth factor receptor (EGFR) and thereby inhibits the initiation of EGFR signal transduction pathways triggered by EGF or TGF-α. Approximately 60% of pancreatic tumors express elevated levels of EGFR and other members of the erbB family of receptors [73]. Inhibition of the EGFR kinase activity with erlotinib has led to positive responses in patients with pancreatic cancer, and has thus gained FDA approval for its use in combination with gemcitabine as a standard therapy [74]. Erlotinib binds to EGFRs on tumor cells as well as other receptor-positive cells within the site. This broad activity may be a positive feature as the importance of targeting cells within the entire tumor site, including supporting stromal cells, was recently revealed in experimental animal tumor models [75]. Tumor cells that express both the erbB- and VEGF-receptors would be doubly targeted in these trials and perhaps more effectively inhibited from further growth.

Another approach to inhibit signal transduction via ligand-triggered receptors is to use specific antibodies to sterically block the receptor itself and prevent binding of its ligand. Alternatively, with two-chain receptors such as EGFR, the antibodies may sterically block the required dimerization of an EGFR chain with either itself (erbB1), or other members of the erbB family of receptor chains, specifically erbB2 (Her2), or erbB3 (Her3), hence preventing the initiation of a complex set of signals transmitted via these receptors into their cells. The antireceptor form of immunotherapy with a humanized anti-EGFR monoclonal antibody, cetuximab, has met with some success in colorectal cancer and is available in clinical trials for patients with pancreatic cancer (Table 3). Cetuximab is a monoclonal antibody that blocks ligand from binding to the EGFR [76]. Again, most current trials combine cetuximab with gemcitabine either alone (NCT00395252) or with other chemotherapeutic agents and either with or without subsequent radiation and/or surgery. The trial NCT00326911 combines the monoclonal antibodies cetuximab with bevacizumab with and without gemcitabine. Since the mode of actions of the tyrosine kinase inhibitor erlotinib and the anti-EGFR antibody cetuximab differ, the outcomes of trials that combine erlotinib with gemcitabine versus cetuximab with gemcitabine, NCT00366457 and NCT00326911, may differ. Furthermore, clinical trials that use both inhibitors are warranted and could yield significantly promising results [77]. The NCT00338039, NCT00448838, and NCT00408564 clinical trials combine cetuximab and gemcitabine with oxaliplatin with or without surgery. The NCT00338039 trial is more complex as it combines cetuximab with gemcitabine and oxaliplatin as induction therapies, then cetuximab concurrent with radiotherapy and capecitabine, followed by maintenance therapy of cetuximab with gemcitabine. Eligible patients in these latter trials are limited to those with locally advanced pancreatic cancer.

Volociximab (M200), another humanized monoclonal antibody, is directed against α5β1, a cell surface integrin, and was used in phase II clinical trials for therapy of pancreatic cancer (Table 3, NCT00401570). The integrin, α5β1, serves as a receptor for fibronectin and is expressed on growing blood vessels and pancreatic cancer epithelial cells. The humanized chimeric volociximab blocks fibronectin from binding to α5β1. The inhibition of α5β1 function in actively proliferating vascular endothelial cells suggested that volociximab might prevent angiogenesis, and therefore that α5β1 might serve as a therapeutic target [78]. This clinical trial has completed enrollment and awaits further analyses before phase III trials are initiated.

One of the molecules defined as a marker specifically expressed in tumor cells and not in differentiated normal cells is mesothelin (Table 1). Mesothelin is a membrane-associated glycoprotein that is involved in cell adhesion and appears to be associated with a variety of cancers including pancreatic cancer. Mesothelin was detected as a target antigen for T-cell—mediated cytotoxicity of lymphocytes isolated from peripheral blood of patients with pancreatic cancer vaccinated with allogeneic tumor cells transfected with GM-CSF [2]. A high-affinity monoclonal antibody was raised against human mesothelin, then humanized for potential therapeutic purposes, MORAb-009. A phase I trial in patients with mesothelin-expressing tumors, including pancreatic cancer, is underway to determine the safety and pharmacokinetics of this antibody (NCT00325494). Preclinical experimental indicators are that MORAb-009 is a potentially useful anti-cancer agent.

Another tumor cell marker discussed earlier is the underglycosylated MUC1 molecule (Tables 1 and 3). Investigators have conjugated radioisotopes yttrium Y^{90} or indium I^{111} to a humanized monoclonal antibody directed against the MUC1 protein backbone (hPAM4). The purposes of current studies are to evaluate safety, biodistribution and targeting of the hPAM4 (NCT00364364) as well as the safety, and dosimetry of conjugated mAb for therapy (NCT00303680). These interesting phase I trials should allow for the determination of the validity of the use of a humanized MUC1 monoclonal antibody for specifically targeting pancreatic tumors with radio-tags.

The final monoclonal antibody discussed here is not directed at pancreatic tumors but at an immunoregulatory molecule expressed on activated T cells, cytotoxic T lymphocyte-associated antigen 4 (CTLA-4) (Table 3, NCT00112580). CTLA-4 is a cell membrane-spanning receptor expressed on activated T cells (CD152) that is triggered by its cognate B7 ligands (CD80, CD86) to down-regulate the cells' immune functions [79]. CTLA-4 is also used by T cells to regulate their own proliferation so that they do not overpopulate the immune system, or give rise to lymphoproliferative diseases. Autonomous regulation of activated T cells via CTLA-4 plays a role in preventing autoimmunity. This became particularly evident in CTLA-4 knock-out mice that lack expression of CTLA-4. Homozygous CTLA-4-deficient animals have lymphoproliferative and autoimmune diseases [80]. The purpose behind the clinical application of an antibody directed against CTLA-4 is to block activation of the CTLA-4 pathway in a variety of disease states. As stated in the introduction, there is substantial evidence that immune T cells are activated against tumor-specific antigens in most patients with pancreatic cancer. Yet, these immune T cells are not capable of eradicating the cancer. In fact, tumor cells can evade and escape activated immune T cells using a number of different mechanisms (Table 4) [57,58].

One mechanism that prevents mature, tumor-specific, immune effector T cells from killing tumor cells is the activation of CTLA-4 on their cell surfaces. The anti-CTLA-4 antibodies block CTLA-4 activation, allowing immune T cells to proliferate, produce cytokines, and function as immune effectors. Because activated, immune T cells migrate into tumors but are down-regulated by tumor cells or their products, one potential mechanism to re-engage immune T cells' function is to block CTLA-4. Ipilimumab (MDX-010) is a fully human, monoclonal antibody directed against CTLA-4 that inhibits the down-regulation and inactivation of immune T cells via CTLA-4. There is evidence from studies of cancers originating in other organ types that this reagent can indeed have beneficial effects in cancer patients [81,82]. However, the value of the anti-CTLA-4 reagent may not be as a single agent; its effects may be more evident in clinical trials where it is used in combination with a tumor vaccine or other drugs expected to activate or expand immune responses to the tumor.

Other immunotherapies under experimental investigation

A number of potentially promising approaches are currently being studied for immunotherapeutic use in a variety of solid tumors, including pancreatic cancer. While an extensive review of all areas of investigation will not be attempted here, those mentioned here should be followed for their potential future inclusion in clinical trials. Dendritic cell vaccines are one example. Investigators have been able to isolate immature dendritic cells and grow them in culture with the cytokines GM-CSF and IL-4 [83]. These immature dendritic cells readily take up molecules added to their cultures, including proteins in cell lysates, apoptotic cells, purified peptides, viral vector constructs, or naked RNA. After allowing time for enzymatic protein processing, the dendritic cells are then induced to mature through the addition of cytokines, including interferon gamma and a variety of other agents. These mature, antigen-presenting dendritic cells can serve to present peptides as vaccines upon administration to histocompatible or autologus recipients. Clinical trials using dendritic cell-based vaccines, including some studies with pancreatic cancer, have been widely reported in cancer literature [84]. T-cell responses to tumor-specific antigens have been demonstrated when these dendritic cell-based vaccines are administered to cancer patients [84–87].

One molecule currently being targeted for therapy by several different approaches, including dendritic cell vaccines, is survivin. Survivin is an intracellular protein involved in cytokinesis and has anti-apoptotic functions [88]. Survivin is overexpressed in a variety of tumors, particularly those of the gastrointestinal tract [89–91]. A number of studies have used dendritic cell-based vaccines of either full-length survivin protein or survivin peptides [92,93]. Indeed, one report is a single case study in which complete remission of liver metastases of pancreatic cancer was observed in a patient whose cancer was refractory to gemcitabine therapy and endured for 8 months following vaccinations of dendritic cells loaded with survivin peptide [93]. In another case, vaccination with dendritic cells loaded with allogeneic lysates of pancreatic tumor cells resulted in stabilization of disease for 6 months [87]. Antigen-specific T cells were demonstrated in another study of patients with pancreatic cancer whose T cells were stimulated with autologous, matured dendritic cells transfected with total tumor mRNA [94]. While these studies suggest that dendritic cell vaccines are a potential approach to therapy, their validity awaits controlled clinical trials.

For T cells to expand and differentiate into immune effector cells, they need to be stimulated with growth factors after TCR recognition of antigen. Interleukin-2 (IL-2) is a cytokine that engages receptors on antigen-activated T cells and drives their proliferation. IL-2 also can counteract some down-regulatory signals that turn off T-cell functions. Low-dose therapy with IL-2 has been shown to be tolerable and to elevate immune responses in patients. In one study, low-dose IL-2 was given preoperatively to a group of patients with pancreatic cancer followed by pancreatico-duodenectomy without any neoadjuvant therapy. The patients receiving preoperative low-dose IL-2 had fewer postoperative complications than a well-matched group of control subjects. Two-year survival of patients receiving low-dose IL-2 was significantly greater (33%) than the control group (10%) [95]. These findings support the argument that the immune system can be modulated effectively to combat tumors.

Patients with pancreatic cancer may also benefit from the use of immune modulators such as drugs that target and activate APCs. One means of APC activation is via Toll-like receptors (TLRs) which are expressed on innate immune and inflammatory cells [96]. A number of companies are developing drugs to serve as specific ligands for the respective TLRs, some of which down-regulate while others up-regulate cellular immune responses. It is particularly intriguing to note recent studies which demonstrate that the small molecule kinase inhibitor, Gleevec (Imatinib Mesylate), by virtue of its inhibition of the PDGF receptor kinase in APCs, can up-regulate immune T-cell activation [97]. Manipulating signal transduction pathways in APCs thus may be a realistic target for cancer therapy. While these are all exciting observations for basic scientists and translational investigators, the challenge for us is to find the right combination of agents to counter the tumors' ability to evade immune effectors, and to bolster tumor-specific immune responses (Table 4). The potential translation of these findings to patients with pancreatic cancer requires further experimentation.

Decisions, decisions: what to do for patients who have pancreatic cancer

Given the statistics of survival data for patients with pancreatic cancer, it is advisable that patients who qualify for inclusion in a clinical trial should be afforded the opportunity to be enrolled in them. The selection of a specific trial among all the choices presented here, and currently identified on the National Cancer Institute's clinical trials Web site (www.clinicaltrials.gov), will depend on the requirements for inclusion or exclusion in the trial and the tools available at the treating institution (Box 1). While the current standard-of-care therapy improves the patients' quality of life, it does not prolong their survival by a substantial amount, and rarely leads to extensive stabilization of disease or a cure. The advantage of clinical trials using immunotherapy as opposed to broadly acting chemotherapeutic drugs is the limitation of serious adverse side effects.

Immunotherapy may give the greatest benefit as postoperative adjuvant therapy, which, if successful, would lead to the eradication of metastatic islands of cells, micronodules, and pancreatic cancer stem cells that may express tumor-specific antigens. Consideration should also be given to preoperative immunotherapy with low-dose IL-2 to make the surgery more tolerable in patients whose pancreatic tumors are deemed resectable. Low-dose IL-2 may have a number of beneficial effects: first, to up-regulate activated anti-tumor-specific T cells; second, to down-regulate anergic or tolerized T cells whose functions have been turned off by tumor products; and third, to alleviate some of the side effects encountered as a result of the surgery itself.

Immunotherapy may also present an advantage in patients with metasta-sized and/or nonresectable tumors. The underlying immunologic concern here is with the suppressive effects of tumor cells on immune cells capable of specifically targeting the tumor — in particular, whether the immunosup-pressive effects can be overcome and tumor-specific T-cell responses

---

Box 1. Considerations for determining immunotherapeutic treatment strategies for patients with pancreatic cancer

1. What is the stage of disease?
A. Is tumor surgically resectable or nonresectable?
   a. If resectable, can preoperative immunotherapy be administered?
   b. If resectable, can adjuvant immunotherapy be administered?
   c. Where adjuvant immunotherapy is administered, can adjuvant radiation therapy be given (ie, examine exclusion and inclusion criteria of clinical trial under consideration)?
   d. Enroll patients in a clinical trial following resection.
   e. Enroll patients in a clinical trial if tumor is nonresectable. The selection of the trial will depend on exclusion and inclusion criteria, and patients' consent.
B. Is tumor localized and/or metastatic?
   a. If localized, can site be reached endoscopically for therapy?
   b. If metastatic, is sufficient time available for development of immune response to be effective?
2. Is immunotherapeutic agent FDA-approved? Is immunotherapeutic agent only available via clinical trials?
3. How does the stage of disease relate to the inclusion versus exclusion criteria for a particular clinical trial?

4. What are the requirements for the clinical trial?
A. Is genotyping a requirement?
   1. Is an adequate quantity of tumor tissue available?
   2. Is laser micro-dissection of tumor from surrounding normal tissue available?
   3. Is a sequencing facility available?
   4. Is there access to GMP laboratory with molecular biology expertise?
B. Are adequate pathways for submission of tissue or blood to reference laboratory in place?

5. Is there access to clinical trials in the institution, or is there access through a subcontracting institution?
A. Does the hospital have an Institutional Review Board?
B. Is there access to a clinical trials data monitoring board?

---

bolstered. For the patient with nonresectable pancreatic cancer, therapy should: kill tumor cells, decrease tumor-derived immunosuppression (or at least its effect on tumor-specific immune cells), and bolster tumor-specific immune responses. Some monotherapies could affect more than one of these three aspects. Immunotherapy that is directed specifically to kill tumor cells with, for example, anti-MUC1 (DOTA hPAM4) and anti-mesothelin (MORab-009) (Table 3) antibodies or cytokines such as TNFerade or OncoVeX vectors (Table 3), may kill tumor cells but may also result in the development of immune responses to the patients' own tumors through the phagocytosis of dead tumor cells and presentation of their personalized tumor antigens in an environment that is supportive of immune T-cell activation. The immunosuppressive aspect, however, must also be addressed. Combining immunotherapies, such as a tumor vaccine containing a dendritic cell activator, with one that overcomes tumor-induced immunosuppression is necessary to create a supportive environment for antigen presentation and for effector T-cell function to develop and be effective. Here, the addition of low-dose IL-2, anti-CTLA-4 (ipilimumab), and/or denileukin diftitox (Ontak) to deplete down-regulatory T cells should be considered [98]. (Denileukin diftitox is a conjugate of an antibody directed against a chain of the IL-2 receptor that is expressed on activated T cells and the toxic domain of diphtheria toxin.) The addition of activators of APC and T-cell function, such as Gleevec and ipilimumab, respectively, to improve immune responses may also provide additional support for immune eradication of tumors. By selecting a combination of reagents to kill tumor cells and to manipulate the immune system to eradicate residual tumor cells and potential cancer stem cells, a long-term survival benefit may be reached in pancreatic cancer. Some of the clinical trials cited here may garner sufficient information to allow rapid progress toward that goal.

References

[1] Plate JM, Harris JE. Immune cell functions in pancreatic cancer. Crit Rev Immunol 2000; 20(5):375–92.
[2] Thomas AM, Santarsiero LM, Lutz ER, et al. Mesothelin-specific CD8+ T- cell responses provide evidence of in vivo cross-priming by antigen-presenting cells in vaccinated pancreatic cancer patients. J Exp Med 2004;200(3):297–306.
[3] Metzgar RS, Gaillard MT, Levine SJ, et al. Antigens of human pancreatic adenocarcinoma cells defined by murine monoclonal antibodies. Cancer Res 1982;42(2):601–8.
[4] Kobari M, Matsuno S, Yamauchi H, et al. Human pancreatic cancer associated antigen detected by monoclonal antibody. Tohoku J Exp Med 1986;148(2):179–95.
[5] Borowitz MJ, Tuck FL, Sindelar WF, et al. Monoclonal antibodies against human pancreatic adenocarcinoma: distribution of DU-PAN-2 antigen on glandular epithelia and adenocarcinomas. J Natl Cancer Inst 1984;72(5):999–1005.
[6] Lan MS, Finn OJ, Fernsten PD, et al. Isolation and properties of a human pancreatic adenocarcinoma-associated antigen, DU-PAN-2. Cancer Res 1985;45(1):305–10.
[7] Kubel R, Buchler M, Baczako K, et al. Immunohistochemistry in pancreatic cancer with new monoclonal antibodies. Langenbecks Arch Chir 1987;371(4):243–52.
[8] Kufe D, Inghirami G, Abe M, et al. Differential reactivity of a novel monoclonal antibody (DF3) with human malignant versus benign breast tumors. Hybridoma 1984;3(3): 223–32.

[9] Lan MS, Khorrami A, Kaufman B, et al. Molecular characterization of a mucin-type antigen associated with human pancreatic cancer: the DU-PAN-2 antigen. Journal of Biological Chemistry 1987;262(26):12863–70.

[10] Satake K, Chung YS, Umeyama K, et al. Diagnostic usefulness and limitation of measuring pancreatic cancer associated antigen, SPan-1, in patients with pancreatic cancer. Gan To Kagaku Ryoho 1989;16(4 Pt 2-1):1139–46.

[11] Kawa S, Kato M, Oguchi H, et al. Preparation of pancreatic cancer-associated mucin expressing CA19-9, CA50, Span-1, sialyl SSEA-1, and Dupan-2. Scand J Gastroenterol 1991;26(9):981–92.

[12] Kiriyama S, Hayakawa T, Kondo T, et al. Usefulness of a new tumor marker, Span-1, for the diagnosis of pancreatic cancer. Cancer 1990;65(7):1557–61.

[13] Wahab ZA, Metzgar RS. Human cytotoxic lymphocytes reactive with pancreatic adenocarcinoma cells. Pancreas 1991;6(3):307–17.

[14] Peiper M, Goedegebuure PS, Eberlein TJ. Generation of peptide-specific cytotoxic T lymphocytes using allogeneic dendritic cells capable of lysing human pancreatic cancer cells. Surgery 1997;122(2):235–41 [discussion: 241–2].

[15] Peiper M, Goedegebuure PS, Linehan DC, et al. The HER2/neu-derived peptide p654-662 is a tumor-associated antigen in human pancreatic cancer recognized by cytotoxic T lymphocytes. Eur J Immunol 1997;27:1115–23.

[16] Qin H, Chen W, Takahashi M, et al. CD4+ T-cell immunity to mutated ras protein in pancreatic and colon cancer patients. Cancer Res 1995;55(14):2984–7.

[17] Rutherford JC, Walters BA, Cavaye G, et al. A modified leukocyte adherence inhibition test in the laboratory investigation of gastrointestinal cancer. Int J Cancer 1977;19(1):43–8.

[18] Tataryn DN, MacFarlane JK, Thomson DM. Leucocyte adherence inhibition for detecting specific tumour immunity in early pancreatic cancer. Lancet 1978;1(8072):1020–2.

[19] Douglass HO Jr, Russo AJ, Howell JH, et al. Selectivity of the micro-leukocyte adherence inhibition assay in pancreatic cancer. Cancer 1979;43(3):1084–8.

[20] Goldrosen MH, Dasmahapatra K, Jenkins D, et al. Microplate leucocyte adherence inhibition (LAI) assay in pancreatic cancer: detection of specific antitumor immunity with patients' peripheral blood cells and serum. Cancer 1981;47(6 Suppl):1614–9.

[21] MacFarlane JK, Thomson DM, Phelan K, et al. Predictive value of tube leukocyte adherence inhibition (LAI) assay for breast, colorectal, stomach and pancreatic cancer. Cancer 1982;49(6):1185–93.

[22] Onji M. Leucocyte adherence inhibition assay for cell-mediated immunity and immunodiagnosis of pancreatic cancer. Gastroenterol J 1984;19(4):328–35.

[23] Meduri F, Doni MG, Merenda R, et al. The role of the leukocyte adherence inhibition (LAI), CA 19-9, and tissue polypeptide antigen (TPA) tests in the diagnosis of pancreatic cancer. Cancer 1989;64(5):1103–6.

[24] Magnani JL, Steplewski Z, Koprowski H, et al. Identification of the gastrointestinal and pancreatic cancer-associated antigen detected by monoclonal antibody 19-9 in the sera of patients as a mucin. Cancer Res 1983;43(11):5489–92.

[25] Ban T, Imai K, Yachi A. Immunohistological and immunochemical characterization of a novel pancreatic cancer-associated antigen MUSE11. Cancer Res 1989;49(24 Pt 1): 7141–6.

[26] Chung YS, Ho JJ, Kim YS, et al. The detection of human pancreatic cancer-associated antigen in the serum of cancer patients. Cancer 1987;60(7):1636–43.

[27] Johnson VG, Schlom J, Paterson AJ, et al. Analysis of a human tumor-associated glycoprotein (TAG-72) identified by monoclonal antibody B72.3. Cancer Res 1986;46(2):850–7.

[28] Gelder FB, Reese CJ, Moossa AR, et al. Purification, partial characterization, and clinical evaluation of a pancreatic oncofetal antigen. Cancer Res 1978;38(2):313–24.

[29] Salazar E, Zaremba S, Arlen PM, et al. Agonist peptide from a cytotoxic t-lymphocyte epitope of human carcinoembryonic antigen stimulates production of tc1-type cytokines

and increases tyrosine phosphorylation more efficiently than cognate peptide. Int J Cancer 2000;85(6):829–38.

[30] Petrulio CA, Kaufman HL. Development of the PANVAC™-VF vaccine for pancreatic cancer. Expert Rev Vaccines 2006;5(1):9–19.

[31] Rasmussen H, Rasmussen C, Lempicki M, et al. TNFerade Biologic: preclinical toxicology of a novel adenovector with a radiation-inducible promoter, carrying the human tumor necrosis factor alpha gene. Cancer Gene Ther 2002;9(11):951–7.

[32] Uyttenhove C, Pilotte L, Theate I, et al. Evidence for a tumoral immune resistance mechanism based on tryptophan degradation by indoleamine 2,3-dioxygenase. Nat Med 2003; 9(10):1269–74.

[33] Gjertsen MK, Bakka A, Breivik J, et al. Vaccination with mutant ras peptides and induction of T-cell responsiveness in pancreatic carcinoma patients carrying the corresponding RAS mutation. Lancet 1995;346:1399–400.

[34] D Laheru CY, B. Biedrzycki, S. Solt, et al. A safety and efficacy trial of lethally irradiated allogeneic pancreatic tumor cells transfected with the GM-CSF gene in combination with adjuvant chemoradiotherapy for the treatment of adenocarcinoma of the pancreas. Paper presented at: Gastrointestinal Cancers Symposium, 2007; Abstract # 106.

[35] Ikemoto T, Yamaguchi T, Morine Y, et al. Clinical roles of increased populations of Foxp3+CD4+ T cells in peripheral blood from advanced pancreatic cancer patients. Pancreas 2006;33(4):386–90.

[36] Hiraoka N, Onozato K, Kosuge T, et al. Prevalence of FOXP3+ regulatory T cells increases during the progression of pancreatic ductal adenocarcinoma and its premalignant lesions. Clin Cancer Res 2006;12(18):5423–34.

[37] Liu VC, Wong LY, Jang T, et al. Tumor evasion of the immune system by converting CD4+CD25- T cells into CD4+CD25+ T regulatory cells: role of tumor-derived TGF-beta. J Immunol 2007;178(5):2883–92.

[38] Fallarino F, Grohmann U, You S, et al. The combined effects of tryptophan starvation and tryptophan catabolites down-regulate T cell receptor zeta-chain and induce a regulatory phenotype in naive T cells. J Immunol 2006;176(11):6752–61.

[39] Terada T, Ohta T, Sasaki M, et al. Expression of MUC apomucins in normal pancreas and pancreatic tumors. J Pathol 1996;180:160–5.

[40] Jerome K, Domenech N, Finn O. Tumor-specific cytotoxic T cell clones from patients with breast and pancreatic adenocarcinoma recognize EBV-immortalized B cells transfected with polymorphic epithelial mucin complementary DNA. J Immunol 1993;151(3): 1654–62.

[41] Barnd DL, Lan MS, Metzgar RS, et al. Specific, MHC-unrestricted recognition of tumor-associated mucins by human cytotoxic T cells. Proc Natl Acad Sci 1989;86:7159–63.

[42] Lan M, Batra S, Qi W, Metzgar R, et al. Cloning and sequencing of a human pancreatic tumor mucin cDNA. J Biol Chem 1990;265(25):15294–9.

[43] Ramanathan RK, Lee KM, McKolanis J, et al. Phase I study of a MUC1 vaccine composed of different doses of MUC1 peptide with SB-AS2 adjuvant in resected and locally advanced pancreatic cancer. Cancer Immunol Immunother 2005;54:254–64.

[44] Yamamoto K, Ueno T, Kawaoka T, et al. MUC1 peptide vaccination in patients with advanced pancreas or biliary tract cancer. Anticancer Res 2005;25(5):3575–9.

[45] Steinman RM. The dendritic cell system and its role in immunogenicity. Annu Rev Immunol 1991;9:271–96.

[46] Shinohara H, Yano S, Bucana CD, et al. Induction of chemokine secretion and enhancement of contact-dependent macrophage cytotoxicity by engineered expression of granulocyte-macrophage colony-stimulating factor in human colon cancer cells. J Immunol 2000; 164(5):2728–37.

[47] McLaughlin JP, Abrams S, Kantor J, et al. Immunization with a syngeneic tumor infected with recombinant vaccinia virus expressing granulocyte-macrophage colony-stimulating

factor (GM-CSF) induces tumor regression and long-lasting systemic immunity. J Immunother 1997;20(6):449–59.

[48] Cresswell P. Antigen processing and presentation. Immunol Rev 2005;207:5–7.

[49] Cresswell P, Ackerman AL, Giodini A, et al. Mechanisms of MHC class I-restricted antigen processing and cross-presentation. Immunol Rev 2005;207:145–57.

[50] Hamblin TJ, Davis Z, Gardiner A, et al. Unmutated IgV(H) genes are associated with a more aggressive form of chronic lymphocytic leukemia. Blood 1999;94(6):1848–54.

[51] Sorlie T, Perou CM, Tibshirani R, et al. Gene expression patterns of breast carcinomas distinguish tumor subclasses with clinical implications. Proc Natl Acad Sci 2001;98(19): 10869–74.

[52] Hruban RH, van Mansfeld AD, Offerhaus GJ, et al. K-ras oncogene activation in adenocarcinoma of the human pancreas. A study of 82 carcinomas using a combination of mutant-enriched polymerase chain reaction analysis and allele-specific oligonucleotide hybridization. Am J Pathol 1993;143(2):545–54.

[53] Hruban RH, Adsay NV, Albores-Saavedra J, et al. Pancreatic intraepithelial neoplasia: a new nomenclature and classification system for pancreatic duct lesions. Am J Surg Pathol 2001;25(5):579–86.

[54] Gjertsen MK, Buanes T, Rosseland AR, et al. Intradermal ras peptide vaccination with granulocyte-macrophage colony-stimulating factor as adjuvant: clinical and immunological responses in patients with pancreatic adenocarcinoma. Int J Cancer 2001;92(3):441–50.

[55] Lu Y, Bellgrau D, Dwyer-Nield LD, et al. Mutation-selective tumor remission with ras-targeted, whole yeast-based immunotherapy. Cancer Res 2004;64(15):5084–8.

[56] Newman SL, Holly A. Candida albicans is phagocytosed, killed, and processed for antigen presentation by human dendritic cells. Infect Immun 2001;69(11):6813–22.

[57] Plate JM, Harris JE. Immunobiotherapy directed against mutated and aberrantly expressed gene products in pancreas cancer. J Cell Biochem 2005;94(6):1069–77.

[58] Rabinovich GA, Gabrilovich D, Sotomayor EM. Immunosuppressive strategies that are mediated by tumor cells. Annual Review of Immunology 2007;25(1):267–96.

[59] Galili U. Autologous tumor vaccines processed to express alpha-gal epitopes: a practical approach to immunotherapy in cancer. Cancer Immunol Immunother 2004;53(11):935–45.

[60] Galili U. Xenotransplantation and ABO incompatible transplantation: the similarities they share. Transfus Apheresis Sci 2006;35(1):45–58.

[61] Zaremba S, Barzaga E, Zhu M, et al. Identification of an enhancer agonist cytotoxic T lymphocyte peptide from human carcinoembryonic antigen. Cancer Res 1997;57(20): 4570–7.

[62] Locker GY, Hamilton S, Harris J, et al. ASCO 2006 update of recommendations for the use of tumor markers in gastrointestinal cancer. J Clin Oncol 2006;24(33):5313–27.

[63] Bernhardt SL, Gjertsen MK, Trachsel S, et al. Telomerase peptide vaccination of patients with non-resectable pancreatic cancer: a dose escalating phase I/II study. Br J Cancer 2006;95(11):1474–82.

[64] Plate JMD, Plate AE, Shott S, et al. Effect of gemcitabine on immune cells in subjects with adenocarcinoma of the pancreas. Cancer Immunol Immunother 2005;54(9):915–25.

[65] Yanagimoto H, Mine T, Yamamoto K, et al. Immunological evaluation of personalized peptide vaccination with gemcitabine for pancreatic cancer. Cancer Sci 2007;98(4): 605–11.

[66] Cardenes HR, Chiorean EG, Dewitt J, et al. Locally advanced pancreatic cancer: current therapeutic approach. Oncologist 2006;11(6):612–23.

[67] Kindler HL, Friberg G, Singh DA, et al. Phase II trial of bevacizumab plus gemcitabine in patients with advanced pancreatic cancer. J Clin Oncol 2005;23(31):8033–40.

[68] Shinkaruk S, Bayle M, Lain G, et al. Vascular endothelial cell growth factor (VEGF), an emerging target for cancer chemotherapy. Curr Med Chem Anticancer Agents 2003;3(2): 95–117.

[69] McMahon G. VEGF receptor signaling in tumor angiogenesis. Oncologist 2000;5(Suppl 1): 3–10.

[70] Cabebe E, Fisher GA. Clinical trials of VEGF receptor tyrosine kinase inhibitors in pancreatic cancer. Expert Opin Invest Drugs 2007;16(4):467–76.

[71] Amoh Y, Li L, Tsuji K, et al. Dual-color imaging of nascent blood vessels vascularizing pancreatic cancer in an orthotopic model demonstrates antiangiogenesis efficacy of gemcitabine. J Surg Res 2006;132(2):164–9.

[72] Rafii S, Avecilla ST, Jin DK. Tumor vasculature address book: identification of stage-specific tumor vessel zip codes by phage display. Cancer Cell 2003;4(5):331–3.

[73] Friess H, Wang L, Zhu Z, et al. Growth factor receptors are differentially expressed in cancers of the papilla of vater and pancreas. Ann Surg 1999;230(6):767–74 [discussion: 774–5].

[74] Moore MJ, Goldstein D, Hamm J, et al. Erlotinib plus gemcitabine compared with gemcitabine alone in patients with advanced pancreatic cancer: a phase III trial of the National Cancer Institute of Canada Clinical Trials Group. J Clin Oncol 2005;23:1.

[75] Zhang B, Bowerman NA, Salama JK, et al. Induced sensitization of tumor stroma leads to eradication of established cancer by T cells. J Exp Med 2007;204(1):49–55.

[76] Mendelsohn J. Targeting the epidermal growth factor receptor for cancer therapy. J Clin Oncol 2002;20(Suppl 1):1s–13s.

[77] Huang S, Armstrong EA, Benavente S, et al. Dual-agent molecular targeting of the epidermal growth factor receptor (EGFR): combining anti-EGFR antibody with tyrosine kinase inhibitor. Cancer Res 2004;64(15):5355–62.

[78] Ramakrishnan V, Bhaskar V, Law DA, et al. Preclinical evaluation of an anti-alpha5beta1 integrin antibody as a novel anti-angiogenic agent. J Exp Ther Oncol 2006;5(4):273–86.

[79] Teft WA, Kirchhof MG, Madrenas J. A molecular perspective of CTLA-4 function. Annu Rev Immunol 2006;24:65–97.

[80] Tivol EA, Borriello F, Schweitzer AN, et al. Loss of CTLA-4 leads to massive lymphoproliferation and fatal multiorgan tissue destruction, revealing a critical negative regulatory role of CTLA-4. Immunity 1995;3(5):541–7.

[81] Phan GQ, Yang JC, Sherry RM, et al. Cancer regression and autoimmunity induced by cytotoxic T lymphocyte-associated antigen 4 blockade in patients with metastatic melanoma. Proc Natl Acad Sci 2003;100(14):8372–7.

[82] Hodi FS, Mihm MC, Soiffer RJ, et al. Biologic activity of cytotoxic T lymphocyte-associated antigen 4 antibody blockade in previously vaccinated metastatic melanoma and ovarian carcinoma patients. Proc Natl Acad Sci 2003;100(8):4712–7.

[83] Zobywalski A, Javorovic M, Frankenberger B, et al. Generation of clinical grade dendritic cells with capacity to produce biologically active IL-12p70. J Transl Med 2007; 5:18.

[84] Ridgway D. The first 1000 dendritic cell vaccines. Cancer Invest 2003;21(6):873–86.

[85] Nair S, Boczkowski D. RNA-transfected dendritic cells. Expert Rev Vaccines 2002;1(4): 507–13.

[86] Heiser A, Maurice MA, Yancey DR, et al. Human dendritic cells transfected with renal tumor RNA stimulate polyclonal T-cell responses against antigens expressed by primary and metastatic tumors. Cancer Res 2001;61(8):3388–93.

[87] Stift A, Friedl J, Dubsky P, et al. In vivo induction of dendritic cell-mediated cytotoxicity against allogeneic pancreatic carcinoma cells. Int J Oncol 2003;22(3):651–6.

[88] Knauer SK, Mann W, Stauber RH. Survivin's dual role: an export's view. Cell Cycle 2007; 6(5):518–21.

[89] Knauer SK, Kramer OH, Knosel T, et al. Nuclear export is essential for the tumor-promoting activity of survivin. FASEB J 2007;21(1):207–16.

[90] Zaffaroni N, Pannati M, Diadone MG. Survivin as a target for new anticancer interventions. J Cell Mol Med 2005;9(2):360–72.

[91] Lopes RB, Gangeswaren R, McNeish IA, et al. Expression of the IAP protein family is dysregulated in pancreatic cancer cells and is important for resistance to chemotherapy. Int J Cancer 2007;120(11):2344–52.

[92] Nagaraj S, Pisarev V, Kinarsky L, et al. Dendritic cell-based full-length survivin vaccine in treatment of experimental tumors. J Immunother 2007;30(2):169–79.

[93] Wobser M, Keikavoussi P, Kunzmann V, et al. Complete remission of liver metastasis of pancreatic cancer under vaccination with a HLA-A2 restricted peptide derived from the universal tumor antigen survivin. Cancer Immunol Immunother 2006;55(10):1294–8.

[94] Kalady MF, Onaitis MW, Emani S, et al. Dendritic cells pulsed with pancreatic cancer total tumor RNA generate specific antipancreatic cancer T cells. J Gastrointest Surg 2004;8(2): 175–81 [discussion: 181–2].

[95] Angelini C, Bovo G, Muselli P, et al. Preoperative interleukin-2 immunotherapy in pancreatic cancer: preliminary results. Hepatogastroenterology 2006;53(67):141–4.

[96] Takeda K, Kaisho T, Akira S. Toll-like receptors. Ann Rev Immunol 2003;21(1):335–76.

[97] Wang H, Cheng F, Cuenca A, et al. Imatinib mesylate (STI-571) enhances antigen-presenting cell function and overcomes tumor-induced CD4+ T-cell tolerance. Blood 2005;105(3): 1135–43.

[98] Barnett B, Kryczek I, Cheng P, et al. Regulatory T cells in ovarian cancer: biology and therapeutic potential. Am J Reprod Immunol 2005;54(6):369–77.

ELSEVIER
SAUNDERS

Surg Oncol Clin N Am
16 (2007) 945–973

SURGICAL
ONCOLOGY CLINICS
OF NORTH AMERICA

Current Immunotherapeutic Strategies in Malignant Melanoma

Nicole M. Agostino, DO[a], Arjumand Ali, MD[b],
Suresh G. Nair, MD[a], Paul J. Mosca, MD, PhD[c],*

[a]*Department of Internal Medicine, Lehigh Valley Hospital and Health Network,
1240 South Cedar Crest Boulevard, Suite 410, Allentown, PA 18103, USA*
[b]*Department of Surgery, Lehigh Valley Hospital and Health Network, 1240 South Cedar
Crest Boulevard, PO Box 689, Allentown, PA 18105–1556, USA*
[c]*Section of Surgical Oncology, Department of Surgery, Lehigh Valley Hospital and Health
Network, 1240 South Cedar Crest Boulevard, Suite 205, Allentown, PA 18103, USA*

Among the most intriguing areas of tumor immunology is that of immunotherapy for the treatment of malignant melanoma. It has been appreciated for many years that melanoma occasionally undergoes spontaneous and sometimes even complete regression [1–3]. This phenomenon suggests that melanomas are relatively immunogenic in comparison with other solid tumors. The possibility that one might be able to use this immunogenicity as a foundation for the development of an alternative treatment modality has fueled interest in immunotherapy for melanoma for several decades.

The concept of treating melanoma with immunotherapy is based on the presumption that melanomas express specific antigens that differ from host proteins in terms of sequence, quantity, or both. In the early 1970s, studies using immunofluorescence techniques led to initial descriptions of melanoma-associated antigens (MAAs). These antigens could elicit the production of melanoma-specific antibodies circulating in the peripheral blood of patients who have the disease [4]. Melanoma-specific antibodies from one patient could recognize melanomas from other patients, indicating the existence of shared tumor antigens [5]. Identification of the first human leukocyte antigen (HLA)–restricted MAA that could be recognized by antigen-specific cytotoxic T lymphocytes (CTLs) represented another major advancement in the field [6]. Investigators found that tumors from patients who have melanoma harbor antigen-specific tumor-infiltrating lymphocytes

* Corresponding author.
E-mail address: paul.mosca@lvh.com (P.J. Mosca).

1055-3207/07/$ - see front matter © 2007 Elsevier Inc. All rights reserved.
doi:10.1016/j.soc.2007.07.010
surgonc.theclinics.com

(TILs) that recognize MAAs [7–9]. Investigators subsequently discovered several different methods for identifying and characterizing MAAs [10–16]; several of these antigens are listed in Table 1 [11–13,17–20].

There are two conceptually distinct approaches to immunotherapy: antigen-specific and antigen-nonspecific. Nonspecific immunotherapies generally modulate the immune system and indirectly enhance antitumor immunity without targeting a specific melanoma antigen. Although the resulting immune response may include an antigen-specific component, this is not dictated by the composition of the therapy itself. In contrast, specific immunotherapies target one or more specific antigenic epitopes.

Surgeons who care for patients who have melanoma must have a basic understanding of immunotherapy for three reasons. First, patients who are ideal candidates for treatment with US Food and Drug Administration (FDA)–approved immunotherapies should be referred to a medical oncologist or other qualified specialist for a discussion regarding the potential benefits and risks associated with these treatment options. Second, patients who have melanoma and may be eligible for clinical trials should be made aware

Table 1
Human melanoma antigens

Melanocyte differentiation antigens		
Gp100	TRP-1	Tyrosinase
MART-1/MelanA	TRP-2	
Cancer testis antigens		
ADAM2	HAGE	PLU-1
AF15q14	HOM-TES-85	SAGE1
BAGE	IL13RA1	SCP1
BORIS	LDHC	SGY1
BRDT	LIP1TSP50	SPA17
CAGE	MAGE family	SPO11
CSAGE	MMA-1	SSX
CTAGE	MORC	TAF7L
CTp11/SPANX	NA88	TDRD1
Dam-6,-10	NXF2	TEX15
E2F-like/HCA661	NY-ESO-1	TPTE
FATE1	NY-SAR-35	TPX1
FTHL17	OY-TES-1	XAGE1
GAGE family	PAGE5	
Tumor-specific antigens		
707-AP	gnT-V	MUM family-1
β-catenin	HPVE7	PRAME
Caspase-8	HSP70-2M	RAGE
CDK-4/m	KIAA0205	SART-2
Widely expressed antigens		
CAMEL	HTERT	RU1/RU2
CEA	P15	SART-31
HER2/neu	PRAME	

Data from Refs. [11–13,17–20].

of this option so that they may make an informed decision regarding participation. Finally, surgeons are likely to be called on increasingly to participate in clinical trials or to cooperate with clinical trial investigators. This may entail proper sequencing of surgery and an established or experimental immunotherapy, the harvesting of biologic specimens for generation of therapeutics or monitoring of the immune response, or playing other key roles in the development and optimal administration of immunologic therapies. This article reviews current approaches to immunotherapy for melanoma in an effort to highlight opportunities for the practicing surgeon to be involved in this evolving therapeutic modality.

Nonspecific immunotherapies

Around 1900, William Coley [21] observed that patients who had cancer and developed infections occasionally exhibited evidence of tumor regression, prompting him to investigate bacterial products ("Coley's toxins") as a potential form of cancer treatment. Since that time, numerous agents that modulate the immune system—biologic response modifiers—have been investigated as potential treatments for melanoma. Many of these, particularly the more crude preparations, such as bacterial products, seem to serve as "danger signals" in that they activate an arm of the immune system that normally serves to signal the presence of foreign pathogens [22]. Many biologic response modifiers have been identified or developed since that time, and significant progress has been made toward understanding the mechanisms of action of these agents.

Toll-like receptor agonists

Toll-like receptors (TLRs) are present on a variety of immune cells, including dendritic cells (DCs), macrophages, granulocytes, and T and B lymphocytes [23–28], and they have even been identified on tumor cells [29]. This family of receptors recognizes a broad array of pathogen-associated molecular patterns (PAMPs) associated with bacteria, fungi, and viruses [23,30,31]. There are at least 10 different TLRs (TLR-1–TLR-10) in human beings [32–36]. These distinct TLRs may form homodimers or heterodimers, and each receptor preferentially recognizes one or more types of ligands. Exogenous ligands include double-stranded RNA, unmethylated DNA, bacterial lipopolysaccharide, staphylococcal lipoteichoic acid, yeast zymosan, and many other PAMP-containing subcellular or viral products. Some TLRs may recognize endogenous molecules, such as heat shock proteins (HSPs) [36]. Although the many immunologic effects mediated or affected by TLRs have not been completely characterized, a major role of this family of receptors is to promote innate immunity. For example, natural killer (NK) cells, which represent one arm of the innate immune system, become activated directly by TLR agonists [37,38]. TLRs also have the potential to influence adaptive immunity, indirectly through an effect mediated by DCs or by direct interaction with T cells or B cells [39,40].

Bacille Calmette-Guérin

Bacille Calmette-Guérin (BCG) consists of a live-attenuated preparation of *Mycobacterium bovis* that seems to act primarily by stimulating TLRs on DCs [4,41,42]. This agent is approved by the FDA for the topical treatment of carcinoma in situ of the urinary bladder, and it has been applied to the treatment of patients who have melanoma for more than 30 years [43–45]. BCG generally has been administered "off-label" as a palliative agent for locoregionally advanced melanoma by the intratumoral (intralesional) route [46] or as an adjuvant agent with other forms of immunotherapy in the context of clinical trials, usually by the intradermal route [47,48]. Although there have been occasional reports of robust and durable clinical responses to BCG treatment in advanced melanoma [42], such responses are rare and have not attracted extensive interest in pursuing the use of this agent as a primary therapy for melanoma. In the adjuvant setting, there are conflicting reports with regard to whether BCG has a significant impact on survival [4,49,50].

Other toll-like receptor agonists

A variety of other TLR agonists have been identified or developed and have received interest as alternative adjuvants in conjunction with experimental immunotherapeutics. A group of synthetic antiviral compounds with TLR-7 agonist activity, the imidazoquinolineamines, include the agent imiquimod (Aldara). Imiquimod is a topical cream that is approved by the FDA for the treatment of actinic keratosis and superficial basal cell carcinoma. CpG-rich oligoDNA molecules have TLR agonist activity and stimulate plasmacytoid DCs by means of TLR-9 [51]. CpG DNA binding to TLR-9 promotes DC survival and expression of major histocompatibility complex (MHC) class II, maturation marker CD83, and costimulatory molecules (CD80, CD86, and CD40) [51]. Interestingly, treatment of plasmacytoid dendritic cells (pDCs) with TLR-7 and TLR-9 agonists has also been shown to enhance a direct cytotoxic effect of pDCs on melanoma target cells [29], apparently through an innate immune system pathway. Data from a recent phase II trial using the TLR-9 stimulating oligonucleotide PF-33512676 in patients who had melanoma was recently reported. Of 20 patients who received PF-3512676 for a mean of 10.9 weeks, 2 patients experienced partial responses (PRs) and 3 patients had stable disease. At the time the study was reported, 1 patient had a PR that was still ongoing at 140 weeks. This method of immune system activation has shown some promise; hence, further studies of TLR agonists in the treatment of melanoma seem warranted.

Cytokines

Granulocyte macrophage colony-stimulating factor

Granulocyte macrophage colony-stimulating factor (GM-CSF) is a cytokine secreted by many cell lines, including macrophages, monocytes, and T lymphocytes. Originally identified in the mid-1980s, its properties include promoting the proliferation of DCs, macrophages, monocytes, and neutrophils [52]. Recombinant human GM-CSF (Leukine, Sargramostim) is approved by the FDA for increasing leukocyte counts after treatment with chemotherapy for leukemia or in the setting of stem cell transplantation. Over the past several years, there has been increasing interest in exploring its value as a potential immune modulator in the treatment of melanoma.

One potential role for GM-CSF is the adjuvant treatment of patients who have melanoma and have no evidence of disease (NED) but are at high risk for recurrence. The presence of lymph node metastasis is a major adverse prognostic factor in malignant melanoma, even in the setting of lymph node micrometastasis detected by lymphatic mapping and sentinel lymph node (SLN) biopsy. Recently, Lee and colleagues [53] of the John Wayne Cancer Institute reported that the presence of residual melanoma at the primary cutaneous site or metastatic melanoma in the SLN is associated with the presence of increased levels of immunosuppressive cytokines in the SLN. They found that preoperative treatment with GM-CSF reversed these changes in cytokine levels and increased the prevalence of T cells and DCs within the SLN.

Another application for GM-CSF is the treatment of metastatic disease. Although intralesional injection of GM-CSF can induce local regression of melanoma deposits, clinically significant systemic antitumor effects are not observed [54,55]. An aerosolized formulation of GM-CSF has been introduced as a potential treatment for pulmonary metastases. In a recent phase I study of this formulation by Rao and colleagues [52], 24 of 40 evaluable patients exhibited stabilization or partial regression of pulmonary metastases and the treatment was well tolerated. Investigators found that GM-CSF enhanced local melanoma-specific CTL activity. Based on the promising results of this study, a multicenter dose-escalation phase I trial was initiated (NCCTG N0071) and is currently underway.

Interleukin-2

Interleukin (IL)-2 is a 15-kilodalton (kd) glycoprotein T-cell growth factor that is produced primarily by activated T helper (Th) lymphocytes [56,57]. IL-2 stimulates the development of CTLs and NK cells, it is a cofactor in the activation of B cells and macrophages, and it plays a role in the generation of CD4+/CD25+ regulatory T lymphocytes (Tregs).

High-dose IL-2 is approved by the FDA for the primary treatment of stage IV melanoma. Rosenberg and colleagues [58] treated 134 patients who had metastatic melanoma with high-dose IL-2 and observed a complete response (CR) in 7% and a PR in 10% of patients. Importantly, the CRs included several durable responses, ranging up to 91 months in that report. Atkins and colleagues [59] reported on 270 patients who had metastatic melanoma and were treated with high-dose IL-2 between 1985 and 1993 at eight different institutions. The overall response rate was 16%, with 17 CRs (6%) and 26 PRs (10%). The major drawbacks of this therapy are the low response rate, toxicity, and cost. Among its toxicities are capillary leak syndrome, hypotension, adult respiratory distress syndrome (ARDS), gastrointestinal toxicity, acute renal failure, infections, and other side effects. In part because of the significant risk for major toxicity, its use is limited to patients with good performance status and organ function and generally at medical centers that specialize in the administration of this agent [57].

As noted in the previous study, a subset of the small percentage of patients who do respond to IL-2 treatment has durable treatment responses measured in years, and some patients seem to have experienced a cure (Fig. 1). Although these patients represent the exceptions, they demonstrate the proof of principle that nonspecific immune modulation of T cells can eradicate melanoma under optimal conditions. The appearance of vitiligo correlates closely with objective clinical response to IL-2 treatment and is presumed to arise from an autoimmune side effect resulting from the cross-reactivity of melanocyte antigens with target MAAs. Rosenberg and White [60] performed a prospective evaluation on patients who had metastatic melanoma and were treated with high-dose IL-2 for the

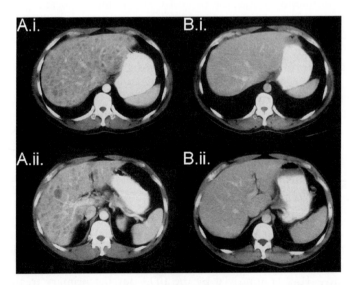

Fig. 1. A 40-year-old man who had stage IV melanoma with numerous liver metastases was treated with six cycles of high-dose IL-2. He experienced a CR and has remained disease-free for more than 7 years. Pretreatment (*A.i.*, *A.ii.*) and posttreatment (*B.i.*, *B.ii.*) intravenous contrast-enhanced abdominal CT scans are shown.

development of vitiligo. In this study, 26% of patients who responded to IL-2 developed vitiligo and vitiligo was not observed in any of the nonresponders to high-dose IL-2. The fact that vitiligo is not observed in patients who have renal cell carcinoma and exhibit a clinical response to IL-2 lends further credence to the proposed mechanism of IL-2 in the treatment of melanoma and the central role of shared melanoma antigens in cancer immunotherapy.

Cytotoxic T-lymphocyte–associated antigen-4–targeted therapy

When DCs present antigens to CTLs, T-cell activation does not occur unless a costimulatory signal ("signal 2") is also present. CD28 is a receptor on T cells that binds to the costimulatory molecules B7.1 (CD80) and B7.2 (CD86) on DCs. Engagement of CD28 with B7.1 and B7.2 promotes T-cell activation, proliferation, and IL-2 production. Additional costimulation is provided by the interaction of CD40 ligand (present on T cells) with CD40 (present on DCs). After activation of CTLs, cytotoxic T-lymphocyte–associated antigen-4 (CTLA-4) is upregulated on the T cells and binds B7.1 and B7.2 with 100-fold greater affinity than CD28. The binding of CTLA-4 to its ligand antagonizes T-cell activation, interferes with IL-2 production and IL-2 receptor expression, and interrupts progression through the cell cycle in activated T cells. This regulatory process prevents uncontrolled expansion of CD8+ T cells and the potentially harmful expansion of self-reactive T cells [61,62].

Because CTLA-4 downregulates activated T cells, an agent with the ability to bind to and block CTLA-4–mediated downregulation could result in the expansion and activation of CTLs, some of which may be directed against melanoma antigens. Ipilimumab (MDX-010) is a human monoclonal antibody that blocks CTLA-4, and thereby activates CTLs. In clinical trial of 14 patients who had metastatic melanoma, ipilimumab was administered in conjunction with a peptide vaccine against two gp100 epitopes [61]. Objective responses were observed in 3 patients (2 with a CR and 1 with a PR). Interestingly, the frequency of grade 3 to 4 autoimmune phenomena was 43% (6 patients), highlighting the central role of CTLA-4 in regulating the ability of the immune system to distinguish self-antigens from foreign antigens. CP-675,206 is a fully human antibody that also binds to and blocks CTLA-4. In a phase I trial with a total of 35 evaluable patients, 3 patients had a CR, 2 had a PR, and 5 experienced disease stabilization for a duration of 7 to 16 months [63]. One patient with a CR had a durable response of nearly 5 years. The treatment was well tolerated in most patients, with the most common severe side effect being grade 3 diarrhea. Although it seems that antibodies targeting CTLA-4 are unlikely to develop into an effective single-agent therapy for melanoma, they could enhance the efficacy of other immunotherapy strategies and are likely to help investigators learn more about the mechanisms regulating antitumor and autoimmune T-cell responsiveness.

Interferons

The interferons (IFNs) are separated into two groups: type I (including α- and β-IFNs) and type II (γ-IFN). In general, IFNs are known to have antiviral and antitumor effects in vivo. IFNs also play a role in linking innate and adaptive immunity. Type I IFNs induce expression of MHC class I, which is present on all nucleated cells in the body and binds antigenic peptide epitopes for presentation to T lymphocytes. α-IFNs have also been shown to promote the maturation of DCs [64–66].

The Eastern Cooperative Oncology Group (ECOG) trial E1684 compared 52 weeks of high-dose IFNα-2b (Intron A; HDI) versus observation and demonstrated a median relapse-free survival (RFS) of 1.72 years for HDI versus 0.98 years for observation ($P = .0023$). The median overall length of survival was 3.82 years versus 2.78 years, respectively ($P = .0237$). This trial led to FDA approval of the HDI regimen as adjuvant therapy for patients who have stage IIB and III melanoma [67]. ECOG trial 1690 randomized patients into an HDI arm, a low-dose IFNα-2b (LDI) arm, or an observation arm. LDI was not associated with an RFS benefit, and neither HDI nor LDI had an impact on overall survival [68]. ECOG trial E1694 compared the ganglioside GM2/keyhole limpet hemocyanin vaccine (GMK) versus HDI. This trial was closed early based on an interim analysis showing that HDI was superior to GMK for relapse and mortality end points [69]. Finally, ECOG trial E2696 was a randomized phase II trial in which patients were treated with GMK versus concurrent HDI, GMK versus sequential HDI, or GMK alone. Both HDI arms had a reduced risk for relapse compared with GMK alone [70].

With the advent of SLN biopsy, subclinical nodal metastatic disease could be detected and the patient population who had stage III melanoma shifted from those with bulky nodal disease to those with nodal micrometastasis. The Sunbelt Melanoma Trial was initiated in 2001 to evaluate the role of HDI in patients who had early nodal disease. Lymph nodes were evaluated by traditional histologic analysis in addition to reverse transcriptase polymerase chain reaction (RT-PCR) analysis if the lymph node was grossly histologically negative for metastatic disease. RT-PCR can detect one melanoma cell among a million normal cells. Patients whose SLN was negative by traditional histology and RT-PCR were observed. Patients whose SLN was negative by traditional histology but positive by RT-PCR were randomized to observation, lymph node dissection only, or lymph node dissection plus 1 month of HDI. Patients whose SLN was the only histologically positive node by traditional analysis were randomized to observation versus HDI. Patients who had more than one node that was positive by traditional histologic analysis were also treated with the 1 month of HDI. Although it has been determined that the method of SLN RT-PCR analysis used in this study provides no additional prognostic information to routine histopathologic examination of SLNs, data regarding the impact of treating patients who have resected stage III melanoma with 1 month of HDI are anxiously awaited [71–73].

In light of the toxicity of IFNα-2b, the possibility that only the first month of high-dose therapy may be all that is needed to reduce the risk for relapse and death has been entertained by other investigators as well. A trial by the Hellenic Cooperative Oncology Group initiated a trial to compare 1 month of HDI treatment compared with the standard 1-year regimen as adjuvant treatment in stage IIB/III melanoma [74]. Thirty-one percent of patients required dose adjustment, mainly in the first month of "induction" therapy, but only 2% required treatment discontinuation. Although the treatment was well tolerated, efficacy results have not yet been reported.

Tumor necrosis factor-α

Another cytokine that has been postulated to facilitate the development of antitumor immunity is tumor necrosis factor-α (TNFα). Although its precise mechanism of action is uncertain, TNFα seems to target the tumor vasculature [75]. Its systemic application has been limited by its significant toxicity. Major side effects include capillary leak syndrome, oliguria, acute renal failure, hypoglycemia, gastrointestinal tract infarction, and disseminated intravascular coagulation. For this reason, interest in this agent has been largely restricted to the context of regional therapy, such as isolated limb perfusion (ILP), typically in conjunction with melphalan (or other cytotoxic agents), for advanced extremity melanoma. Unfortunately, even the leakage of TNFα into the systemic circulation can be life threatening. In the prospective multicenter study ACOSOG Z0020, 133 patients were randomized to receive melphalan alone or melphalan plus TNFα [76]. The study was terminated early after interim review by the data safety monitoring committee because of increased toxicity in the TFNα arm. After treatment of 124 evaluable patients, the response rates were similar (69% versus 64% overall response rate at 3 months [$P = .435$]), but 16% of patients experienced grade 4 adverse events in the TNFα group compared with 4% in the melphalan-alone group ($P = .0436$). Despite these results, ILP with TNFα-containing drug regimens continues to receive support in Europe, with some reports suggesting that toxicity may be reduced with lower dose regimens [77–80]. Although TNFα has some biologic activity in malignant melanoma, it is not likely to become a major player in treatment regimens until the advent of a delivery system that affords a substantial reduction in toxicity.

Interleukin-12

In animal models, IL-12 has been shown to decrease tumor burden and prevent metastases in renal cell cancer, sarcomas, mammary cancer, and bladder cancer. The antitumor effects involve cell-mediated tumoricidal activity and inhibition of angiogenesis [66]. Phase I studies of IL-12 in human beings have been completed, and phase II studies are currently underway. In the setting of metastatic melanoma, IL-12, alone or in conjunction with IFNα-2b or IL-2, has exhibited limited biologic activity with occasional minor responses [81–84]. In light of its limited activity as a single agent, IL-12 might be most effective as an adjuvant agent in conjunction with specific immunotherapy or other treatment modalities.

Other nonspecific immunotherapies

Fusion proteins

As mechanisms underlying the development of antitumor immunity are increasingly elucidated at the molecular level, opportunities for the development of bi- or multifunctional fusion molecules abound. This strategy is attractive because proper selection of active moieties could theoretically produce a synergistic effect on immunomodulation and because the creation of novel therapeutics has important ramifications in terms of intellectual property and patent protection. Stagg and colleagues [85], for example, constructed a GM-CSF–IL-2 fusion cDNA and expressed it in a murine melanoma cell line. The fusion cDNA exhibited synergistic biologic activity relative to cells expressing GM-CSF and IL-2 individually in a whole-cell vaccine model.

Regulatory T cells are CD4+/CD25+/FoxP3+ T lymphocytes that seem to be important for controlling autoreactive immune effector cells and maintaining immunologic homeostasis [86]. Studies in murine models have shown that Tregs impair antitumor CTL activity and that Treg depletion in vivo augments antitumor immunity [87–90]. *Denileukin diftitox* (ONTAK) is a fusion protein of IL-2 and diphtheria toxin A that is designed to produce a cytotoxic effect on T lymphocytes with a high level of expression of the IL-2 receptor (IL-2R) [91,92]. This agent is approved by the FDA for the treatment of cutaneous T-cell lymphoma. Because CD25+ Tregs are known to have a high level of IL-2R expression, there has been interest in exploring whether there is the potential to induce antitumor CTL activity through elimination of Tregs. Attia and colleagues [93] treated 12 patients who had metastatic melanoma with ONTAK and found neither a reduction in Treg frequency nor regression of melanoma. Whether an agent that targets Tregs more specifically and effectively than ONTAK would exhibit significant clinical antitumor activity against melanoma is unclear, but the central role of these cells in immunoregulation seems to justify further research in this arena.

Allovectin-7

Melanoma may adapt and change its cell surface proteins to evade the host immune system. One mechanism of immunologic escape involves a reduction in the expression of MHC class I molecules on the cell surface, enabling tumor cells to evade cell-mediated immunity. Allovectin-7 is a novel type of gene therapy that targets this escape mechanism. It comprises a DNA plasmid construct encoding the genes for an allogeneic MHC class I protein (HLA-B7) and β_2-microglobulin complex with a cationic lipid mixture that facilitates the plasmid's uptake by tumor cells. This plasmid also includes unmethylated CpG motifs to enhance the immune response further. In a phase II clinical trial of Allovectin-7 in patients who had metastatic melanoma, investigators observed a systemic response in 11% and disease stabilization in 19% using an intent-to-treat analysis [94]. The treatment was well tolerated, and major side effects were primarily associated with biopsy or injection procedures. Phase III trials comparing Allovectin-7 plus dacarbazine versus dacarbazine alone are currently under way.

Combination therapies

Biochemotherapy (chemoimmunotherapy) refers to strategies in which biologic response modifiers are combined with systemic chemotherapy. For a more comprehensive review of this topic, the reader is referred to several previously published review articles [95–99]. Briefly, some phase II trials examining biochemotherapy regimens have demonstrated promising biologic activity in advanced melanoma, with reported overall response rates as high as 52% in stage IV disease [100–103]. IFNα-2b has been used as monotherapy or in conjunction with traditional chemotherapy as primary treatment for metastatic melanoma. An overview of trials from 1984 through 1989 in which IFNα-2b was used as a single agent for stage IV melanoma showed a mean response rate of 15% (range: 6%–27%). Reported response duration ranges from 1 month to 60+ months. Mixed results were observed when IFNα-2b was combined with a variety of chemotherapeutic regimens. Hahka-Kemppinen and colleagues [104] used combination therapy with dacarbazine, vincristine, lomustine, and IFNα-2b and achieved PR rates of 27% and CR rates of 41%, with a median response duration of 10.2 months. Vuoristo and colleagues [105] used combination therapy with dacarbazine, vincristine, bleomycin, lomustine, and IFNα-2b with an 18% PR rate, 14% CR rate, and median response durations of 9 months and 6 months, respectively. A major concern regarding biochemotherapy is increased toxicity relative to immunotherapy alone without a comparable increase in efficacy [99,101,106,107]; hence, the use of biochemotherapy for the treatment of melanoma remains controversial.

Specific immunotherapies

Specific immunotherapy refers to those immunologic strategies that target one or more specific antigens. The discovery that melanomas express shared antigens sparked a resurgence of interest in specific immunotherapy over the past 2 to 3 decades (Fig. 2). Currently relevant primarily in the context of specific (as opposed to nonspecific) immunotherapy strategies is the distinction between active versus passive approaches. Passive (adoptive) immunotherapies involve the provision of the actual effector molecules (eg, antibodies) or cells (eg, T cells) that directly target tumor cells. In contrast, active immunotherapy induces the patient's own immune system to

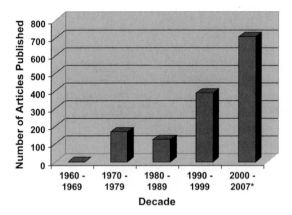

Fig. 2. The past 3 decades have seen a dramatic surge of interest in melanoma vaccine research, as evidenced, in part, by a dramatic increase in the number of articles published on the topic (Ovid Medline search on April 7, 2007: abstracts containing terms *melanoma and* [*vaccine* or *active specific immunotherapy* or *specific active immunotherapy*]). *Includes published articles through the fourth week of March 2007.

generate a melanoma-specific immune response. Active specific immunotherapy generally refers to cancer vaccines. Despite several advances, this approach has been hampered consistently by poor clinical efficacy. Consequently, investigators have examined a wide array of specific immunotherapy platforms and have increasingly incorporated one or more adjuvant agents to augment immune responsiveness. Several different nonspecific immune modulators, some of which have been discussed in the previous section, have been used as adjuvants. This section describes a variety of specific immunotherapies that have been investigated for the treatment of melanoma.

Specific active immunotherapy

Specific active immunotherapy for melanoma refers to the use of a melanoma-specific vaccine for the primary or adjuvant treatment of melanoma. There are some fundamental differences between cancer vaccines and traditional vaccines against infectious pathogens. Vaccines against infectious diseases target foreign antigens, which are highly immunogenic and usually are able to induce protective immunity after an appropriate immunization dose and schedule. This is in contrast to cancer vaccines, which primarily target overexpressed, selectively expressed, or mutated self-antigens and are inherently less immunogenic compared with most foreign pathogens. Furthermore, cellular immunity—particularly MAA-specific CTL responses—rather than humoral immunity is believed to represent an essential component of clinically meaningful antitumor immunity. Induction of MAA-specific CTL activity necessitates a series of immunologic events that lead to the formation of an immunologic synapse at the DC-CTL interface

[108,109]. DCs must not only present MAA peptide–MHC class I complexes to CTLs, but they must do so in conjunction with costimulatory molecules, such as B7.1, B7.2, and CD40. In addition, DCs must secrete adequate quantities of Th1-promoting cytokines (eg, IL-12) to create a Th1 bias in the polarity of the T-cell response. It seems that tolerance rather than immunity may result if key signals do not occur in the appropriate manner.

Melanoma vaccines have taken many forms through the course of their evolution; a comprehensive discussion of cancer vaccine strategies is beyond the scope of this review (please refer to other articles [17,110–112]). Such strategies may target defined antigens—meaning that the specific antigens present in (or encoded by) the vaccine are known—or undefined antigens. The latter category includes vaccines incorporating cell lysates, irradiated whole cells, or cellular DNA or RNA, for example. Examples of defined-antigen vaccine formulations comprising specific MAAs include oligopeptides; proteins; recombinant DNA–containing preparations; and carbohydrate-containing antigens, such as gangliosides. Several of these are discussed briefly here.

Peptide vaccines

Protein-based vaccines provide multiple epitopes without the disadvantage of HLA restriction. Production of large enough quantities of MAA proteins for vaccine formulation is less practical and desirable in terms of immunologic monitoring relative to preparation of oligopeptide-based vaccines; hence, the major emphasis has been on the latter. Several immunodominant peptide epitopes have been sequenced and characterized. The synthesis and purification of MAA peptides on a large scale for preparation of melanoma vaccines is generally feasible from technical and financial standpoints. Although peptides do not represent a highly immunogenic form of antigen, they do not require antigen processing by DCs and they are readily amenable to immunologic monitoring because of their defined nature. In addition, the immunogenicity of some MAA peptide epitopes has been enhanced with single amino acid substitutions (eg, gp100:209–217[210M]) [113]. One disadvantage of peptide-based vaccines is that, for practical reasons, only patients with more common HLA types and for whom HLA-restricted peptides are available (eg, HLA A1, A2, A3) are candidates for treatment with most preparations. As new immunodominant class I and class II restricted epitopes are identified, multiepitope vaccine preparations that are suitable for patients with a broader array of HLA types should become increasingly available.

Numerous peptide-based vaccines have been examined in the context of small clinical trials, and, although immunologic responses have been observed, major clinical responses have been infrequent [66]. This has prompted interest in identifying more effective adjuvant agents, combining multiple antigenic peptides, incorporating unrelated helper peptides that enhance CD4+ T-cell responses, and exploring agents that activate CTLs

[114–118]. In a phase II trial of 56 patients who had metastatic melanoma, ipilimumab was combined with a vaccine containing two HLA-A*0201– restricted gp100 melanoma peptides [62,119]. Data reported from this trial have thus far revealed two CRs that have persisted at 30 and 31 months and five PRs that have persisted from 4 to more than 34 months. Interestingly, induction of durable objective responses correlated with the induction of autoimmunity. Cooperative group trial ECOG E1602, currently underway, is a randomized, controlled, multicenter trial examining the immunologic response to a multiepitope peptide vaccine. In this protocol, patients who have measurable stage IV melanoma are treated with 12 HLA-A1–, -A2–, or -A3–restricted melanoma peptides and six helper peptides and with GM-CSF and the oil-based vaccine adjuvant montanide ISA-51.

Nucleic acid vaccines

Vaccination with genetic material encoding tumor antigens represents an alternative to vaccination with antigens themselves. Although an undefined-antigen preparation can be derived from tumor cell DNA or RNA, a defined-antigen preparation can be generated through recombinant molecular techniques. Using the latter approach, constructs may be developed that encode not only the MAA(s) of interest but costimulatory molecules, cytokines, or other factors that promote the induction of antitumor immunity. One vector for delivery of genetic material is plasmid DNA. Plasmid DNA vaccines are usually injected intramuscularly, allowing the plasmids to be taken up by host myocytes, which then produce the encoded antigen. The antigen is then processed by DCs and presented to T cells. Because plasmid DNA is derived from bacteria, it contains unmethylated CpG repeats that could contribute to immunogenicity by activation of DC TLRs. A phase I study was recently reported in which 12 patients who had high-risk resected melanoma received intramuscular injections of a plasmid-based vaccine encoding Mart-1 and a control plasmid encoding hepatitis B surface antigen (HBsAg) [120]. Although the treatment was well tolerated, there were no clinical responses, nor were there antibody or T-cell responses against Mart-1 or HBsAg.

An alternative approach to the delivery of genetic material is to use viral vectors. Constructs encoding the same antigen(s) may be developed from heterologous viral vectors and administered sequentially in a "prime-boost" fashion. An advantage of the prime-boost strategy is that the deleterious effect of neutralizing antibodies on vaccine efficacy can be mitigated. Jager and colleagues [121] recently reported on the treatment of patients who had a variety of solid tumor types, including melanoma, with a prime-boost strategy that incorporated a vaccinia construct and a fowlpox construct, each encoding the antigen NY-ESO-1. Although there were no major clinical responses, the vaccine was tolerated well and humoral and CTL responses against multiple NY-ESO-1 epitopes were observed.

Heat shock proteins

HSPs are molecular chaperones that are upregulated when cells are exposed to thermal stress. HSPs facilitate folding, assembly, or disassembly of proteins. Certain proteins, when unfolded, expose parts of their structure that can trigger apoptosis in the cell. HSPs also possess inflammatory qualities, including activation and maturation of DCs and induction of cytokine and chemokine release. When an HSP is conjugated with a peptide and is taken up by a DC, the HSP enhances presentation of that peptide in association with the MHC complex [122]. This has attracted interest in HSP-containing cancer vaccines. Pilla and colleagues [123] examined the activity of autologous "personalized" tumor-derived HSP gp96 peptide complexes (Oncophage) in patients who had stage IV melanoma. The vaccine was administered in conjunction with GM-CSF and IFNα-2b. Of 38 patients enrolled, 18 patients who had measurable disease and at least four weekly injections were considered evaluable. Although no clinical responses were noted (only disease stabilization), toxicity was mild and 5 of 17 patients tested had evidence of an HLA class I–restricted T-cell response by enzyme-linked immunospot (ELISpot) assay. An alternative approach that is currently in development is to construct hybrid peptides that contain an MHC class I–binding epitope and an HSP-binding moiety, a strategy that has been shown to enhance immunogenicity [122]. This technology could enhance the potency of defined-antigen multivalent peptide melanoma vaccines.

Whole tumor cell vaccines

Whole-cell vaccines may be autologous or allogeneic. Although the autologous approach is desirable, because the vaccine contains all the antigens relevant to a patient's tumor, preparation of autologous tumor vaccines is cumbersome and may not be feasible in a substantial proportion of patients. In contrast, allogeneic vaccines generally originate from melanoma cell lines cultivated from tumors of unrelated patients. A distinct practical advantage is that the antigenic properties of an allogeneic melanoma vaccine derived from established cell lines can be thoroughly characterized, and such a vaccine can be cultivated in large quantities in a highly reproducible manner. An example of this is an irradiated, polyvalent, whole-cell melanoma vaccine (Canvaxin) developed by Morton and colleagues [124]. Canvaxin seemed promising in phase II studies as an adjuvant therapy in the setting of completely resected melanoma with high risk for relapse. Unfortunately, each of two phase III trials—examining the value of adjuvant Canvaxin in completely resected stage III melanoma and (in a separate trial) completely resected stage IV melanoma—showed no improvement in disease-free or overall survival [125]. Therefore, in the absence of a major improvement in formulation (eg, demonstration of clinically significant biologic activity with a superior adjuvant), allogeneic whole-cell melanoma vaccine preparations are unlikely to receive significant emphasis over the ensuing years.

Dendritic cell vaccines

Because of the central role of DCs in the priming of antigen-specific T-cell immunity, the preparation of customized DC-based vaccines is an attractive approach to specific immunotherapy. The ability to generate and manipulate large numbers of DCs ex vivo made this a feasible vaccine platform [126]. A wide variety of DC-based vaccines have been tested in early-phase clinical trials of patients who have advanced melanoma and have included DCs loaded with peptides, tumor lysates, autologous tumor RNA, and other forms of MAAs [127–135]. In general, although DC-based vaccines have the potential to induce robust MAA-specific immune responses, the clinical impact has been disappointing. An exciting preclinical development is the generation of MAA peptide- or protein-loaded DCs that are genetically modified with adenoviral constructs encoding IL-18 and the IL-12 p70 subunit [136]. These DCs have been shown to induce strongly Th1 biased T-cell responses in vitro against MAAs, such as MAGE-A6. Although DC-based vaccines are cumbersome to prepare, the ability to manipulate them ex vivo to induce MAA-specific immune responses and to provide a customized milieu of regulatory signals could translate into clinically meaningful antitumor immunity.

Dendritic cell–melanoma fusion ("dendritoma") vaccines

One problem with irradiated tumor cell vaccines is that they do not contain high levels of MHC class I molecules or costimulatory molecules, a limitation that could hamper immune activation. DCs, conversely, must be properly loaded with MAAs, and this presents a host of technical considerations that may have an adverse impact on vaccine effectiveness. An exciting strategy that overcomes many of these problems is a vaccine platform based on the fusion of DCs with irradiated autologous melanoma cells. This approach has been developed and applied to patients who have advanced melanoma [137–142]. In a recent study by Wei and colleagues, 10 patients who had metastatic melanoma were treated daily for 5 days with subcutaneous injections of autologous dendritomas plus low-dose IL-2, followed by up to five additional injections of dendritomas alone at 3-month intervals [138]. The vaccine was well tolerated, with all grade 3 or higher toxicities being attributable to the IL-2. Eight of 9 patients had immunologic responses. There was one CR and two mixed responses, and 2 patients had disease stabilization (with durations of 4 and 9 months). The applicability of this therapy may be limited, in part, by the number of patients for whom dendritomas can be generated, but early results seem to show enough promise to warrant further investigation into the potential role of this strategy in the treatment of melanoma.

Barriers to generating successful melanoma vaccines

Despite the development of increasingly sophisticated melanoma vaccines and the successful induction of MAA-specific immune responses in some studies, robust clinical responses are uncommon. One fundamental problem is that the ideal surrogate biomarker for the clinical efficacy of cancer vaccines remains unknown. For example, it is not even certain that the measurement of peripheral blood T-cell responses, which represents the metric for many standard immunologic monitoring techniques, accurately reflects the clinically relevant antitumor T-cell response to a melanoma vaccine. Slingluff and colleagues [143] have developed a method for measuring the MAA-specific T-cell response within the SLN draining the melanoma vaccine site (the "sentinel immunized node"). They found that peptide-specific T-cell responses could be identified in only 42% of patients' peripheral blood lymphocytes (PBLs) but in 80% of sentinel immunized nodes. This illustrates the complexity of selecting appropriate biomarkers for melanoma vaccine efficacy and the key role of surgeons in facilitating the proper immunologic monitoring of specific active immunotherapy.

Still more importantly, the key variables regarding vaccine administration, such as the specific antigen(s), vaccine type, vaccine formulation (including adjuvant[s]), dose, dosing frequency, and route of administration, remain largely undefined (Fig. 3). For example, despite the phenomenon of epitope spreading [144] after MAA peptide vaccination, targeting a single peptide epitope is unlikely to produce a robust clinical antitumor response because of antigen escape and other mechanisms of resistance. Conversely, the use of highly complex or even undefined forms of MAAs (eg, whole tumor cells, tumor lysates) dilutes out immunodominant epitopes and results in the expansion of a large number of "competing" T cells that recognize irrelevant antigens. How to find the perfect balance between these two extremes remains a mystery. During the next decade, a major focus of research is likely to be the characterization and optimization of these variables.

Specific adoptive immunotherapy

Adoptive molecular immunotherapy

Several monoclonal antibodies targeting specific antigens have been shown to be useful adjuncts to treatment of other tumors, such as trastuzumab (Herceptin) for breast cancer and rituximab (Rituxan) for B-cell lymphoma [145,146]. Although there are no FDA-approved MAA-specific antibodies for the treatment of melanoma, there is interest in developing antibody-based therapies in this disease. Ganglioside-directed antibodies have received the greatest attention. Choi and colleagues [147] recently reported the results of a phase I trial of IL-2 in conjunction with two ganglioside-directed antibodies: one chimeric antibody (ch14.18) against GD2 and one murine antibody (R24) against GD.sub.3 ganglioside. Immunologic effects included the induction of anti-idiotype antibodies against ch14.18 in 6 patients. Augmentation of lymphokine-activated killer (LAK) cell activity and antibody-dependent cell-mediated cytotoxicity was also observed. Of 23 patients who had melanoma and were enrolled in the study, 2 had

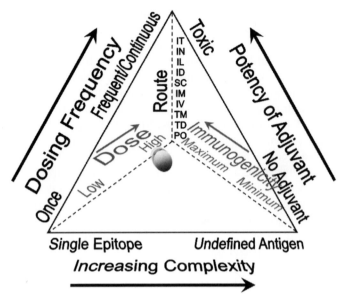

Fig. 3. Optimizing cancer vaccines: an nth dimensional problem. One of the barriers to progress toward the development of clinically effective melanoma vaccines is that many variables regarding vaccine preparation and administration remain poorly understood. Several potentially important factors are shown in this figure, which, for simplicity, depicts the complexity of solving a multidimensional optimization problem, the solution of which is denoted by the blue ovoid figure lying within the pyramidal space. In reality, because of the complexity of the immunologic mechanisms underlying antitumor immunity in human beings, it is doubtful that all the critical variables that must be optimized to achieve maximal vaccine effectiveness have even been recognized yet. Therefore, the challenge of developing effective melanoma vaccines may be likened to solving an nth dimensional mathematic problem. ID, intradermal; IL, intralymphatic; IM, intramuscular; IN, intranodal; IT, intratumoral (intralesional); IV, intravenous; PO, per os (orally); SC, subcutaneous; TM, transmucosal; TD, transdermal.

a PR and 4 had stable disease. This work helped to lay the foundation for the development of fusion proteins called immunocytokines—cytokines that have been fused with antibodies against MAAs to direct their activity specifically to tumor cells. One such fusion protein is a GD2-specific antibody–IL-2 fusion protein (ch14.18-IL-2). The biologic activity of this agent is currently being examined by Albertini at the University of Wisconsin in the setting of advanced unresectable melanoma (NCI-6304, ClinicalTrials.gov NCT00109863).

Adoptive cellular immunotherapy

Adoptive cellular immunotherapy is a strategy involving the administration of immune effector cells—most notably, activated tumor-reactive T cells—to the patient who has melanoma. The early stages of development of adoptive cell transfer began with LAK cells, a nonspecific adoptive immunotherapy consisting of activated NK cells. LAK cells were created by stimulating PBLs with a T-cell growth factor that was later determined to be IL-2 [148,149]. With the recognition that TILs could be harvested from melanoma deposits and expanded ex vivo with IL-2, researchers turned their attention to using TILs for adoptive cell transfer [150].

From 1992 to 2001, Ridolfi and colleagues [151] treated 25 patients who had completely resected stage III and IV melanoma with adoptive immunotherapy using TILs. The expanded TILs were reinfused back into patients on day 1 of a 5-day cycle of continuous infusion high-dose IL-2. Treatment was continued for 6 months unless unacceptable side effects occurred. Eight (36.3%) of 22 evaluable patients were disease-free after a median follow-up of 5 years.

In an effort to enhance the effectiveness of TIL therapy, Dudley and colleagues [152] administered lymphodepleting nonmyeloablative chemotherapy before TIL administration to eliminate suppressor T cells and to decrease competition by endogenous lymphocytes for homeostatic regulatory cytokines. Thirty-five patients who had metastatic melanoma that was refractory to standard treatments, including high-dose IL-2, were first given nonmyeloablative lymphodepleting chemotherapy consisting of 2 days of cyclophosphamide followed by 5 days of fludarabine. Patients were then given an infusion of tumor-reactive lymphocytes and high dose IL-2. After 15 patients were enrolled, a modification was made to the trial to include vaccination with the MART-1 or gp100 peptide if the TILs the patients received were MART-1 or gp100 specific. Eighteen (35%) of 51 patients experienced an objective response, with three CRs and 15 PRs. Toxicity of the treatment included opportunistic infections; fludarabine-related side effects; and IL-2–associated toxicities, such as autoimmune phenomena (eg, vitiligo, uveitis). Three of these patients required a second course of treatment to obtain an objective response. Peptide vaccination after TIL administration had no effect on treatment efficacy. Response duration lasted from 2 months to more than 2 years. Immunocytochemical analysis of relapsing patients showed loss of antigen expression by tumors, loss of HLA class I antigen, and decreased expression of the MART-1 antigen, whereas other differentiation antigens were not affected. This illustrates that TILs exert a significant selective pressure on the expression pattern of tumor cell populations.

Genetically modified T cells

To be a candidate for adoptive cellular therapy with TILs, a patient must meet several requirements. First, the patient must have a particular HLA type. A tumor must be accessible for surgical resection or biopsy, and viable TILs must be generated from the tumor in adequate numbers. The TILs must recognize MAAs and must have tumoricidal activity. Only a few patients meet these criteria. Recently, tumor-reactive T cells have been generated through gene transfer technology [153]. Morgan and colleagues [154] reported on 15 patients who had metastatic melanoma and were treated with adoptive transfer of autologous T lymphocytes that were genetically modified with a retroviral vector encoding a Mart-1–specific T-cell receptor (TCR). They observed durable engraftment of genetically modified T cells as long as 1 year after adoptive transfer. Two patients experienced regression of melanoma.

Another approach to "designer T-cell" therapy has been developed and is also in the early stages of testing. These T cells express chimeric immuno-globulin T-cell receptor complexes (IgTCRs), which were created by joining the cell-signaling portion of the TCR with the antigen recognition domain of an antibody. This enables T cells to target specific tumor antigens in an MHC-unrestricted fashion, rendering this a viable treatment option for virtually all patients. Activation of the IgTCR induces production of IL-2, IFN, GM-CSF, and TNFα [155,156]. In vitro studies targeting the melanoma antigen GD3 or high-molecular-weight (HMW) MAA have been promising [157–159]. The ability to incorporate key accessory proteins, such as costimulatory molecules, into these constructs represents an exciting strategy for producing highly potent melanoma-reactive CTLs against MAAs of interest.

Summary

Immunotherapy for the treatment of malignant melanoma has been a ripe area of research since the 1970s, and interest in this modality only continues to grow. Two immunotherapies remain approved by the FDA for the treatment of melanoma: IFNα-2b for the adjuvant treatment of patients who have high-risk resected stage II and III melanoma and IL-2 for the primary treatment of patients who have stage IV melanoma. Because their application is limited by significant toxicity and modest biologic activity, both are the subject of some controversy. Nonetheless, some patients who receive IL-2 experience dramatic and durable responses, and this represents a proof of principle that immunotherapy can serve as a highly effective treatment modality in the setting of advanced melanoma.

Studies of specific and nonspecific immunotherapy strategies have shown some promise. These two areas are gradually evolving into two facets of a single modality. In particular, many of the "nonspecific" immune modulators are increasingly being used as a means of providing the molecular signals required to program immune cells to mount a clinically significant melanoma-specific immune response. A variety of specific immunotherapies have been investigated in human beings. Although they generally have not induced robust clinical responses, these strategies allow investigators to study melanoma-specific immune responses in a precise manner. It is likely only a matter of time before there is enough information available to design clinically effective immunotherapies targeting the appropriate antigenic epitopes for each patient.

Progress in immunotherapy for melanoma is critically dependent on the participation of surgeons. Surgeons represent the front line of medical care for patients who have high-risk resectable melanomas. Many such patients are candidates or may become candidates for established or experimental immunotherapies. The ability of surgeons to participate actively in or to facilitate the development, administration, or monitoring of immunotherapies for patients who have melanoma should undoubtedly have a major impact on the future success of this treatment modality. Melanoma immunotherapy represents an opportunity for surgeons to shun a strictly technical role in the care of patients who have cancer and assume an active role in developing new therapeutic options for patients who have a potentially disabling and life-threatening disease.

References

[1] Chong CA, Gregor RJ, Augsburger JJ, et al. Spontaneous regression of choroidal melanoma over 8 years. Retina 1989;9(2):136–8.

[2] Shields CL, Piccone MR, Fung KL, et al. Spontaneous regression of metastatic cutaneous melanoma to the choroid. Retina 2002;22(6):806–8.

[3] King M, Spooner D, Rowlands DC. Spontaneous regression of metastatic malignant melanoma of the parotid gland and neck lymph nodes: a case report and a review of the literature. Clin Oncol (R Coll Radiol) 2001;13(6):466–9.

[4] Morton DL, Eilber FR, Holmes EC, et al. BCG immunotherapy of malignant melanoma: summary of a seven-year experience. Ann Surg 1974;180(4):635–43.

[5] Darrow TL, Slingluff CL Jr, Seigler HF. The role of HLA class I antigens in recognition of melanoma cells by tumor-specific cytotoxic T lymphocytes. Evidence for shared tumor antigens. J Immunol 1989;142(9):3329–35.

[6] van der Bruggen P, Traversari C, Chomez P, et al. A gene encoding an antigen recognized by cytolytic T lymphocytes on a human melanoma. Science 1991;254(5038):1643–7.

[7] Kawakami Y, Zakut R, Topalian SL, et al. Shared human melanoma antigens. Recognition by tumor-infiltrating lymphocytes in HLA-A2.1-transfected melanomas. J Immunol 1992; 148(2):638–43.

[8] Topalian SL, Hom SS, Kawakami Y, et al. Recognition of shared melanoma antigens by human tumor-infiltrating lymphocytes. J Immunother 1992;12(3):203–6.

[9] Hom SS, Schwartzentruber DJ, Rosenberg SA, et al. Specific release of cytokines by lymphocytes infiltrating human melanomas in response to shared melanoma antigens. J Immunother 1993;13(1):18–30.

[10] Storkus WJ, Zeh HJ 3rd, Maeurer MJ, et al. Identification of human melanoma peptides recognized by class I restricted tumor infiltrating T lymphocytes. J Immunol 1993;151(7): 3719–27.

[11] Rosenberg SA. A new era for cancer immunotherapy based on the genes that encode cancer antigens. Immunity 1999;10(3):281–7.

[12] Chen YT, Scanlan MJ, Sahin U, et al. A testicular antigen aberrantly expressed in human cancers detected by autologous antibody screening. Proc Natl Acad Sci USA 1997;94(5): 1914–8.

[13] Sahin U, Tureci O, Schmitt H, et al. Human neoplasms elicit multiple specific immune responses in the autologous host. Proc Natl Acad Sci USA 1995;92(25):11810–3.

[14] Cox AL, Skipper J, Chen Y, et al. Identification of a peptide recognized by five melanoma-specific human cytotoxic T cell lines. Science 1994;264(5159):716–9.

[15] Topalian SL, Rivoltini L, Mancini M, et al. Human CD4+ T cells specifically recognize a shared melanoma-associated antigen encoded by the tyrosinase gene. Proc Natl Acad Sci USA 1994;91(20):9461–5.

[16] Parkhurst MR, Fitzgerald EB, Southwood S, et al. Identification of a shared HLA-A*0201-restricted T-cell epitope from the melanoma antigen tyrosinase-related protein 2 (TRP2). Cancer Res 1998;58(21):4895–901.

[17] Spagnoli GC, Adamina M, Bolli M, et al. Active antigen-specific immunotherapy of melanoma: from basic science to clinical investigation. World J Surg 2005;29(6):692–9.

[18] Renkvist N, Castelli C, Robbins PF, et al. A listing of human tumor antigens recognized by T cells. Cancer Immunol Immunother 2001;50(1):3–15.

[19] Simpson AJ, Caballero OL, Jungbluth A, et al. Cancer/testis antigens, gametogenesis and cancer. Nat Rev Cancer 2005;5(8):615–25.

[20] Epping MT, Bernards R. A causal role for the human tumor antigen preferentially expressed antigen of melanoma in cancer. Cancer Res 2006;66(22):10639–42.

[21] Coley WB. Late results of the treatment of inoperable sarcoma by the mixed toxins of erysipelas and bacillus prodigiosus. Am J Med Sci 1906;131:375–430.

[22] Gallucci S, Matzinger P. Danger signals: SOS to the immune system. Curr Opin Immunol 2001;13(1):114–9.

[23] Hsu LC, Park JM, Zhang K, et al. The protein kinase PKR is required for macrophage apoptosis after activation of Toll-like receptor 4. Nature 2004;428(6980):341–5.

[24] Hattar K, Grandel U, Moeller A, et al. Lipoteichoic acid (LTA) from Staphylococcus aureus stimulates human neutrophil cytokine release by a CD14-dependent, Toll-like-receptor-independent mechanism: autocrine role of tumor necrosis factor-[alpha] in mediating LTA-induced interleukin-8 generation. Crit Care Med 2006;34(3):835–41.

[25] Haselmayer P, Tenzer S, Kwon BS, et al. Herpes virus entry mediator synergizes with Toll-like receptor mediated neutrophil inflammatory responses. Immunology 2006;119(3):404–11.

[26] Pasare C, Medzhitov R. Control of B-cell responses by Toll-like receptors. Nature 2005;438(7066):364–8.

[27] Ruprecht CR, Lanzavecchia A. Toll-like receptor stimulation as a third signal required for activation of human naive B cells. Eur J Immunol 2006;36(4):810–6.

[28] Peng G, Guo Z, Kiniwa Y, et al. Toll-like receptor 8-mediated reversal of CD4+ regulatory T cell function. Science 2005;309(5739):1380–4.

[29] Chaperot L, Blum A, Manches O, et al. Virus or TLR agonists induce TRAIL-mediated cytotoxic activity of plasmacytoid dendritic cells. J Immunol 2006;176(1):248–55.

[30] Horng T, Barton GM, Flavell RA, et al. The adaptor molecule TIRAP provides signalling specificity for Toll-like receptors. Nature 2002;420(6913):329–33.

[31] Hacker H, Redecke V, Blagoev B, et al. Specificity in Toll-like receptor signalling through distinct effector functions of TRAF3 and TRAF6. Nature 2006;439(7073):204–7.

[32] Zhou X-X, Jia W-H, Shen G-P, et al. Sequence variants in toll-like receptor 10 are associated with nasopharyngeal carcinoma risk. Cancer Epidemiol Biomarkers Prev 2006;15(5):862–6.

[33] Kollisch G, Kalali BN, Voelcker V, et al. Various members of the Toll-like receptor family contribute to the innate immune response of human epidermal keratinocytes. Immunology 2005;114(4):531–41.

[34] Schaefer TM, Fahey JV, Wright JA, et al. Innate immunity in the human female reproductive tract: antiviral response of uterine epithelial cells to the TLR3 agonist poly (I:C). J Immunol 2005;174(2):992–1002.

[35] Beutler B, Hoebe K, Georgel P, et al. Genetic analysis of innate immunity: identification and function of the TIR adapter proteins. Adv Exp Med Biol 2005;560:29–39.

[36] Tsan MF, Gao B. Endogenous ligands of Toll-like receptors. J Leukoc Biol 2004;76(3):514–9.

[37] Lauzon NM, Mian F, MacKenzie R, et al. The direct effects of Toll-like receptor ligands on human NK cell cytokine production and cytotoxicity. Cell Immunol 2006;241(2):102–12.

[38] Sivori S, Falco M, Della Chiesa M, et al. CpG and double-stranded RNA trigger human NK cells by Toll-like receptors: induction of cytokine release and cytotoxicity against tumors and dendritic cells. Proc Natl Acad Sci USA 2004;101(27):10116–21.

[39] Qian C, Jiang X, An H, et al. TLR agonists promote ERK-mediated preferential IL-10 production of regulatory dendritic cells (diffDCs), leading to NK-cell activation. Blood 2006; 108(7):2307–15.

[40] Delale T, Paquin A, Asselin-Paturel C, et al. MyD88-dependent and -independent murine cytomegalovirus sensing for IFN-alpha release and initiation of immune responses in vivo. J Immunol 2005;175(10):6723–32.

[41] Seigler HF, Shingleton WW, Pickrell KL. Intralesional BCG, intravenous immune lymphocytes, and immunization with neuraminidase-treated tumor cells to manage melanoma; a clinical assessment. Plast Reconstr Surg 1975;55(3):294–8.

[42] Mastrangelo MJ, Bellet RE, Berkelhammer J, et al. Regression of pulmonary metastatic disease associated with intralesional BCG therapy of intracutaneous melanoma metastases. Cancer 1975;36(4):1305–8.

[43] Baker MA, Taub RN. BCG in malignant melanoma. Lancet 1973;1(7812):1117–8.

[44] Nathanson L. Regression of intradermal malignant melanoma after intralesional injection of Mycobacterium bovis strain BCG. Cancer Chemother Reports - Part 1 1972;56(5): 659–65.

[45] Bluming AZ, Vogel CL, Ziegler JL, et al. Immunological effects of BCG in malignant melanoma: two modes of administration compared. Ann Intern Med 1972;76(3):405–11.

[46] Mastrangelo MJ, Sulit HL, Prehn LM, et al. Intralesional BCG in the treatment of metastatic malignant melanoma. Cancer 1976;37(2):684–92.

[47] Ariyan S, Kirkwood JM, Mitchell MS, et al. Intralymphatic and regional surgical adjuvant immunotherapy in high-risk melanoma of the extremities. Surgery 1982;92(3):459–63.

[48] Livingston PO. Approaches to augmenting the immunogenicity of melanoma gangliosides: from whole melanoma cells to ganglioside-KLH conjugate vaccines. Immunol Rev 1995; 145:147–66.

[49] Kolmel KF, Grange JM, Krone B, et al. Prior immunisation of patients with malignant melanoma with vaccinia or BCG is associated with better survival. A European Organization for Research and Treatment of Cancer cohort study on 542 patients. Eur J Cancer 2005;41(1):118–25.

[50] Agarwala SS, Neuberg D, Park Y, et al. Mature results of a phase III randomized trial of bacillus Calmette-Guerin (BCG) versus observation and BCG plus dacarbazine versus BCG in the adjuvant therapy of American Joint Committee on Cancer stage I-III melanoma (E1673): a trial of the Eastern Oncology Group. Cancer 2004;100(8):1692–8.

[51] Krug A, Towarowski A, Britsch S, et al. Toll-like receptor expression reveals CpG DNA as a unique microbial stimulus for plasmacytoid dendritic cells which synergizes with CD40 ligand to induce high amounts of IL-12. Eur J Immunol 2001;31(10):3026–37.

[52] Rao RD, Anderson PM, Arndt CA, et al. Aerosolized granulocyte macrophage colony-stimulating factor (GM-CSF) therapy in metastatic cancer. Am J Clin Oncol 2003;26(5): 493–8.

[53] Lee JH, Torisu-Itakara H, Cochran AJ, et al. Quantitative analysis of melanoma-induced cytokine-mediated immunosuppression in melanoma sentinel nodes. Clin Cancer Res 2005; 11(1):107–12.

[54] Nasi ML, Lieberman P, Busam KJ, et al. Intradermal injection of granulocyte-macrophage colony-stimulating factor (GM-CSF) in patients with metastatic melanoma recruits dendritic cells. Cytokines Cell Mol Ther 1999;5(3):139–44.

[55] Si Z, Hersey P, Coates AS. Clinical responses and lymphoid infiltrates in metastatic melanoma following treatment with intralesional GM-CSF. Melanoma Res 1996;6(3): 247–55.

[56] Atkins MB, Lotze MT, Dutcher JP, et al. High-dose recombinant interleukin 2 therapy for patients with metastatic melanoma: analysis of 270 patients treated between 1985 and 1993. J Clin Oncol 1999;17(7):2105–16.

[57] Tarhini AA, Agarwala SS. Interleukin-2 for the treatment of melanoma. Curr Opin Investig Drugs 2005;6(12):1234–9.

[58] Rosenberg SA, Yang JC, Topalian SL, et al. Treatment of 283 consecutive patients with metastatic melanoma or renal cell cancer using high-dose bolus interleukin 2. JAMA 1994;271(12):907–13.

[59] Atkins MB, Kunkel L, Sznol M, et al. High-dose recombinant interleukin-2 therapy in patients with metastatic melanoma: long-term survival update. Cancer J Sci Am 2000;6(Suppl 1): S11–4.

[60] Rosenberg SA, White DE. Vitiligo in patients with melanoma: normal tissue antigens can be targets for cancer immunotherapy. J Immunother Emphasis Tumor Immunol 1996; 19(1):81–4.

[61] Phan GQ, Yang JC, Sherry RM, et al. Cancer regression and autoimmunity induced by cytotoxic T lymphocyte-associated antigen 4 blockade in patients with metastatic melanoma. Proc Natl Acad Sci USA 2003;100(14):8372–7.

[62] Morse MA. Technology evaluation: ipilimumab, Medarex/Bristol-Myers Squibb. Curr Opin Mol Ther 2005;7(6):588–97.

[63] Ribas A, Camacho LH, Lopez-Berestein G, et al. Antitumor activity in melanoma and anti-self responses in a phase I trial with the anti-cytotoxic T lymphocyte-associated antigen 4 monoclonal antibody CP-675,206. J Clin Oncol 2005;23(35):8968–77.

[64] Pfeffer LM, Dinarello CA, Herberman RB, et al. Biological properties of recombinant alpha-interferons: 40th anniversary of the discovery of interferons. Cancer Res 1998;58(12): 2489–99.

[65] Dunn GP, Koebel CM, Schreiber RD. Interferons, immunity and cancer immunoediting. Nat Rev Immunol 2006;6(11):836–48.

[66] Morse MA, Lyerly HK, Clay TM, et al. Immunotherapy of surgical malignancies. Curr Probl Surg 2004;41(1):15–132.

[67] Kirkwood JM, Strawderman MH, Ernstoff MS, et al. Interferon alfa-2b adjuvant therapy of high-risk resected cutaneous melanoma: the Eastern Cooperative Oncology Group trial EST 1684. J Clin Oncol 1996;14(1):7–17.

[68] Kirkwood JM, Ibrahim JG, Sondak VK, et al. High- and low-dose interferon alfa-2b in high-risk melanoma: first analysis of intergroup trial E1690/S9111/C9190. J Clin Oncol 2000;18(12):2444–58.

[69] Kirkwood JM, Ibrahim JG, Sosman JA, et al. High-dose interferon alfa-2b significantly prolongs relapse-free and overall survival compared with the GM2-KLH/QS-21 vaccine in patients with resected stage IIB-III melanoma: results of intergroup trial E1694/S9512/C509801. J Clin Oncol 2001;19(9):2370–80.

[70] Kirkwood JM, Ibrahim J, Lawson DH, et al. High-dose interferon alfa-2b does not diminish antibody response to GM2 vaccination in patients with resected melanoma: results of the multicenter Eastern Cooperative Oncology Group phase II trial E2696. J Clin Oncol 2001;19(5):1430–6.

[71] McMasters KM. The Sunbelt Melanoma Trial. Ann Surg Oncol 2001;8(9 Suppl):41S–3S.

[72] McMasters KM, Noyes RD, Reintgen DS, et al. Lessons learned from the Sunbelt Melanoma Trial. J Surg Oncol 2004;86(4):212–23.

[73] Scoggins CR, Ross MI, Reintgen DS, et al. Prospective multi-institutional study of reverse transcriptase polymerase chain reaction for molecular staging of melanoma. J Clin Oncol 2006;24(18):2849–57.

[74] Gogas H, Bafaloukos D, Ioannovich J, et al. Tolerability of adjuvant high-dose interferon alfa-2b: 1 month versus 1 year—a Hellenic Cooperative Oncology Group study. Anticancer Res 2004;24(3b):1947–52.

[75] Menon C, Iyer M, Prabakaran I, et al. TNF-alpha downregulates vascular endothelial Flk-1 expression in human melanoma xenograft model. Am J Physiol Heart Circ Physiol 2003; 284(1):H317–29.

[76] Cornett WR, McCall LM, Petersen RP, et al. Randomized multicenter trial of hyperthermic isolated limb perfusion with melphalan alone compared with melphalan plus tumor

necrosis factor: American College of Surgeons Oncology Group trial Z0020. J Clin Oncol 2006;24(25):4196–201.

[77] Hayes AJ, Neuhaus SJ, Clark MA, et al. Isolated limb perfusion with melphalan and tumor necrosis factor alpha for advanced melanoma and soft-tissue sarcoma. Ann Surg Oncol 2007;14(1):230–8.

[78] Grunhagen DJ, de Wilt JH, van Geel AN, et al. Isolated limb perfusion for melanoma patients—a review of its indications and the role of tumour necrosis factor-alpha. Eur J Surg Oncol 2006;32(4):371–80.

[79] Grunhagen DJ, van Etten B, Brunstein F, et al. Efficacy of repeat isolated limb perfusions with tumor necrosis factor alpha and melphalan for multiple in-transit metastases in patients with prior isolated limb perfusion failure. Ann Surg Oncol 2005;12(8):609–15.

[80] Rossi CR, Foletto M, Mocellin S, et al. Hyperthermic isolated limb perfusion with low-dose tumor necrosis factor-alpha and melphalan for bulky in-transit melanoma metastases. Ann Surg Oncol 2004;11(2):173–7.

[81] Bajetta E, Del Vecchio M, Mortarini R, et al. Pilot study of subcutaneous recombinant human interleukin 12 in metastatic melanoma. Clin Cancer Res 1998;4(1):75–85.

[82] Gollob JA, Veenstra KG, Parker RA, et al. Phase I trial of concurrent twice-weekly recombinant human interleukin-12 plus low-dose IL-2 in patients with melanoma or renal cell carcinoma. J Clin Oncol 2003;21(13):2564–73.

[83] Alatrash G, Hutson TE, Molto L, et al. Clinical and immunologic effects of subcutaneously administered interleukin-12 and interferon alfa-2b: phase I trial of patients with metastatic renal cell carcinoma or malignant melanoma. J Clin Oncol 2004;22(14):2891–900.

[84] Lee P, Wang F, Kuniyoshi J, et al. Effects of interleukin-12 on the immune response to a multipeptide vaccine for resected metastatic melanoma. J Clin Oncol 2001;19(18): 3836–47.

[85] Stagg J, Wu JH, Bouganim N, et al. Granulocyte-macrophage colony-stimulating factor and interleukin-2 fusion cDNA for cancer gene immunotherapy. Cancer Res 2004; 64(24):8795–9.

[86] Knutson KL, Disis ML, Salazar LG. CD4 regulatory T cells in human cancer pathogenesis. Cancer Immunol Immunother 2007;56(3):271–85.

[87] Nagai H, Horikawa T, Hara I, et al. In vivo elimination of CD25+ regulatory T cells leads to tumor rejection of B16F10 melanoma, when combined with interleukin-12 gene transfer. Exp Dermatol 2004;13(10):613–20.

[88] Turk MJ, Guevara-Patino JA, Rizzuto GA, et al. Concomitant tumor immunity to a poorly immunogenic melanoma is prevented by regulatory T cells. J Exp Med 2004; 200(6):771–82.

[89] Jones E, Dahm-Vicker M, Simon AK, et al. Depletion of CD25+ regulatory cells results in suppression of melanoma growth and induction of autoreactivity in mice. Cancer Immunity 2002;2:1–12.

[90] Sutmuller RP, van Duivenvoorde LM, van Elsas A, et al. Synergism of cytotoxic T lymphocyte-associated antigen 4 blockade and depletion of CD25(+) regulatory T cells in antitumor therapy reveals alternative pathways for suppression of autoreactive cytotoxic T lymphocyte responses. J Exp Med 2001;194(6):823–32.

[91] Turturro F. Denileukin diftitox: a biotherapeutic paradigm shift in the treatment of lymphoid-derived disorders. Expert Rev Anticancer Ther 2007;7(1):11–7.

[92] Foss F. Clinical experience with denileukin diftitox (ONTAK). Semin Oncol 2006;33 (1 Suppl 3):S11–6.

[93] Attia P, Maker AV, Haworth LR, et al. Inability of a fusion protein of IL-2 and diphtheria toxin (Denileukin Diftitox, DAB389IL-2, ONTAK) to eliminate regulatory T lymphocytes in patients with melanoma. J Immunother 2005;28(6):582–92.

[94] Galanis E. Technology evaluation: Allovectin-7, Vical. Curr Opin Mol Ther 2002;4(1): 80–7.

[95] Atkins MB. Cytokine-based therapy and biochemotherapy for advanced melanoma. Clin Cancer Res 2006;12(7 Pt 2):2353s–8s.

[96] Keilholz U. Biochemotherapy of melanoma. Forum (Genova) 2003;13(2):158–65 [quiz 189].

[97] Alexandrescu DT, Dutcher JP, Wiernik PH. Metastatic melanoma: is biochemotherapy the future? Med Oncol 2005;22(2):101–11.

[98] Buzaid AC. Biochemotherapy for advanced melanoma. Crit Rev Oncol Hematol 2002; 44(1):103–8.

[99] O'Day SJ, Kim CJ, Reintgen DS. Metastatic melanoma: chemotherapy to biochemotherapy. Cancer Control 2002;9(1):31–8.

[100] Neri B, Vannozzi L, Fulignati C, et al. Long-term survival in metastatic melanoma patients treated with sequential biochemotherapy: report of a phase II study. Cancer Invest 2006; 24(5):474–8.

[101] Lewis KD, Robinson WA, McCarter M, et al. Phase II multicenter study of neoadjuvant biochemotherapy for patients with stage III malignant melanoma. J Clin Oncol 2006; 24(19):3157–63.

[102] Ron IG, Sarid D, Ryvo L, et al. A biochemotherapy regimen with concurrent administration of cisplatin, vinblastine, temozolomide (Temodal), interferon-alfa and interleukin-2 for metastatic melanoma: a phase II study. Melanoma Res 2006;16(1):65–9.

[103] Gonzalez Cao M, Puig S, Malvehy J, et al. Biochemotherapy with low doses of subcutaneous interleukin-2 in patients with melanoma: results of a phase II trial. Clin Transl Oncol Official Publ Fed Spanish Oncol Soc Natl Cancer Inst Mexico 2005;7(6):250–4.

[104] Hahka-Kemppinen M, Muhonen T, Virolainen M, et al. Response of subcutaneous and cutaneous metastases of malignant melanoma to combined cytostatic plus interferon therapy. Br J Dermatol 1995;132(6):973–7.

[105] Vuoristo MS, Grohn P, Kellokumpu-Lehtinen P, et al. Intermittent interferon and polychemotherapy in metastatic melanoma. J Cancer Res Clin Oncol 1995;121(3):175–80.

[106] Eton O, Legha SS, Bedikian AY, et al. Sequential biochemotherapy versus chemotherapy for metastatic melanoma: results from a phase III randomized trial. J Clin Oncol 2002; 20(8):2045–52.

[107] Lewis KD, Gibbs P, O'Day S, et al. A phase II study of biochemotherapy for advanced melanoma incorporating temozolomide, decrescendo interleukin-2 and GM-CSF. Cancer Invest 2005;23(4):303–8.

[108] Krummel MF, Davis MM. Dynamics of the immunological synapse: finding, establishing and solidifying a connection. Curr Opin Immunol 2002;14(1):66–74.

[109] Jansson A, Barnes E, Klenerman P, et al. A theoretical framework for quantitative analysis of the molecular basis of costimulation. J Immunol 2005;175(3):1575–85.

[110] Ghiringhelli F, Zitvogel L. Vaccine strategies against melanoma. Medecine Sciences (Paris) 2006;22(2):183–7.

[111] Kaplan JM. New cancer vaccine approaches. Drugs of Today 2004;40(11):913–29.

[112] Mocellin S, Rossi CR, Nitti D. Cancer vaccine development: on the way to break immune tolerance to malignant cells. Exp Cell Res 2004;299(2):267–78.

[113] Dudley ME, Ngo LT, Westwood J, et al. T-cell clones from melanoma patients immunized against an anchor-modified gp100 peptide display discordant effector phenotypes. Cancer J 2000;6(2):69–77.

[114] Topalian SL, Gonzales MI, Parkhurst M, et al. Melanoma-specific CD4+ T cells recognize nonmutated HLA-DR-restricted tyrosinase epitopes. J Exp Med 1996;183(5):1965–71.

[115] Kobayashi H, Kokubo T, Sato K, et al. CD4+ T cells from peripheral blood of a melanoma patient recognize peptides derived from nonmutated tyrosinase. Cancer Res 1998;58(2): 296–301.

[116] Zarour HM, Kirkwood JM, Kierstead LS, et al. Melan-A/MART-1(51-73) represents an immunogenic HLA-DR4-restricted epitope recognized by melanoma-reactive CD4(+) T cells. Proc Natl Acad Sci USA 2000;97(1):400–5.

[117] Manici S, Sturniolo T, Imro MA, et al. Melanoma cells present a MAGE-3 epitope to CD4(+) cytotoxic T cells in association with histocompatibility leukocyte antigen DR11. J Exp Med 1999;189(5):871–6.

[118] Chaux P, Vantomme V, Stroobant V, et al. Identification of MAGE-3 epitopes presented by HLA-DR molecules to CD4(+) T lymphocytes. J Exp Med 1999;189(5): 767–78.

[119] Attia P, Phan GQ, Maker AV, et al. Autoimmunity correlates with tumor regression in patients with metastatic melanoma treated with anti-cytotoxic T-lymphocyte antigen-4. J Clin Oncol 2005;23(25):6043–53.

[120] Triozzi PL, Aldrich W, Allen KO, et al. Phase I study of a plasmid DNA vaccine encoding MART-1 in patients with resected melanoma at risk for relapse. J Immunother 2005;28(4): 382–8.

[121] Jager E, Karbach J, Gnjatic S, et al. Recombinant vaccinia/fowlpox NY-ESO-1 vaccines induce both humoral and cellular NY-ESO-1-specific immune responses in cancer patients. Proc Natl Acad Sci USA 2006;103(39):14453–8.

[122] Flechtner JB, Cohane KP, Mehta S, et al. High-affinity interactions between peptides and heat shock protein 70 augment CD8+ T lymphocyte immune responses. J Immunol 2006; 177(2):1017–27.

[123] Pilla L, Patuzzo R, Rivoltini L, et al. A phase II trial of vaccination with autologous, tumor-derived heat-shock protein peptide complexes Gp96, in combination with GM-CSF and interferon-alpha in metastatic melanoma patients. Cancer Immunol Immunother 2006;55(8): 958–68.

[124] Morton DL, Hsueh EC, Essner R, et al. Prolonged survival of patients receiving active immunotherapy with Canvaxin therapeutic polyvalent vaccine after complete resection of melanoma metastatic to regional lymph nodes. Ann Surg 2002;236(4):438–48.

[125] Morton DL. Multicenter double-blind phase 3 trial of Canvaxin vs placebo as post surgical adjuvant in metastatic melanoma. Paper presented at Society of Surgical Oncology 59th Annual Cancer Symposium. San Diego (CA), March 24, 2006.

[126] Osada T, Clay TM, Woo CY, et al. Dendritic cell-based immunotherapy. Int Rev Immunol 2006;25(5–6):377–413.

[127] Vilella R, Benitez D, Mila J, et al. Pilot study of treatment of biochemotherapy-refractory stage IV melanoma patients with autologous dendritic cells pulsed with a heterologous melanoma cell line lysate. Cancer Immunol Immunother 2004;53(7):651–8.

[128] Salcedo M, Bercovici N, Taylor R, et al. Vaccination of melanoma patients using dendritic cells loaded with an allogeneic tumor cell lysate. Cancer Immunol Immunother 2006;55(7): 819–29.

[129] Linette GP, Zhang D, Hodi FS, et al. Immunization using autologous dendritic cells pulsed with the melanoma-associated antigen gp100-derived G280-9V peptide elicits CD8+ immunity. Clin Cancer Res 2005;11(21):7692–9.

[130] Kyte JA, Mu L, Aamdal S, et al. Phase I/II trial of melanoma therapy with dendritic cells transfected with autologous tumor-mRNA. Cancer Gene Ther 2006;13(10):905–18.

[131] Grover A, Kim GJ, Lizee G, et al. Intralymphatic dendritic cell vaccination induces tumor antigen-specific, skin-homing T lymphocytes. Clin Cancer Res 2006;12(19):5801–8.

[132] Fay JW, Palucka AK, Paczesny S, et al. Long-term outcomes in patients with metastatic melanoma vaccinated with melanoma peptide-pulsed CD34(+) progenitor-derived dendritic cells. Cancer Immunol Immunother 2006;55(10):1209–18.

[133] Dillman R, Selvan S, Schiltz P, et al. Phase I/II trial of melanoma patient-specific vaccine of proliferating autologous tumor cells, dendritic cells, and GM-CSF: planned interim analysis. Cancer Biother Radiopharm 2004;19(5):658–65.

[134] Di Pucchio T, Pilla L, Capone I, et al. Immunization of stage IV melanoma patients with Melan-A/MART-1 and gp100 peptides plus IFN-alpha results in the activation of specific CD8 (+) T cells and monocyte/dendritic cell precursors. Cancer Res 2006;66(9): 4943–51.

[135] Banchereau J, Ueno H, Dhodapkar M, et al. Immune and clinical outcomes in patients with stage IV melanoma vaccinated with peptide-pulsed dendritic cells derived from CD34+ progenitors and activated with type I interferon. J Immunother 2005;28(5):505–16.

[136] Vujanovic L, Ranieri E, Gambotto A, et al. IL-12p70 and IL-18 gene-modified dendritic cells loaded with tumor antigen-derived peptides or recombinant protein effectively stimulate specific Type-1 CD4+ T-cell responses from normal donors and melanoma patients in vitro. Cancer Gene Ther 2006;13(8):798–805.

[137] Krause SW, Neumann C, Soruri A, et al. The treatment of patients with disseminated malignant melanoma by vaccination with autologous cell hybrids of tumor cells and dendritic cells. J Immunother 2002;25(5):421–8.

[138] Wei Y, Sticca RP, Holmes LM, et al. Dendritoma vaccination combined with low dose interleukin-2 in metastatic melanoma patients induced immunological and clinical responses. Int J Oncol 2006;28(3):585–93.

[139] Trefzer U, Herberth G, Wohlan K, et al. Tumour-dendritic hybrid cell vaccination for the treatment of patients with malignant melanoma: immunological effects and clinical results. Vaccine 2005;23(17–18):2367–73.

[140] Neves AR, Ensina LF, Anselmo LB, et al. Dendritic cells derived from metastatic cancer patients vaccinated with allogeneic dendritic cell-autologous tumor cell hybrids express more CD86 and induce higher levels of interferon-gamma in mixed lymphocyte reactions. Cancer Immunol Immunother 2005;54(1):61–6.

[141] Trefzer U, Herberth G, Wohlan K, et al. Vaccination with hybrids of tumor and dendritic cells induces tumor-specific T-cell and clinical responses in melanoma stage III and IV patients. Int J Cancer 2004;110(5):730–40.

[142] Haenssle HA, Krause SW, Emmert S, et al. Hybrid cell vaccination in metastatic melanoma: clinical and immunologic results of a phase I/II study. J Immunother 2004;27(2): 147–55.

[143] Slingluff CL Jr, Petroni GR, Yamshchikov GV, et al. Clinical and immunologic results of a randomized phase II trial of vaccination using four melanoma peptides either administered in granulocyte-macrophage colony-stimulating factor in adjuvant or pulsed on dendritic cells. J Clin Oncol 2003;21(21):4016–26.

[144] Chiong B, Wong R, Lee P, et al. Characterization of long-term effector-memory T-cell responses in patients with resected high-risk melanoma receiving a melanoma peptide vaccine. J Immunother 2004;27(5):368–79.

[145] Baselga J, Perez EA, Pienkowski T, et al. Adjuvant trastuzumab: a milestone in the treatment of HER-2-positive early breast cancer. Oncologist 2006;11(Suppl 1):4–12.

[146] Held G, Poschel V, Pfreundschuh M. Rituximab for the treatment of diffuse large B-cell lymphomas. Expert Rev Anticancer Ther 2006;6(8):1175–86.

[147] Choi BS, Sondel PM, Hank JA, et al. Phase I trial of combined treatment with ch14.18 and R24 monoclonal antibodies and interleukin-2 for patients with melanoma or sarcoma. Cancer Immunol Immunother 2006;55(7):761–74.

[148] Grimm EA, Ramsey KM, Mazumder A, et al. Lymphokine-activated killer cell phenomenon. II. Precursor phenotype is serologically distinct from peripheral T lymphocytes, memory cytotoxic thymus-derived lymphocytes, and natural killer cells. J Exp Med 1983;157(3): 884–97.

[149] Lindemann A, Herrmann F, Oster W, et al. Lymphokine activated killer cells. Blut 1989; 59(4):375–84.

[150] Dudley ME, Wunderlich JR, Shelton TE, et al. Generation of tumor-infiltrating lymphocyte cultures for use in adoptive transfer therapy for melanoma patients. J Immunother 2003;26(4):332–42.

[151] Ridolfi L, Ridolfi R, Riccobon A, et al. Adjuvant immunotherapy with tumor infiltrating lymphocytes and interleukin-2 in patients with resected stage III and IV melanoma. J Immunother 2003;26(2):156–62.

[152] Dudley ME, Wunderlich JR, Yang JC, et al. Adoptive cell transfer therapy following non-myeloablative but lymphodepleting chemotherapy for the treatment of patients with refractory metastatic melanoma. J Clin Oncol 2005;23(10):2346–57.

[153] Johnson LA, Heemskerk B, Powell DJ Jr, et al. Gene transfer of tumor-reactive TCR confers both high avidity and tumor reactivity to nonreactive peripheral blood mononuclear cells and tumor-infiltrating lymphocytes. J Immunol 2006;177(9):6548–59.

[154] Morgan RA, Dudley ME, Wunderlich JR, et al. Cancer regression in patients after transfer of genetically engineered lymphocytes. Science 2006;314(5796):126–9.

[155] Ma Q, DeMarte L, Wang Y, et al. Carcinoembryonic antigen-immunoglobulin Fc fusion protein (CEA-Fc) for identification and activation of anti-CEA immunoglobulin-T-cell receptor-modified T cells, representative of a new class of Ig fusion proteins. Cancer Gene Ther 2004;11(4):297–306.

[156] Ma Q, Safar M, Holmes E, et al. Anti-prostate specific membrane antigen designer T cells for prostate cancer therapy. Prostate 2004;61(1):12–25.

[157] Yun CO, Nolan KF, Beecham EJ, et al. Targeting of T lymphocytes to melanoma cells through chimeric anti-GD3 immunoglobulin T-cell receptors. Neoplasia 2000;2(5):449–59.

[158] Reinhold U, Liu L, Ludtke-Handjery HC, et al. Specific lysis of melanoma cells by receptor grafted T cells is enhanced by anti-idiotypic monoclonal antibodies directed to the scFv domain of the receptor. J Investigative Dermatology 1999;112(5):744–50.

[159] Abken H, Hombach A, Heuser C, et al. A novel strategy in the elimination of disseminated melanoma cells: chimeric receptors endow T cells with tumor specificity. Recent Results Cancer Res 2001;158:249–64.

ELSEVIER
SAUNDERS

Surg Oncol Clin N Am
16 (2007) 975–986

SURGICAL
ONCOLOGY CLINICS
OF NORTH AMERICA

Current Immunotherapeutic Strategies in Renal Cell Carcinoma

Robert J. Amato, DO

*Genitourinary Oncology Program, The Methodist Hospital Research Institute,
6560 Fannin, Suite 2050, Houston, TX 77030, USA*

Despite a better understanding of the biology of renal cancer, an estimated 51,190 individuals (31,590 men and 19,600 women) will be diagnosed with the disease and 12,890 individuals will die of it in 2007 [1]. Although renal cancer is more common in men [1], its incidence among women has risen over the past three decades [2]. Most renal malignancies originate in the lining of proximal tubules and are of the type known as renal cell carcinoma (RCC) (alternative terms include clear-cell cancer and renal adenocarcinoma) [3]. Most RCCs appear clear or granular under a light microscope and are often associated with von Hippel-Lindau tumor suppressor gene inactivation [3,4].

Disease progression after initial therapy is a problem. Although early-stage RCCs can be treated successfully with radical or nephron-sparing nephrectomy, metastasis still occurs in an estimated 20% to 30% of cases [5]. By some estimates, up to half of all RCCs are locally advanced or metastatic and symptomatic at presentation [5,6], resulting in poor 5-year survival outcomes [5]. Unlike many other malignancies, RCC is refractory to chemotherapy and hormone therapy [7]. In the 1980s, immunotherapy with nonspecific agents, such as interleukin-2 (IL-2) and interferon-α (IFN-α), was introduced.

Since the early 1990s, high-dose IL-2 has been considered the standard immunotherapy for advanced RCC, eliciting response rates superior to those of chemotherapy when administered alone (10%–20%) or in combination (20%–30%) [7]. It has not significantly improved long-term survival, however [7–11], even when conventional high-dose IL-2 regimens are replaced with low-dose IL-2 alone or in combination with IFN-α [12].

Consequently, clinical investigations have branched off in several new directions. Some studies are aimed at identifying predictors of IL-2

E-mail address: ramato@tmh.tmc.edu

1055-3207/07/$ - see front matter © 2007 Elsevier Inc. All rights reserved.
doi:10.1016/j.soc.2007.07.006

therapeutic response (eg, carbonic anhydrase IX [CA9] overexpression) that might be used to optimize patient selection [8,9,13]. Recent rapid advances in understanding key tumorigenesis-related mechanisms (ie, inappropriate signal transduction, angiogenesis, and dysfunctional immune regulation) have led to the development of new agents more specific to RCC. Several of these advances have been shepherded successfully through preclinical and clinical testing. Examples include molecularly targeted agents, such as monoclonal antibodies, tyrosine kinase inhibitors (eg, sunitinib and sorafenib), and mammalian target of rapamycin inhibitors (eg, temsirolimus). Recently, the US Food and Drug Administration (FDA) approved sunitinib, sorafenib, and temsirolimus for use against advanced RCC. Tumor-specific vaccines are also being designed and evaluated.

Some, but not all, of these newer agents have improved significantly upon the established therapies (Table 1), and efforts are underway to improve efficacy even further by combining them. This article covers important immunotherapies that are currently being used or investigated in RCC.

Monoclonal antibodies

Monoclonal antibody therapies are already approved for hematologic and breast cancers [14–16]. None is yet approved for RCC, but several have been evaluated in this setting. Cetuximab (Erbitux) and panitumumab (ABX-EGF) target the epidermal growth factor receptor, which is

Table 1
Current immunotherapies for advanced renal cell carcinoma

Agent	Mechanism of action/molecular target	Development stage
High-dose IL-2	Cytokine	FDA approved
Bevacizumab	Monoclonal antibody: binds circulating VEGF	Phase III
Panitumumab	Monoclonal antibody: binds EGFR	Phase II
cG250	Monoclonal antibody: binds chimeric G250 antigen	Phase II
Sunitinib	Small molecule: multitargeted tyrosine kinase inhibitor	FDA approved
Temsirolimus (Torisel, CCI-779)	Small molecule: kinase inhibitor of mTOR	FDA approved
Dendritic cells	Vaccine: raises antitumor immune responses	Phase I
HSPPC-96	Vaccine: raises antitumor immune responses to tumor antigen-presenting cells	Phase III
CA9	Vaccine: raises antitumor responses to tumor antigen-presenting cells	Phase I
MVA-5T4 (TroVax)	Vaccine: raises immune responses to tumor cells presenting oncofetal antigen 5T4	Phase III

Abbreviations: EGFR, epidermal growth factor receptor; mTOR, mammalian target of rapamycin; VEGF, vascular endothelial growth factor.

inappropriately activated in many cancers, associated with aggressive disease, and frequently overexpressed in RCC [17,18]. Bevacizumab (Avastin) targets vascular endothelial growth factor [19] and has been shown to improve overall survival of patients with metastatic colorectal cancer by inhibiting tumor angiogenesis [20]. Chimeric G250 (cG250) recognizes the tumor-specific, heat-sensitive surface antigen carbonic anhydrase IX (CA9), which is overexpressed on malignant but not normal renal cells.

Promising preclinical studies have shown IFN-α and IFN-γ to up-regulate G250 activity and a chimeric monoclonal antibody to G250 to induce antibody-dependent cellular cytotoxicity [21]. In a small dose escalation study that involved 12 patients, 6-week cycles of radiolabeled cG250 antibody administered at doses of 5, 10, 25, or 50 mg/m^2 were relatively safe and effective. Adverse effects were few (most notably, severe infusion-related sacral pain in one case and a human antichimeric antibody response requiring treatment discontinuation in another), and the overall response rate was good (complete response in one case and stable disease in eight) [22]. In an ongoing randomized, double-blind, placebo-controlled phase III trial, cG50 is being evaluated as adjuvant therapy in a large population of patients at high risk for relapse after surgical treatment of nonmetastatic RCC [23].

Reports of mutation-induced vascular endothelial growth factor overproduction in RCCs have led to attempts to inhibit tumor angiogenesis by neutralizing circulating vascular endothelial growth factor. In a randomized phase II trial of bevacizumab, 116 patients previously treated with IL-2 were randomly assigned to receive placebo, low-dose antibody (3 mg/kg) or high-dose antibody (10 mg/kg) intravenously every 2 weeks [19]. Bevacizumab was well tolerated at high and low doses and—despite an anomalous increase in plasma vascular endothelial growth factor levels that the investigators attributed to poor clearance of inactivated antibody-bound factor—demonstrated good clinical activity. Bevacizumab therapy also significantly increased time to progression by 2.55-fold ($P<.001$) and 1.26-fold ($P = .053$), respectively, when compared with placebo and improved estimated progression-free survival at 4 months (64% [high-dose] versus 39% [low-dose] versus 20% [placebo]). On the other hand, neither the high nor low dose significantly enhanced overall survival (see Table 1).

Bevacizumab was deemed worthy of further clinical study in phase III trials. This promise was highlighted recently in the remarkable case of a 14-year-old girl whose previously unresectable and IL-2–resistant RCC shrank enough to be safely resected after 7 months of bevacizumab treatment [24]. In a recently reported, placebo-controlled phase III trial of bevacizumab and IFN-α2a as combination first-line therapy for metastatic RCC, the well-tolerated addition of bevacizumab significantly improved the objective response rate (30.6% versus 12.4%, $P<.0001$) and progression-free survival (10.2 versus 5.4 months, $P<.0001$) [25]. The combination was also well tolerated.

Small molecule inhibitors

Tyrosine kinase inhibitors

Two tyrosine kinase inhibitors—sunitinib and sorafenib—have been approved by the FDA for treatment of advanced RCC. Both agents selectively inhibit receptor tyrosine kinases associated with angiogenesis and cell proliferation. In a double-blind, randomized, placebo-controlled, crossover phase III trial in patients with metastatic RCC, sorafenib significantly prolonged progression-free survival (median time to progression, 5.5 months versus 2.8 months for placebo [$P<.01$]; hazard ratio, 0.44) and lowered the risk of death ($P = .02$; hazard ratio, 0.72) [26]. In a randomized, phase III trial that compared 6-week cycles of sunitinib versus IFN-α as first-line therapy in patients with previously untreated clear-cell metastatic RCC, sunitinib produced significantly better objective response rates (31% versus 6% [$P<.001$]) and longer progression-free survival (median, 11 months versus 5 months [$P<.001$]; hazard ratio, 0.42) while also improving self-reported quality of life [27]. Sunitinib is currently recommended as first-line therapy and sorafenib as second-line therapy [28].

Another promising inhibitory molecule is the multitarget tyrosine kinase receptor inhibitor axitinib (AG-013736). In phase II trials, it has demonstrated antitumor (ie, antiangiogenic) activity against cytokine-refractory and sorafenib-refractory metastatic renal cell cancers [29,30].

Temsirolimus (Torisel, CCI-779)

The rapamycin derivative and cell-cycle inhibitor temsirolimus (formerly known as CCI-779) suppresses tumor growth and proliferation by inhibiting the mammalian target of rapamycin [31,32], thereby indirectly down-regulating the expression of key cell-cycle proteins and arresting tumor cells in the G1 phase.

In a double-blind, phase II randomized study, 111 patients (many of them recipients of previous cytokine therapy) were randomly assigned to receive temsirolimus at weekly doses of 25, 75, or 250 mg [33]. Although well tolerated except for some episodes of hyperglycemia and anemia, CCI-779 did not remarkably affect overall response rates, time to progression, or survival even at the higher doses. Objective responses were achieved in 7% (one complete response and seven partial responses) and minor responses in 26% of cases, the median time to progression was 5.8 months, and the median survival was 15 months.

In a subsequent phase III randomized trial, 626 patients with treatment-naïve metastatic RCC were randomly assigned to receive temsirolimus alone, IFN-α alone, or both in combination [34]. Overall survival was significantly better in the group that received temsirolimus alone than in the groups that received the combination or IFN-α alone (median, 7.3 versus 8.4 versus 10.9 months). That this survival benefit was obtained in patients with advanced metastatic tumors suggests that temsirolimus might provide an even greater benefit to patients with less extensive metastatic disease.

On the basis of this phase III trial, temsirolimus has been approved by the FDA for use against advanced RCC [35]. It had been on the FDA's fast track for development as second-line therapy for IL-2–refractory RCC since early 2002 and as first-line therapy for advanced RCC since late 2004 [36]. It joins sunitinib as the only other molecularly targeted therapy currently recommended as first-line therapy for advanced RCC (sorafenib is recommended as second-line therapy) and as another sorely needed addition to the slowly expanding arsenal of anti-RCC treatments [28].

Immunotherapeutic and immunochemotherapeutic combinations

Several combination therapies for advanced RCC have been evaluated clinically. Many have included IFN-α and IL-2 in varying doses in an effort to achieve greater efficacy than the standard high-dose IL-2 immunotherapy. Some have gone further to include 5-fluorouracil (5-FU) in a less toxic but potentially less effective therapeutic cocktail [8,37]. Several combinations have included thalidomide, an extremely teratogenic but potent immunomodulatory and antiangiogenic agent that has been relatively well tolerated and effective when used as a single agent against metastatic RCC [38–40].

Combination therapy with low-dose IL-2 and IFN-α may be clinically beneficial in patients with metastatic RCC, although there have been conflicting clinical reports. According to a recent Japanese feasibility study in previously nephrectomized patients with metastatic RCC, this regimen safely produced objective responses (one complete response and five partial responses) in half of evaluable cases (50% [6/12]) and a median durable response of 13.5 months [41]. The potential for achieving further clinical benefit by adding radiation therapy to this combination is underscored by the report of a durable (16-month) complete response to radiation therapy in a 59-year-old man whose postnephrectomy lung metastases had resisted treatment with low-dose IL-2 and IFN-α [42]. In a recent Italian trial in patients with operable nonmetastatic RCC, the combination of adjuvant low-dose IL-2 and IFN-α seemed to reduce the risk of disease recurrence at 5 years after diagnosis [43].

On the other hand, in a randomized phase III trial that involved 192 patients with metastatic RCC, combination of low-dose IL-2 and IFN-α did not seem to significantly improve response rates, response duration, or survival [12]. Contrary to the perceived inferiority of high-dose IL-2 [44], the high-dose regimen resulted in much better survival, thus buttressing—at least for the time being—its continued use as first-line immunotherapy in CA9-positive cases of advanced clear-cell RCC [12].

Dendritic cell vaccines

Improved understanding of the biology and immunologic role of dendritic cells (DCs) and continuing optimization of their immunostimulatory function have cleared the way for standardized clinical trials of DC vaccination in RCC [45]. Suggestions for optimizing DC vaccination have included defining better antigen sources, devising more efficient means of antigen loading, using DCs that secrete biologically active IL-12, and combining DC vaccination with therapies that address immune suppression [46]. Theoretically, sequentially combining a tumor lysate-stimulated DC vaccine with subsequent cytokine therapy may beneficially alter the aberrant intratumoral balance between proinflammatory and immunoregulatory pathways to activate other immunocytotoxic pathways and overcome the cytokine resistance of RCC [47].

In a phase I feasibility trial, 20 patients with metastatic RCC received subcutaneous injections of a vaccine made up of DCs derived from peripheral blood monocytes pulsed with the HLA-A2-binding MUC1 peptides. Vaccinations were administered once every 2 weeks for 8 weeks and then monthly thereafter until disease progression. After the fifth vaccination, patients also began receiving 3 weekly injections of low-dose IL-2. The vaccine was well tolerated and elicited metastatic regression and objective responses in 6 patients (complete in 1, partial in 2, mixed response in 2, and stable disease in 1). Four patients enjoyed stable disease for up to 14 months. MUC1-specific T-cell responses detected in vivo in the peripheral blood monocytes of the 6 objective responders demonstrated the immunostimulatory and clinical efficacy of this DC vaccine [48].

Cancer vaccines

Being extremely immunogenic, RCCs are presumably predisposed to tumor vaccination. Several tumor-associated antigen vaccines are being developed and evaluated for use against RCC. This process has been helped along by the identification of particular antigens overexpressed on the surface of tumors and by the availability of safe recombinant viral vectors for delivering tumor-associated antigens to target cells [49].

Heat-shock protein-peptide complexes-96

Patient-specific vaccines have been developed using the heat-shock protein-peptide complexes (HSPPC-96) that form between heat-shock proteins and tumor antigen peptides [50]. Although purification of these complexes from individual tumors can be significantly hampered by differences in the protease content of different tissues, the potent antitumor responses to be elicited on antigen-presenting cells (DCs or macrophages) make their isolation worthwhile [51].

In a phase II efficacy study, HSPPC-96 was injected at a dose of 25 μg once a week for 4 weeks and then every 2 weeks until disease progression. Patients were evaluated for progression at 10 weeks and then every 8 weeks thereafter. In cases of disease progression, IL-2 was added to the treatment regimen at a dose of 11 million U and given in 8-week cycles (5 days per week for 4 consecutive weeks followed by 4 weeks of rest). No adverse events were reported. Of 61 patients who received at least one vaccine dose, 1 achieved a complete response (and remained disease free at 2.5 years), 2 achieved a partial response, and 18 had stable disease. Of 16 patients whose disease progressed, 7 achieved stable disease in response to subsequent IL-2 treatment. Median progression-free survival for patients treated with only vaccine was 18 weeks, compared with 25 weeks for patients who received the vaccine and IL-2. Two years after initial vaccination, 30% of patients remained alive [52]. These encouraging findings, especially with regard to stable disease, have led to larger, multicenter phase III clinical trials currently underway [51].

Carbonic anhydrase IX

Carbonic anhydrase IX (CA9) is ubiquitously expressed in RCC. Its overexpression in RCC seems to correlate with significantly higher rates of response to IL-2–based therapy and subsequent survival [53]. In a phase I trial, 23 patients with progressive, HLA-A24–positive cytokine-refractory metastatic RCC were injected with CA9-derived peptides every 2 weeks and then evaluated every 3 months [54]. The vaccinations were well tolerated and eventually elicited immunostimulatory responses followed by gradual increases in levels of cytotoxic T lymphocyte and peptide-reactive serum IgG. Partial objective responses (ie, disappearance or shrinking of metastatic lesions) were achieved in 3 patients, and stable disease that lasted more than 6 months (median, 12.2 months) was achieved in 6 patients. The overall median survival time was 21 months (range, 5–35 months). These findings warrant further trials of CA9 vaccination in patients who have metastatic RCC.

Modified vaccinia Ankara-5T4 (TroVax)

The gene-based tumor vaccine MVA-5T4 (TroVax) consists of an extremely weakened vaccinia virus (modified vaccinia Ankara [MVA]) that expresses the oncofetal antigen 5T4. 5T4 is expressed on a wide variety of human adenocarcinomas, including RCCs and colorectal cancers, but not to any significant extent on healthy human tissues. Preclinical studies in mice [55] and early clinical trials in patients with late-stage colorectal cancer [49] have shown that MVA-5T4 can elicit powerful immune responses and improve clinical outcomes (ie, time to progression and overall survival). In a small phase I trial that combined MVA-5T4 and high-dose IL-2 therapy, 25 patients with metastatic RCC were vaccinated once every 3 weeks (for a total of three vaccinations) and treated with high-dose IL-2 after the second and third vaccinations; the combination safely increased MVA-5T4 antibody levels in all cases [56].

Subsequent clinical trials of MVA-5T4 in advanced RCC are currently underway, including a small, single-center phase II safety and efficacy trial of MVA-5T4 in combination with low-dose IL-2 and an international, placebo-controlled, randomized phase III study in which MVA-5T4 is being added to standard first-line therapy (both are listed at the National Institutes of Health's clinicaltrials.gov Web site). Preliminary results of the phase II trial indicated that the combination has been well tolerated by the 10 patients treated so far and elicited early signs of clinical responses in some cases [57]. Also underway is a small, single-center phase II trial of MVA-5T4 in combination with low-dose IFN-α in patients who have metastatic RCC. Initiated in November 2006, the phase III trial, designated the TroVax Renal Immunotherapy Survival Trial, has been enrolling patients to receive standard therapy (IL-2, IFN-α, or sunitinib) followed by vaccination with TroVax or a placebo. It is expected that the combination therapy will enhance survival and warrant the vaccine's registration in the United States before the decade is over. The results of a recently completed preliminary trial of MVA 5T4 alone or in combination with IL-2 or IFN suggested that patients with locally advanced or metastatic clear-cell RCCs are more likely to experience a clinically beneficial response and that combination with standard cytokine therapy may enhance the vaccine's potency [58].

New research avenues

Despite a better understanding of the molecular biology of RCC and the increasing ability to target immunotherapeutic agents more specifically at such tumors, clinical response rates remain modest and, except in the case of thalidomide, no better than those achieved in historical controls. The reasons for this therapeutic impasse are unclear. Perhaps dosing at the cellular level has been suboptimal, signaling pathways are more complex than previously thought, or appropriate therapeutic targets are made essentially inaccessible by their existence in slightly different isoforms. Then again, differences between individual patients may be at fault. It may be necessary to tweak the design of some agents so as to improve their targeting, further optimize dosing schedules, and establish which immunotherapeutic-containing combinations might produce better clinical results.

It also may be necessary to fine-tune the design of such trials by optimizing patient selection (eg, enrolling functionally active, nephrectomized patients with relatively well-contained and well-controlled metastases) and using tumor response criteria that are more specifically appropriate for trials of immunotherapy [59]. Although combination regimens (eg, thalidomide and IL-2) have produced the best objective response rates, the rate of stable disease has been relatively constant across trials, regardless of regimen. This outcome has led some researchers to suggest that long-term stable disease— rather than objective responses such as time to progression and survival— may be a more appropriate and useful endpoint in clinical trials of some antiangiogenic agents and in trials involving cytokine-refractory patients [60]. One recent systematic review noted that "remission rate" (ie, response rate) is a poor surrogate marker or intermediate outcome for survival in patients with advanced RCC [61]. Studies aimed at validating stable disease as a measure of antitumor activity seem warranted.

Summary

Advanced RCC remains resistant to drug-, hormone-, and cytokine-based therapies. Promising new immunotherapeutic approaches include monoclonal antibodies, tyrosine kinase inhibitors, mammalian target of rapamycin inhibition, DCs, and tumor antigen vaccines. Some—but not all— of these approaches have produced clinical responses significantly superior to those of previous standard therapies, and most are well tolerated and elicit relatively high rates of stable disease. Two recently approved kinase inhibitors (ie, the tyrosine kinase inhibitor sunitinib and the mammalian target of rapamycin inhibitor temsirolimus) are recommended for use as first-line therapies against RCC. An additional approved tyrosine kinase inhibitor, sorafenib, is recommended as second-line therapy. More clinical research on these agents and their use in combination, especially sequentially, is warranted.

Acknowledgments

The author thanks Rose Salazar and Laura Riojas for their assistance in the preparation of this article.

References

[1] Ries LAG, Melbert D, Krapcho M, et al, editors. SEER Cancer Statistics Review, 1975–2004. Bethesda (MD): National Cancer Institue; 2007. Available at: http://seer.cancer.gov/csr/1975_2004/. Accessed May 21, 2007.

[2] Chow WH, Devesa SS, Warren JL, et al. Rising incidence of renal cell cancer in the United States. JAMA 1999;28:1628–31.

[3] Amato RJ. Chemotherapy for renal cell carcinoma. Semin Oncol 2000;27:177–86.

[4] George DJ, Kaelin WG Jr. The von Hippel-Lindau protein, vascular endothelial growth factor, and kidney cancer. N Engl J Med 2003;349:419–21.

[5] Godley PA, Taylor M. Renal cell carcinoma. Curr Opin Oncol 2001;13:199–203.

[6] Bleumer I, Oosterwijk E, De Mulder P, et al. Immunotherapy for renal cell carcinoma. Eur Urol 2003;44:65–75.

[7] Motzer RJ, Mazumdar M, Bacik J, et al. Effect of cytokine therapy on survival for patients with advanced renal cell carcinoma. J Clin Oncol 2000;18:1928–35.

[8] McDermott DF, Atkins MB. Application of IL-2 and other cytokines in renal cancer. Expert Opin Biol Ther 2004;4(4):455–68.

[9] McDermott DF, Atkins MB. Interleukin-2 therapy of metastatic renal cell carcinoma: predictors of response. Semin Oncol 2006;33(5):583–7.

[10] McDermott DF, Regan MM, Atkins MB. Interleukin-2 therapy of metastatic renal cell carcinoma: update of phase III trials. Clin Genitourin Cancer 2006;5(2):114–9.

[11] Halbert RJ, Figlin RA, Atkins MB, et al. Treatment of patients with metastatic renal cell cancer: a RAND appropriateness panel. Cancer 2006;107(10):2375–83.

[12] McDermott DF, Regan MM, Clark JI, et al. Randomized phase III trial of high-dose interleukin-2 versus subcutaneous interleukin-2 and interferon in patients with metastatic renal cell carcinoma. J Clin Oncol 2005;23(1):133–41.

[13] Rini BI. Current status and future directions of molecular markers in renal cell carcinoma. Curr Opin Urol 2006;16(5):332–6.

[14] Herceptin [package insert]. South San Francisco (CA): Genentech, Inc.; 2002.

[15] Rituxan (Rituximab) [package insert]. San Diego (CA): IDEC Pharmaceuticals Corp. and Genentech, Inc.; 2002.

[16] Zevalin [package insert]. San Diego (CA): IDEC Pharmaceuticals Corp.; 2002.

[17] Lager DJ, Slagel DD, Palechek PL. The expression of epidermal growth factor receptor and transforming growth factor alpha in renal cell carcinoma. Mod Pathol 1994;7: 544–8.

[18] Mendelsohn J, Baselga J. Status of epidermal growth factor receptor antagonists in the biology and treatment of cancer. J Clin Oncol 2003;21:2787–99.

[19] Yang JC, Haworth L, Sherry RM, et al. A randomized trial of bevacizumab, an anti-vascular endothelial growth factor antibody, for metastatic renal cancer. N Engl J Med 2003;349: 427–34.

[20] Genentech. Pipeline–clinical trials–avastin. Available at: http://www.gene.com/gene/ pipeline/status/oncology/avastin/index.jsp. Accessed May 21, 2007.

[21] Liu Z, Smyth FE, Renner C, et al. Anti-renal cell carcinoma chimeric antibody G250: cytokine enhancement of in vitro antibody-dependent cellular cytotoxicity. Cancer Immunol Immunother 2003;51:171–7.

[22] Wiseman GA, Scott AM, Lee F, et al. Chimeric G250 (cG250) monoclonal antibody phase I dose escalation trial in patients with advanced renal cell carcinoma (RCC) [abstract 1027]. Proceedings of the American Society for Clinical Oncology 2001;20:257.

[23] Lam JS, Leppert JT, Belldegrun AS, et al. Adjuvant therapy of renal cell carcinoma: patient selection and therapeutic options. BJU Int 2005;96:483–8.

[24] Joshi DD, Banerjee T. Vascular endothelial growth factor (VEGF) receptor antibody bevacizumab (avastin) induces regression of renal cell carcinoma in an adolescent resulting in residual tumorectomy. Pediatr Blood Cancer 2007; [Epub ahead of print].

[25] Escudier B, Koralewski P, Pluzanska A, et al. A randomized, controlled, double-blind phase III study (AVOREN) of bevacizumab/interferon-α2a vs placebo/interferon- α2a as first-line therapy in metastatic renal cell carcinoma [abstract 3]. J Clin Oncol 2007 ASCO Annual Meeting Proceedings 2007;25(18S):3.

[26] Escudier B, Eisen T, Stadler WM. Sorafenib in advanced clear-cell renal-cell carcinoma. N Engl J Med 2007;356(2):125–34.

[27] Motzer RJ, Hutson TE, Tomczak P, et al. Sunitinib versus interferon alpha in metastatic renal-cell carcinoma. N Engl J Med 2007;356(2):115–24.

[28] Ljunberg B, Hanbury DC, Kuczyk MA, et al. Guidelines on renal cell carcinoma. Arnhem (Netherlands): European Association of Urology; 2007.

[29] Rini B, Rixe O, Bukowski R, et al. AG-013736, a multi-target tyrosine kinase receptor inhibitor, demonstrates anti-tumor activity in a Phase 2 study of cytokine-refractory, metastatic renal cell cancer (RCC) [abstract 4509]. J Clin Oncol 2005 ASCO Annual Meeting Proceedings 2005;23(16S Part I):4509.

[30] Rini BI, Wilding GT, Hudes G, et al. Axitinib (AG-013736; AG) in patients (pts) with metastatic renal cell cancer (RCC) refractory to sorafenib [abstract 5032]. J Clin Oncol 2007 ASCO Annual Meeting Proceedings 2007;25(18S):5032.

[31] Huang S, Houghton PJ. Targeting mTOR signaling for cancer therapy. Curr Opin Pharmacol 2003;3:371–7.

[32] Dutcher JP, Hudes G, Motzer R. Preliminary report of a phase 1 study of intravenous (IV) CCI-779 given in combination with interferon (IFN) to patients with advanced renal cell carcinoma (RCC) [abstract 854]. Proceedings of the American Society for Clinical Oncology 2003;22:213.

[33] Atkins MB, Hidalgo M, Stadler WM, et al. Randomized phase II study of multiple dose levels of CCI-779, a novel mammalian target of rapamycin kinase inhibitor, in patients with advanced refractory renal cell carcinoma. J Clin Oncol 2004;22(5):909–18.

[34] Hudes G, Carducci M, Tomczak P, et al. Temsirolimus, interferon alpha, or both for advanced renal-cell carcinoma. N Engl J Med 2007;356(22):2271–81.

[35] US Food and Drug Administration. FDA approves new drug for advanced kidney cancer. Available at: http://www.fda.gov/bbs/topics/NEWS/2007/NEW01644.html. Accessed June 8, 2007.

[36] Temsirolimus: CCI 779, CCI-779, cell cycle inhibitor-779. Drugs R D 2004;5(6):363–7.

[37] Demidov L, Kharkevich G, Tsimafeyeu I. A randomized prospective study of low-dose interleukin-2 (IL-2) in combination with interferon-alpha (IFN) and 5-fluorouracil (5-FU) for metastatic renal cell carcinoma: final results [abstract 15643]. J Clin Oncol 2007 ASCO Annual Meeting Proceedings 2007;25(18S):15643.

[38] Amato RJ. Thalidomide therapy for renal cell carcinoma. Crit Rev Oncol Hematol 2003;46: 59–65.

[39] Daliani DD, Papandreou CN, Thall PF, et al. A pilot study of thalidomide in patients with progressive metastatic renal cell carcinoma. Cancer 2002;95:758–65.

[40] Eisen T. Phase II results of a phase II/III study comparing thalidomide with medroxyprogesterone in patients with metastatic renal cell carcinoma [abstract 1606]. Proceedings of the American Society for Clinical Oncology 2003;22:400.

[41] Miyake H, Hara I, Sakai I, et al. Clinical outcome of combined immunotherapy with low-dose interleukin-2 and interferon-alpha for Japanese patients with metastatic renal cell carcinoma who had undergone radical nephrectomy: a preliminary report. Int J Clin Oncol 2005;10(5):338–41.

[42] Sawada N, Fukasawa M, Araki I, et al. Multifocal metastases of recurrent renal cell carcinoma successfully treated with a combination of low dose interleukin-2, alpha-interferon and radiotherapy. Int J Urol 2005;12(11):994–5.

[43] Passalaqua R, Buzio C, Buti S, et al. Adjuvant low-dose interleukin-2 (IL2) plus interferon-alpha (IFN) in operable renal cell cancer (RCC): a phase III, randomized, multicenter, independent trial of the Italian Oncology Group for Clinical Research (GOIRC) [abstract LBA5028]. J Clin Oncol 2007 ASCO Annual Meeting Proceedings 2007;25(18S):LBA5028.

[44] Alikhan M, Spencer HJ, Kohli M. High-dose interleukin-2 may not be superior to low-dose interleukin-2 plus interferon. J Clin Oncol 2005;23(25):6267–8 [author reply 6268–9].

[45] Tuyaerts S, Aerts JL, Corthals J, et al. Current approaches in dendritic cell generation and future implications for cancer immunotherapy. Cancer Immunol Immunother 2007;56(10): 1513–37.

[46] Schendel DJ. Dendritic cell vaccine strategies for renal cell carcinoma. Expert Opin Biol Ther 2007;7(2):221–32.

[47] Ernstoff MS, Crocenzi TS, Seigne JD, et al. Developing a rational tumor vaccine therapy for renal cell carcinoma: immune yin and yang. Clin Cancer Res 2007;13(2 Pt 2):733s–40s.

[48] Wierecky J, Muller MR, Wirths S, et al. Immunologic and clinical responses after vaccinations with peptide-pulsed dendritic cells in metastatic renal cancer patients. Cancer Res 2006; 66(11):5910–8.

[49] Harrop R, Connolly N, Redchenko I, et al. Vaccination of colorectal cancer patients with modified vaccinia Ankara delivering the tumor antigen 5T4 (TroVax) induces immune responses which correlate with disease control: a phase I/II trial. Clin Cancer Res 2006; 12(11 Pt 1):3416–24.

[50] Amato R, Murray L, Wood L, et al. Active specific immunotherapy in patients with renal cell carcinoma (RCC) using autologous tumor derived heat shock protein–peptide complex-96 (HSPP-96) vaccine [abstract 1278]. Proceedings of the American Society for Clinical Oncology 1999;18:332a.

[51] Cancer vaccine: Antigenics. BioDrugs 2002;16:72–4.

[52] Assikis VJ, Daliani D, Pagliaro L, et al. Phase II study of an autologous tumor derived heat shock protein–peptide complex vaccine (HSPPC-96) for patients with metastatic renal cell carcinoma (mRCC) [abstract 1552]. Proceedings of the American Society for Clinical Oncology 2003;22:386.

[53] Atkins M, Regan M, McDermott D, et al. Carbonic anhydrase IX expression predicts outcome of interleukin 2 therapy for renal cancer. Clin Cancer Res 2005;11(10):3714–21.

[54] Uemura H, Fujimoto K, Tanaka M, et al. A phase I trial of vaccination of CA9-derived peptides for HLA-A24-positive patients with cytokine-refractory metastatic renal cell carcinoma. Clin Cancer Res 2006;12(6):1768–75.

[55] Harrop R, Ryan MG, Myers KA, et al. Active treatment of murine tumors with a highly attenuated vaccinia virus expressing the tumor associated antigen 5T4 (TroVax) is CD4+ T cell dependent and antibody mediated. Cancer Immunol Immunother 2006;55(9):1081–90.

[56] Kaufman HL, Deraffele G, Mitcham J, et al. A phase I clinical trial of MVA expressing 5T4 and high-dose interleukin-2 (IL-2) for metastatic renal cell carcinoma [abstract 12500]. J Clin Oncol 2006 ASCO Annual Meeting Proceedings 2006;24(18S):12500.

[57] Gary A, Marsh L, McDonald M, et al. A phase II trial to assess the activity of MVA5T4 plus interleukin-2 in patients (Pts) with metastatic renal cell carcinoma (MRCC) [abstract 14642]. J Clin Oncol 2006 ASCO Annual Meeting Proceedings 2006;24(18S):14642.

[58] Cao A, Hernandez-McClain J, Willis J, et al. Activity of MVA 5T4 alone or in combination with either interleukin-2 (IL-2) or interferon-α (IFN) in patients (Pts) with metastatic renal cell cancer (MRCC) [abstract 3069]. J Clin Oncol 2007 ASCO Annual Meeting Proceedings 2007;25(18S):3069.

[59] Wysocki PJ, Zolnierek J, Szczylik C, et al. Recent developments in renal cell cancer immunotherapy. Expert Opin Biol Ther 2007;7(5):727–37.

[60] Motzer RJ, Berg W, Ginsberg M, et al. Phase II trial of thalidomide for patients with advanced renal cell carcinoma. J Clin Oncol 2002;20:302–6.

[61] Coppin C, Porzsolt F, Awa A, et al. Immunotherapy for advanced renal cell cancer. Cochrane Database Syst Rev 2005;1:CD001425.

SURGICAL
ONCOLOGY CLINICS
OF NORTH AMERICA

ELSEVIER
SAUNDERS

Surg Oncol Clin N Am
16 (2007) 987–1004

Current Immunotherapeutic Strategies for Central Nervous System Tumors

Medina C. Kushen, MD, Adam M. Sonabend, MD,
Maciej S. Lesniak, MD*

*Neurosurgical Oncology and The University of Chicago Brain Tumor Center,
Section of Neurosurgery, MC 3026, The University of Chicago Hospital,
5841 South Maryland Avenue, Chicago, IL 60637, USA*

Immune system and the central nervous system

The immune system has the ability to recognize and destroy foreign cells via two separate modalities: innate and adaptive immunity. The innate component consists of macrophages, natural killer cells, monocytes, and granulocytes, which identify molecular patterns involved in cellular transformation and release various cytokines and inflammatory mediators. The innate response lacks the memory capability for foreign antigens, a feature present in adaptive immune response. This latter component of the immune system also features specificity for foreign antigens, which is imparted by the presence of receptors on lymphocytes. Antigen-presenting cells also play a role in the adaptive response—they engulf foreign antigens and present them to the lymphocytes in the context of major histocompatibility complex (MHC). CD4+ T cells bear receptors that recognize antigens in the context of MHC class II molecules, which then enables them to release cytokines and further activate CD8+ lymphocytes (CTLs) or B cells. CTLs are part of cell-mediated immunity and are capable of eliminating cells presented in the context of MHC class I molecules via apoptosis or perforin-mediated cell lysis [1]. It is widely accepted that T-cell–mediated immunity plays a vital role in the antitumor response, particularly when it comes to central nervous system (CNS) tumors [2].

This work was supported by a grant from the National Institutes of Neurological Disorders and Stroke (K08 NS046430 [ML]) and the Elsa U. Pardee Foundation (ML).

* Corresponding author.

E-mail address: mlesniak@surgery.bsd.uchicago.edu (M.S. Lesniak).

B cells are involved in release of immunoglobulins and as such are part of the humoral immune system. This latter system is not a significant part of immune response to CNS tumors, because antibodies largely interact with soluble antigens and are not fully capable of responding to cytoplasmic tumor antigens. Immunoglobulins also poorly penetrate the blood-brain barrier [3].

The brain historically has been considered an "immune privileged" site [4]. This theory was based on the lack of organized lymphoid tissue or lymphatic drainage within the brain. The presence of the blood-brain barrier and scarcity of MHC expression by neurons and astrocytes also led to this assumption [1]. Such considerations alter the immune response in the CNS; however, they do not render it completely immune privileged. It is known that lymphocytes are present within the brain during infections and neoplastic processes, and glioma cells are capable of expressing various tumor-associated antigens. The immune-privileged state is overcome during such processes, and the immune responses within the CNS are finely regulated. Antigen-presenting cells are still necessary for the immune response to be mounted within the brain, although the exact mechanism of this process has not been fully elucidated.

The most likely antigen-presenting cells within the CNS are microglia [5] because they express MHC class I and II molecules and other costimulatory factors [6]. Dendritic cells also play a part in antigen presentation within CNS, as demonstrated by primate studies of experimental allergic encephalomyelitis [7]. Immune modulation within the brain with up-regulation of MHC antigens takes place at sites of injury and after exposure to cytokines [8]. Experimental evidence indicates that human glioma cells express CD 95 and Fas ligand, which enables them to interact with T cells and initiate apoptosis [9,10]. These cells also present tumor-associated antigens, which are capable of producing immune responses.

It has been shown that brain tumor–specific T cells are primed within cervical lymph nodes [11]. Despite the blood-brain barrier, multiple types of lymphoid cells have been found within brain parenchyma during disease processes [12–14], which is possibly explained by the presence of proinflammatory cytokines affecting the blood-brain barrier [15]. There is also evidence that astrocytes exert immunosuppressive function under normal conditions, which may produce an anti-inflammatory state via repression of microglia [5,16].

Current strategies against malignant gliomas

Malignant gliomas have an intrinsic capability to evade the immune response, a finding caused by several factors. First, the level of MHC class I expression in glioma is low [17]; however, the process can be up-regulated by interferon-γ (IFN- γ) [8]. Second, certain receptors on natural killer cells enable them to lyse tumor cells that intrinsically express low levels of MHCs [18]. Glioma cells also express human leukocyte antigen-G, which is a nontypical class I MHC molecule [19]. Expression of human leukocyte antigen-G has been shown to lessen the susceptibility of tumor cells to immune responses [20]. Gliomas also can affect immune system constituents via secretion of certain tumor factors, which results in dysregulation of antigen-presenting cells function and T cell receptor signaling [21,22]. Among the better characterized immunosuppressive factors identified to date, transforming growth factor beta 2 (TGF-β2) is notably overexpressed in patients with glioblastoma multiforme (GBM) and as such has arisen as the most likely candidate for immunosuppressive properties of gliomas [23,24]. TGF-β2 hinders the cytotoxic response of glioma cells to lymphocytes, interleukin (IL)-2 receptor induction, natural killer cell activity, and cytokine production [25–27]. Another contributing factor to TGF-β2's ability to suppress gliomas' immune response is via down-regulation of human leukocyte antigen–DR expression on tumor cells, which is an important MHC antigen [28]. TGF-β2 also may promote growth of glioma cells, which results in angiogenesis and stromal growth [29]. TGF-β2 antagonists are currently being investigated and have so far been demonstrated to inhibit proliferation of glioma cells. In addition to TGF-β2, another factor may be responsible for human leukocyte antigen–DR down-regulation, prostaglandin E2 [30]. This cytokine is also capable of decreasing lymphokine activated killer cell activity, thereby contributing to the ability of malignant gliomas to evade immune response [31].

Recent advances in research on antigen presentation, specific cytokines, and T-cell cytotoxicity have given new direction to immunotherapeutic strategies against CNS tumors. Evidence of CNS manifestations after peripheral vaccination with brain-specific antigens in experimental allergic encephalomyelitis and paraneoplastic cerebellar degeneration models also have led to a search for possible immunotherapy regimens for management of malignant gliomas [32]. Current directions in immunotherapy investigations include the use of various cytokines, dendritic cells, viral and peptide vaccines, and toxins.

Cytokines

Cytokines augment T-cell activation and MHC antigen expression. Antitumor effects mediated by expression of cytokines in cancer models have been demonstrated with IL-2, -4, -12, and -23, IFN-α, and granulocytes-macrophage colony stimulating factor (GM-CSF) [33–40]. Cytokine gene therapy for malignant glioma has been investigated as a tool for enhancement of T-cell activity and antigen-presenting cell activation. Preclinical studies using peripheral cytokine-secreting vaccines have been shown to be efficacious against glioma in animal models, thereby leading to investigation of these cytokines in human studies [41].

Dillman and colleagues [42] performed a study using IL-2 to generate autologous lymphokine activated killer cells. After generation, these lymphokine activated killer cells were injected intratumorally. That trial included 40 patients with GBM. The patients were compared with historical controls. Besides a positive conclusion regarding the safety of this approach, a clinical benefit was documented. The median survival after the therapy was 9 months, and the 1-year survival rate was 34%. Nine patients survived beyond 1 year, and 3 patients survived beyond 2 years. Control patients had a median survival of 13.6 months from their initial diagnosis, with a 2-year survival rate of 20%; for the 31 patients who underwent lymphokine activated killer cell placement during the course of their disease, median survival was 17.5 months and the 2-year survival rate was 31% (p = 0.012). Other studies using lymphokine activated killer cells could not reproduce these encouraging outcomes, and one study reported considerable toxicity [42].

IL-2 also has been used in clinical studies with cytotoxic T lymphocytes [43]. Initially, five patients with recurrent glioma were treated with intracavitary CTLs and IL-2. Alloreactive CTLs were sensitized to the MHC proteins of the patients, thereby offering selective destruction of glioma cells that express MHC. The treatment was well tolerated. The trial included two patients with GBM (both subsequently died), two patients with anaplastic oligodendroglioma (no evidence of tumor at 28 and 30 months' follow-up), and one patient with anaplastic astrocytoma (AA) (no evidence of tumor at 28 months). A larger phase I trial using CTLs is currently in the planning stages.

Colombo and colleagues [44] described another trial using IL-2 as a transgene. In this case, the cytokine was tested in combination with herpes simplex virus-tyrosine kinase transgene; the genes were carried by a retrovirus on vector-producing cells. Twelve patients with recurrent GBM were enrolled. Treatment consisted of intratumoral injection of the construct followed by systemic administration of acyclovir. The treatment was well tolerated. Although none of the patients achieved a complete response, 2 had a partial response, 4 had a minor response, 4 had stable disease, and 2 had progressive disease. Of the 2 patients who showed a 50% reduction of mass size, 1 presented with a mass in the corpus callosum; this patient underwent stereotactic injection of the construct. After treatment, the patient experienced clinical improvement and regression of the tumor mass, as demonstrated by MRI performed 1 month after completion of treatment. The patient died of pulmonary embolism 11 months after the treatment. The second patient who achieved partial response presented with GBM in the corpus callosum and a second small lesion in the left temporal lobe. The patient underwent intratumoral treatment of the corpus callosum lesion and subsequently experienced improvement of the neurologic symptoms. Follow-up by MRI showed regression not only of the injected mass but also of the temporal lesion. Unfortunately, the patient showed tumor relapse and died 13 months after the therapy.

Okada and colleagues [45] described a case in which IL-4 was used to treat recurrent GBM. The IL-4 transgene was expressed by transfected fibroblasts. The therapy consisted of the combination of transfected fibro-blasts and irradiated autologous glioma cells injected intradermally. With regard to the immune response related to treatment, infiltration of dendritic cells (CD 1a+), CD4+, and CD8+ T cells was demonstrated at sites of in-jection. These cells increased proportionally to the amount of IL-4 produced at each of the injection sites. The patient demonstrated partial clinical and radiologic response, as demonstrated by temporary symptomatic improve-ment and considerable resolution of enhancement and peritumoral edema relative to the pretreatment MRI. Treatment was well tolerated, and the patient survived 10 months after initiation of this treatment.

IL-12 also has been tested in treatment of patients with gliomas. Kikuchi and colleagues [46] conducted a study that included 15 patients with AA, an-aplastic oligoastrocytoma, and GBM. Treatment consisted of subcutaneous administration of recombinant IL-12 in combination with a fusion of autol-ogous dendritic and glioma cells. In 2 patients, augmentation of CD8+ cytolytic activity on glioma cells was documented after treatment. With regards to clinical responses, 4 of 15 patients experienced deterioration in symptoms (3 patients had worsening of the level of consciousness at the end of first course of vaccination, and 1 patient's presenting symptom of hemiparesis worsened during the study). In these 4 patients, therapy was discontinued and steroids were administered. In the remaining 11 patients, clinical symptoms did not worsen during therapy. Radiologic findings showed that 4 patients had more than 50% reduction in size of tumors, as documented by follow-up MRI. The clinical trial demonstrated that using a fusion product of dendritic and glioma cells with IL-12 resulted in no serious side effects and measurable radiographic response in four tumors.

IFN-α was tested in a phase III clinical trial for patients with high-grade gliomas [47]. The study included 360 patients with AA, anaplastic oligoden-droglioma, GBM, and gliosarcoma. Of the 360 patients, only 214 met the eligibility criteria for further evaluation. The patients were initially treated with radiation and β-chloro-nitrosourea (carmustine). After radiotherapy, patients without disease progression were stratified and randomized into two groups: β-chloro-nitrosourea (carmustine) and β-chloro-nitrosourea (carmustine) plus INF-α. Unfortunately, there was no difference in response rates between the two treatment arms in the final evaluation [47].

Table 1 summarizes the most recent clinical trials that use various cytokine-based regimens against CNS tumors. More studies using various cytokine-based protocols are currently underway, and given the encourag-ing results of animal studies, the hope for such approaches is appealing.

Dendritic cells

Dendritic cells are hematopoietically derived leukocytes involved in immune surveillance [48,49]. They are effective antigen-presenting cells and as such have been the target of investigation for possible antiglioma

Table 1
Current clinical trials in cytokine therapies for central nervous system tumors

Cytokine/cell used	Study description	Route of administration	n	Tumor	Outcome	Reference
IL-2/HSV-tk transgenes on retroviral vector-producing cells and ganciclovir	Phase II	Intratumoral	12	Recurrent GBM	Safety was demonstrated. Tumor responses in 50% of cases Intratumoral and plasma Th1 cytokine levels were noted	[44]
IL-2 generated LAK cells	Phase I	Intratumoral	40	GBM	Safety was demonstrated; median survival increased	[42]
IL-2 with CTLs	Phase I	Intratumoral	5	GBM, AOA, AA	Mild toxicity	[43]
IL-4 expressed by transfected fibroblasts/irradiated autologous glioma cells	Phase I	Intradermal	1	Recurrent GBM	Infiltration of CD4, CD8 and CD1a cells at injection sites 10 months survival after treatment	[45]
IL-12/fusion of dendritic and glioma cells	Phase I	Subcutaneous	15	Malignant gliomas (GBM, AA, AOA)	No serious adverse effects were observed In four patients, MRI showed >50% reduction in tumor size	[46]
IFN-α/BCNU and radiation	Phase III	Subcutaneous	275	AA, AO, GBM, and gliosarcoma	Patients receiving IFN-α experienced more fever, chills, myalgias, and neurocortical symptoms, including somnolence, confusion, and exacerbation of neurologic deficits There was no significant difference with regard to time to disease progression or overall survival between the two groups	[47]

Abbreviations: AO, anaplastic oligodendroglioma; AOA, anaplastic oligoastrocytoma; BCNU, β-chloro-nitrosourea (carmustine); HSV-tk, herpes simplex virus-tyrosine kinase; LAK, lymphokine-activated killer cells.

treatment strategies. Under normal conditions, dendritic cells are absent from the brain parenchyma; they are, however, found within CNS under inflammatory conditions, most likely attracted by specific chemokines released by tissue astrocytes and microglia [50].

Several issues must be resolved before large-scale clinical use of dendritic cells. First, an appropriate source of dendritic cells must be elucidated, whether it is direct isolation from patient-derived tumor antigens or from in vitro–derived dendritic cells. Second, mature and immature dendritic cells have different antitumor properties, and optimal level of maturity is still not clear [51]. Dendritic cell maturation is enhanced by addition of TNF-α [52], and clinical trials have shown that mature dendritic cells are better at generating CTL responses in malignant melanoma [53]. Antigen-loading strategies present a third topic of investigation. Possible options include tumor-derived mRNA [54,55], tumor cell lysates [56–58], and whole tumor peptides [59]. Finally, optimal route of administration and co-administration of cytokines are further topics that arise with the use of dendritic cells. Intravenous injection results in movement of dendritic cells to reticular organs, whereas intradermal administration leads to homing of dendritic cells to local lymph nodes [60]. Both routes can be beneficial, as the former results in Th2 activation of IL-10 and antibodies, whereas the latter results in Th1 activation of IL-2 [61,62]. Adjuvant administration of cytokines, such as IL-12 [63] and IFN-α [64], has shown promising results in animal experiments and is currently a topic of investigation for human trials.

Genetically engineered dendritic cells are the next venue of research [65]. This strategy involves introduction of genes that encode tumor antigens or certain cytokines into dendritic cells [66]. Candidate genes include GM-CSF, IFN-α, IL-12, and IL-18, because transfection with these cytokine genes is expected to enhance the function of dendritic cells.

The use of dendritic cells for treatment of brain tumors also has been tested in human trials. One of the treatments tested was the injection of a fusion product of dendritic cells and autologous glioma cells [52]. Fusion cells were injected intradermally close to a cervical lymph node in eight patients with malignant gliomas. All patients received these cells every 3 weeks for a minimum of three and a maximum of seven immunizations. With regards to the antitumoral immune response, five patients were assessed. In four of five patients, immunization led to a modest rise in CD16+ and CD56+ cells in peripheral blood lymphocytes. Peripheral blood mononuclear cells also were incubated with irradiated autologous glioma and supernatants were harvested. In six cases analyzed, the concentration of IFN-γ in the supernatant increased after immunization. Clinical results showed that there were no serious adverse effects and two partial responses [52].

Dendritic cells also have been injected after exposure to tumoral antigens ex vivo. The rationale for this strategy was to promote tumoral antigenic presentation to trigger cellular immune response. Dendritic cells pulsed with peptides from patient's tumors have been tested in trials for malignant gliomas [67,68]. One of these trials evaluated five patients with GBM and AA [67]. In this study, dendritic cells were injected intradermally and intracranially. The mean number of vaccinations was 3.7 times intradermally (close to a cervical lymph node) and 3.2 times intratumorally via an Ommaya reservoir. With regards to the mounting of antitumoral response, the number of CD56+ cells in blood increased after treatment. T-cell–mediated antitumor activity also was enhanced—as evaluated by the ELISPOT assay after vaccination—in two of five tested patients. Three patients showed delayed-type hypersensitivity reactivity to the autologous tumor lysate, two patients had a minor clinical response, and two had an increased ELISPOT result. Intratumoral CD4+ and CD8+ T-cell infiltration was detected in two patients who underwent reoperation after vaccination. On the other hand, radiographic outcomes included two minor responses and four cases in which no change was appreciated [67].

Another study included nine patients with GBM and AA who were treated with intradermal vaccinations of peptide-pulsed dendritic cells [68]. The peptides were obtained by eluting autologous glioma cells. In this study, the treatment was administrated biweekly. Treatment-related immune responses included systemic cytotoxicity in four of seven tested patients. Robust intratumoral cytotoxic and memory T-cell infiltration was detected in two of four patients who underwent reoperation after vaccination. With regards to clinical results, the study demonstrated this treatment regimen to be safe because no major side effects were observed [68]. Increase in survival was also demonstrated; median survival times for the study and control groups were 455 and 257 days, respectively [68].

Table 2 summarizes current clinical trial using dendritic cell-based approaches for CNS tumors [52,67,68]. Partial responses were observed in some trials, whereas two of the trials were also able to demonstrate increased survival. Dendritic cell–based approach is clearly a promising strategy in immunotherapeutic modalities against gliomas.

Viral vectors and peptide vaccines

Several viral vectors have shown promising results with regard to their potential to enhance immunotherapy of malignant gliomas. Replication-competent and replication-incompetent viruses have been used, with the latter group demonstrating more effective transgene expression. Herpesvirus, adenovirus, vaccinia, reovirus, and New Castle disease viruses have been used in various clinical studies. As an augmentation tool for immunotherapy, viral vectors have been used to deliver certain cytokines to brain tumors [69–71].

Herpes simplex virus/IL-4 combination was shown to augment the oncolytic effect of the virus when compared with herpes simplex virus used alone in animal models [72]. Such beneficial effects were also observed in studies of herpes simplex virus with IL-12, IL-2, and TNF-α [73,74]. Human studies

Table 2
Current clinical trials using dendritic cell vaccines for central nervous system tumors

Cell/vaccination strategy	Study description	Route of administration	n	Tumor	Outcome	Reference
Fusions of dendritic and glioma cells	Phase I	Intradermal	8	Malignant gliomas	No serious adverse effects; two partial responses	[52]
DCs pulsed with tumor lysate	Phase I/II	Intradermal and intracranial	5	GBM, AA	Treatment was well tolerated. Two minor responses and four no-change cases evaluated by radiologic findings; T-cell–mediated antitumor activity in two of five tested patients; three patients showed delayed-type hypersensitivity reactivity to the autologous tumor lysate, two of whom had a minor clinical response	[67]
DCs with peptide eluted from tumor cells	Phase I	Intradermal	9	GBM, AA	Evidence of intratumoral infiltration; increased survival	[68]

Abbreviation: DCs, dendritic cells.

are needed to confirm these encouraging combination regimens for targeting malignant gliomas.

The amplification of epidermal growth factor receptor (EGFR) gene is present in approximately 40% of gliomas and is most frequently associated with EGFRvIII (variant III) gene rearrangement. Attenuated measles vaccines displaying EGFRvIII have potent antitumor activity in GBM but have no significant toxicity on normal cells [75]. Investigations are ongoing to explore efficacy of EGFRvIII-retargeted oncolytic measles virus vaccines in human trials. Of note, the EGFRvIII peptide also has been used as an antigen to elicit antitumoral immune response. A phase I study was conducted with this peptide as a vaccine (study presented at the American Society of Clinical Oncology Meeting 2006). This trial consisted in vaccinating 12 patients who had newly diagnosed GBM with an EGFRvIII peptide vaccine. The study demonstrated minimal toxicity and showed that this vaccine generates cellular and humoral immune response against this peptide. With respect to clinical outcome, median time to progression from surgery for vaccinated patients was 12 months, which suggested a therapeutic benefit when compared with that of an historical matched control cohort that had a median time to progression of 7.1 months ($n = 39$) ($P = .0058$). Among the recurrent tumors that were evaluated by immunohistochemistry, 100% lacked expression of EGFRvIII, which suggested that treatment might have eliminated EFGRvIII+ cells.

Peptide vaccines directed at IL-13 receptor α-2 (IL-13Rα2) have been investigated as potential tools against glioma cells [76]. These receptors are highly expressed in most malignant gliomas, which makes them an attractive target for vaccination. Preclinical studies have found that vaccines that contain IL-13Rα2 are highly immunogenic and are effective at expanding tumor-reactive CTLs [77].

Toxins

Convection-enhanced delivery of toxins has been the topic of extensive and encouraging research in glioma therapies. The technique implies administration of fusion proteins under image guidance with the aid of positive pressure microinfusion [78,79]. Currently investigated toxins include bacteria-derived products, such as diphtheria and *Pseudomonas* exotoxin, which are fused to a carrier ligand that can recognize a tumor cell-surface marker [80]. The rationale for selecting a specific cytokine derives from the fact that certain cytokine receptors are overexpressed in brain tumors; thus, the toxic complex preferentially binds to tumor cells.

A dose-escalation trial of intratumoral administration of IL-4 *Pseudomonas* exotoxin (NBI-3001) in patients with recurrent malignant glioma was conducted. Thirty-one patients with grade 3 and 4 astrocytoma were studied (25 with GBM, 6 with AA). Patients were assigned to one of four dose groups. NBI-3001 was administered via convection-enhanced delivery intratumorally using stereotactically placed catheters. In this study, no drug-related systemic toxicity was noted. Some CNS-related adverse effects were present. Grade 3 or 4 toxicity was seen in 39% of patients in all dose groups and 22% of patients at the maximum tolerated dose; no deaths were attributable to treatment. With regards to clinical efficacy, median survival was 8.2 months overall, with a median survival of 5.8 months for the patients who had GBM. Six-month survival rates were 52% and 48%, respectively. Post-treatment MRI showed decreased signal intensity within the tumor consistent with tumor necrosis in many patients [81].

Neurotoxicity of this agent is a concern that needs to be addressed. A case report of a patient who had recurrent GBM that followed the same protocol from this study was published in 2004 [82]. The maximal dose was used. The agent was injected intracranially by high-flow bulk infusion. Side effects included seizures, clinical signs of meningeal reaction, hydrocephalus, increase in motor deficits, severely impaired vision in both eyes, and bilateral hearing loss [81]. On the other hand, a follow-up MRI 4 weeks after the toxin infusion demonstrated necrosis with shrinkage of tumor; months later, the tumor had shrunk and almost disappeared, leaving less than 5% residual contrast enhancement surrounded by scar. Follow-up MRI confirmed the durable tumor response. Three years after the toxin infusion, the patient presented with a local recurrence and died 4 months later. Despite toxicity, the patient survived 3 years after treatment with this toxin [81].

Another study investigated the safety and activity of directly infusing IL-4(38-37)-PE38KDEL, a chimeric protein composed of circularly permuted IL-4 and a truncated form of *Pseudomonas* exotoxin, into recurrent malignant high-grade gliomas [83]. In this case, IL-4 toxin complex was infused over a 4- to 8-day period into gliomas of nine patients via one to three stereotactically placed catheters. No apparent systemic toxicity occurred in any patient. The infusion of IL-4 toxin in six of nine patients showed glioma necrosis, as evidenced by diminished enhancement on MRI. On the other hand, seven of nine patients underwent craniotomy because of increased intracranial pressure after the beginning of infusion. In six of these seven patients, partial to extensive tumor necrosis with edema was confirmed pathologically. Local toxicity seemed attributable mainly to tumor necrosis or occasionally to the volume of infusion. With regards to the two patients who did not undergo surgery, MRI showed gadolinium enhancement in one patient and the other patient showed extensive necrosis of tumor leading to complete remission. That patient remained disease free 18 months after the procedure [83].

Some studies have tested the ability of IL-13 to target toxins into gliomas [84]. This strategy is based on taking advantage of the overexpression of IL-13α2 receptor on these tumors [85]. IL13PE38QQR is a recombinant toxin composed of the enzymatically active portion of *Pseudomonas* exotoxin A conjugated with human IL-13. A report on preliminary results

Table 3
Current clinical trials in toxin therapies for central nervous system tumors

Ligand/toxin	Study description by authors	Route of administration	n	Tumor	Outcome	Reference
IL-4/*Pseudomonas* toxin	Case report	Intracranial	1	Recurrent GBM	Some permanent neurologic side effects resulted from toxin infusion, survived 3 years after toxin infusion	[81]
IL-4/*Pseudomonas* toxin	Open-label, dose-escalation trial	Intracranial	31	Recurrent malignant glioma, (grades 3 and 4 astrocytoma)	Acceptable safety and toxicity, no drug-related systemic toxicity, treatment-related neurotoxicity	[82,87]
IL-4/*Pseudomonas* toxin	Phase I	Intracranial	9	Recurrent GBM	Occasional increase in intracranial pressure attributed to volume of infusion, otherwise well tolerated	[83]
IL-13/*Pseudomonas* toxin	Phase I	Intracranial	46	Recurrent malignant glioma	Well-tolerated with corticosteroid prophylaxis, occasional prolongation of survival times has been observed	[84]
TGF-α/*Pseudomonas* toxin	Case report	Intracranial	1	Recurrent GBM	Clinical improvement, tumor has not progressed for >43 months	[86]

from three phase I studies that tested this strategy was published [84]. These studies were conducted on 46 patients with recurrent malignant gliomas. The trials suggested that intratumoral infusion with or without resection is fairly well tolerated. Postresection infusion into the peritumoral brain parenchyma also seems to be well tolerated. Histopathologic tumor effect was seen at drug concentrations of 0.5 to 2 μg/mL. A phase III study of IL-13 and *Pseudomonas* toxin was recently performed and showed no therapeutic benefit of this system.

The fusion protein TGF-α/*Pseudomonas* exotoxin was demonstrated to bind EGFR on human glioma cells. This construct, TP-38, was tested in one patient who had recurrent bifrontal GBM that was refractory to other treatments [86]. The treatment was administered via two multiport pediatric ventricular catheters placed stereotactically into the left and right frontal cortices, respectively. Twenty milliliters of TP-38 were infused through each catheter. The TP-38 concentration was 25 ng/mL, which resulted in a total delivered TP-38 dose of 1 mg. No significant increases in intracranial pressure were observed throughout the duration of the infusion. The patient tolerated the TP-38 infusion without complication and was discharged. After therapy, she improved clinically, was weaned off steroids and anticonvulsants, and experienced a progressive decrease in enhancing tumor volume. At the time of publication the patient remained without progression for 43 months after TP-38 therapy. The results of this case remain to be corroborated in further studies, but the clinical response and tolerability of this treatment are encouraging [86].

Table 3 presents a summary of recent clinical trials using cytokine/toxin constructs [87].

Summary

As a result of enormous progress in tumor immunobiology, immunotherapeutic approaches to treatment of CNS tumors have entered an exciting phase of research. Many novel strategies are currently being investigated in human trials and already have been found safe and efficacious in preliminary studies. Dendritic cell–based approaches seem promising for increasing survival in patients who have glioma. Peptide vaccine and various cytokine-based protocols are currently in different stages of investigation. Development of effective immunotherapy protocols is the goal of current research. The progress is being hampered by our lack of full understanding of glioma-specific antigens, the heterogeneity of tumor cells, and the poor understanding of the exact mechanisms of glioma-induced immunosuppression. The potential for immunotherapeutic strategies in treatment of CNS tumors, as an adjunct to the current regimens or as a stand-alone approach, is tangible; however, the challenges of applying our knowledge of laboratory research to patient care remain real and formidable.

References

[1] Janeway C, Travers P, Walport M. Immunobiology: the immune system in health and disease. New York: Current Biology Publications; 1999.

[2] Holladay FP, Heitz T, Wood GW. Antitumor activity against established intracerebral gliomas exhibited by cytotoxic T lymphocytes, but not by lymphokine-activated killer cells. J Neurosurg 1992;77(5):757–62.

[3] Prins RM, Liau LM. Immunology and immunotherapy in neurosurgical disease. Neurosurgery 2003;53(1):144–52 [discussion: 144–52].

[4] Lampson BC. Basic principles of CNS immunology. Philadelphia: WB Saunders; 2002.

[5] Aloisi F, Ria F, Penna G, et al. Microglia are more efficient than astrocytes in antigen processing and in Th1 but not Th2 cell activation. J Immunol 1998;160(10):4671–80.

[6] Aloisi F. Immune function of microglia. Glia 2001;36(2):165–79.

[7] de Vos AF, van Meurs M, Brok HP, et al. Transfer of central nervous system autoantigens and presentation in secondary lymphoid organs. J Immunol 2002;169(10):5415–23.

[8] Sethna MP, Lampson LA. Immune modulation within the brain: recruitment of inflammatory cells and increased major histocompatibility antigen expression following intracerebral injection of interferon-gamma. J Neuroimmunol 1991;34(2–3):121–32.

[9] Parney IF, Farr-Jones MA, Chang LJ, et al. Human glioma immunobiology in vitro: implications for immunogene therapy. Neurosurgery 2000;46(5):1169–77 [discussion: 1169–78].

[10] Weller M, Frei K, Groscurth P, et al. Anti-Fas/APO-1 antibody-mediated apoptosis of cultured human glioma cells: induction and modulation of sensitivity by cytokines. J Clin Invest 1994;94(3):954–64.

[11] Walker PR, Calzascia T, Schnuriger V, et al. The brain parenchyma is permissive for full antitumor CTL effector function, even in the absence of CD4 T cells. J Immunol 2000;165(6):3128–35.

[12] Hickey WF, Hsu BL, Kimura H. T-lymphocyte entry into the central nervous system. J Neurosci Res 1991;28(2):254–60.

[13] Perry VH, Anthony DC, Bolton SJ, et al. The blood-brain barrier and the inflammatory response. Mol Med Today 1997;3(8):335–41.

[14] Dix AR, Brooks WH, Roszman TL, et al. Immune defects observed in patients with primary malignant brain tumors. J Neuroimmunol 1999;100(1–2):216–32.

[15] Gordon FL, Nguyen KB, White CA, et al. Rapid entry and downregulation of T cells in the central nervous system during the reinduction of experimental autoimmune encephalomyelitis. J Neuroimmunol 2001;112(1–2):15–27.

[16] Matsumoto Y, Ohmori K, Fujiwara M. Immune regulation by brain cells in the central nervous system: microglia but not astrocytes present myelin basic protein to encephalitogenic T cells under in vivo-mimicking conditions. Immunology 1992;76(2):209–16.

[17] Ito A, Shinkai M, Honda H, et al. Augmentation of MHC class I antigen presentation via heat shock protein expression by hyperthermia. Cancer Immunol Immunother 2001;50(10):515–22.

[18] Prins RM, Liau LM. Cellular immunity and immunotherapy of brain tumors. Front Biosci 2004;9:3124–36.

[19] Wiendl H, Mitsdoerffer M, Hofmeister V, et al. A functional role of HLA-G expression in human gliomas: an alternative strategy of immune escape. J Immunol 2002;168(9):4772–80.

[20] Wiendl H, Mitsdoerffer M, Weller M. Hide-and-seek in the brain: a role for HLA-G mediating immune privilege for glioma cells. Semin Cancer Biol 2003;13(5):343–51.

[21] Morford LA, Elliott LH, Carlson SL, et al. T cell receptor-mediated signaling is defective in T cells obtained from patients with primary intracranial tumors. J Immunol 1997;159(9):4415–25.

[22] Prins RM, Graf MR, Merchant RE. Cytotoxic T cells infiltrating a glioma express an aberrant phenotype that is associated with decreased function and apoptosis. Cancer Immunol Immunother 2001;50(6):285–92.

[23] Olofsson A, Miyazono K, Kanzaki T, et al. Transforming growth factor-beta 1, -beta 2, and -beta 3 secreted by a human glioblastoma cell line: identification of small and different forms of large latent complexes. J Biol Chem 1992;267(27):19482–8.

[24] Kuppner MC, Hamou MF, Sawamura Y, et al. Inhibition of lymphocyte function by glioblastoma-derived transforming growth factor beta 2. J Neurosurg 1989;71(2):211–7.

[25] Kehrl JH, Roberts AB, Wakefield LM, et al. Transforming growth factor beta is an important immunomodulatory protein for human B lymphocytes. J Immunol 1986;137(12):3855–60.

[26] Rook AH, Kehrl JH, Wakefield LM, et al. Effects of transforming growth factor beta on the functions of natural killer cells: depressed cytolytic activity and blunting of interferon responsiveness. J Immunol 1986;136(10):3916–20.

[27] Kehrl JH, Wakefield LM, Roberts AB, et al. Production of transforming growth factor beta by human T lymphocytes and its potential role in the regulation of T cell growth. J Exp Med 1986;163(5):1037–50.

[28] Zuber P, Kuppner MC, De Tribolet N. Transforming growth factor-beta 2 down-regulates HLA-DR antigen expression on human malignant glioma cells. Eur J Immunol 1988;18(10): 1623–6.

[29] Jensen RL. Growth factor-mediated angiogenesis in the malignant progression of glial tumors: a review. Surg Neurol 1998;49(2):189–95 [discussion: 196].

[30] Kuppner MC, Sawamura Y, Hamou MF, et al. Influence of PGE2- and cAMP-modulating agents on human glioblastoma cell killing by interleukin-2-activated lymphocytes. J Neurosurg 1990;72(4):619–25.

[31] Yamanaka R, Tanaka R, Yoshida S, et al. Suppression of TGF-beta1 in human gliomas by retroviral gene transfection enhances susceptibility to LAK cells. J Neurooncol 1999;43(1): 27–34.

[32] Krakowski ML, Owens T. The central nervous system environment controls effector CD4+ T cell cytokine profile in experimental allergic encephalomyelitis. Eur J Immunol 1997; 27(11):2840–7.

[33] Glick RP, Lichtor T, de Zoeten E, et al. Prolongation of survival of mice with glioma treated with semiallogeneic fibroblasts secreting interleukin-2. Neurosurgery 1999;45(4):867–74.

[34] Okada H, Giezeman-Smits KM, Tahara H, et al. Effective cytokine gene therapy against an intracranial glioma using a retrovirally transduced IL-4 plus HSVtk tumor vaccine. Gene Ther 1999;6(2):219–26.

[35] Dranoff G. GM-CSF-secreting melanoma vaccines. Oncogene 2003;22(20):3188–92.

[36] Sampath P, Hanes J, DiMeco F, et al. Paracrine immunotherapy with interleukin-2 and local chemotherapy is synergistic in the treatment of experimental brain tumors. Cancer Res 1999; 59(9):2107–14.

[37] Ferrantini M, Giovarelli M, Modesti A, et al. IFN-alpha 1 gene expression into a metastatic murine adenocarcinoma (TS/A) results in CD8+ T cell-mediated tumor rejection and development of antitumor immunity: comparative studies with IFN-gamma-producing TS/A cells. J Immunol 1994;153(10):4604–15.

[38] Hiroishi K, Tuting T, Tahara H, et al. Interferon-alpha gene therapy in combination with CD80 transduction reduces tumorigenicity and growth of established tumor in poorly immunogenic tumor models. Gene Ther 1999;6(12):1988–94.

[39] Lo CH, Lee SC, Wu PY, et al. Antitumor and antimetastatic activity of IL-23. J Immunol 2003;171(2):600–7.

[40] Tahara H, Zitvogel L, Storkus WJ, et al. Effective eradication of established murine tumors with IL-12 gene therapy using a polycistronic retroviral vector. J Immunol 1995;154(12): 6466–74.

[41] Okada H, Pollack IF. Cytokine gene therapy for malignant glioma. Expert Opin Biol Ther 2004;4(10):1609–20.

[42] Dillman RO, Duma CM, Schiltz PM, et al. Intracavitary placement of autologous lymphokine-activated killer (LAK) cells after resection of recurrent glioblastoma. J Immunother 2004;27(5):398–404.

[43] Kruse CA, Cepeda L, Owens B, et al. Treatment of recurrent glioma with intracavitary alloreactive cytotoxic T lymphocytes and interleukin-2. Cancer Immunol Immunother 1997; 45(2):77–87.

[44] Colombo F, Barzon L, Franchin E, et al. Combined HSV-TK/IL-2 gene therapy in patients with recurrent glioblastoma multiforme: biological and clinical results. Cancer Gene Ther 2005;12(10):835–48.

[45] Okada H, Lieberman FS, Edington HD, et al. Autologous glioma cell vaccine admixed with interleukin-4 gene transfected fibroblasts in the treatment of recurrent glioblastoma: preliminary observations in a patient with a favorable response to therapy. J Neurooncol 2003; 64(1–2):13–20.

[46] Kikuchi T, Akasaki Y, Abe T, et al. Vaccination of glioma patients with fusions of dendritic and glioma cells and recombinant human interleukin 12. J Immunother 2004;27(6): 452–9.

[47] Buckner JC, Schomberg PJ, McGinnis WL, et al. A phase III study of radiation therapy plus carmustine with or without recombinant interferon-alpha in the treatment of patients with newly diagnosed high-grade glioma. Cancer 2001;92(2):420–33.

[48] Steinman RM. The dendritic cell system and its role in immunogenicity. Annu Rev Immunol 1991;9:271–96.

[49] Steinman RM, Pack M, Inaba K. Dendritic cells in the T-cell areas of lymphoid organs. Immunol Rev 1997;156:25–37.

[50] Gourmala NG, Buttini M, Limonta S, et al. Differential and time-dependent expression of monocyte chemoattractant protein-1 mRNA by astrocytes and macrophages in rat brain: effects of ischemia and peripheral lipopolysaccharide administration. J Neuroimmunol 1997;74(1–2):35–44.

[51] Grabbe S, Kampgen E, Schuler G. Dendritic cells: multi-lineal and multi-functional. Immunol Today 2000;21(9):431–3.

[52] Kikuchi T, Akasaki Y, Irie M, et al. Results of a phase I clinical trial of vaccination of glioma patients with fusions of dendritic and glioma cells. Cancer Immunol Immunother 2001;50(7): 337–44.

[53] Jonuleit H, Giesecke A, Kandemir A, et al. Induction of tumor peptide-specific cytotoxic T cells under serum-free conditions by mature human dendritic cells. Arch Dermatol Res 2000; 292(7):325–32.

[54] Ashley DM, Faiola B, Nair S, et al. Bone marrow-generated dendritic cells pulsed with tumor extracts or tumor RNA induce antitumor immunity against central nervous system tumors. J Exp Med 1997;186(7):1177–82.

[55] Boczkowski D, Nair SK, Snyder D, et al. Dendritic cells pulsed with RNA are potent antigen-presenting cells in vitro and in vivo. J Exp Med 1996;184(2):465–72.

[56] Aoki H, Mizuno M, Natsume A, et al. Dendritic cells pulsed with tumor extract-cationic liposome complex increase the induction of cytotoxic T lymphocytes in mouse brain tumor. Cancer Immunol Immunother 2001;50(9):463–8.

[57] Heimberger AB, Crotty LE, Archer GE, et al. Bone marrow-derived dendritic cells pulsed with tumor homogenate induce immunity against syngeneic intracerebral glioma. J Neuroimmunol 2000;103(1):16–25.

[58] Ni HT, Spellman SR, Jean WC, et al. Immunization with dendritic cells pulsed with tumor extract increases survival of mice bearing intracranial gliomas. J Neurooncol 2001;51(1):1–9.

[59] Lassmann H, Schmied M, Vass K, et al. Bone marrow derived elements and resident microglia in brain inflammation. Glia 1993;7(1):19–24.

[60] Fossum S. Lymph-borne dendritic leucocytes do not recirculate, but enter the lymph node paracortex to become interdigitating cells. Scand J Immunol 1988;27(1):97–105.

[61] Everson MP, McDuffie DS, Lemak DG, et al. Dendritic cells from different tissues induce production of different T cell cytokine profiles. J Leukoc Biol 1996;59(4):494–8.

[62] Morikawa Y, Tohya K, Ishida H, et al. Different migration patterns of antigen-presenting cells correlate with Th1/Th2-type responses in mice. Immunology 1995;85(4):575–81.

[63] Yamanaka R, Yajima N, Tsuchiya N, et al. Administration of interleukin-12 and -18 enhancing the antitumor immunity of genetically modified dendritic cells that had been pulsed with semliki forest virus-mediated tumor complementary DNA. J Neurosurg 2002; 97(5):1184–90.

[64] Insug O, Ku G, Ertl HC, et al. A dendritic cell vaccine induces protective immunity to intracranial growth of glioma. Anticancer Res 2002;22(2A):613–21.

[65] Nishioka Y, Hirao M, Robbins PD, et al. Induction of systemic and therapeutic antitumor immunity using intratumoral injection of dendritic cells genetically modified to express interleukin-12. Cancer Res 1999;59(16):4035–41.

[66] Yamanaka R, Zullo SA, Ramsey J, et al. Marked enhancement of antitumor immune responses in mouse brain tumor models by genetically modified dendritic cells producing semliki forest virus-mediated interleukin-12. J Neurosurg 2002;97(3):611–8.

[67] Yamanaka R, Abe T, Yajima N, et al. Vaccination of recurrent glioma patients with tumour lysate-pulsed dendritic cells elicits immune responses: results of a clinical phase I/II trial. Br J Cancer 2003;89(7):1172–9.

[68] Yu JS, Wheeler CJ, Zeltzer PM, et al. Vaccination of malignant glioma patients with peptide-pulsed dendritic cells elicits systemic cytotoxicity and intracranial T-cell infiltration. Cancer Res 2001;61(3):842–7.

[69] Miyatake S, Martuza RL, Rabkin SD. Defective herpes simplex virus vectors expressing thymidine kinase for the treatment of malignant glioma. Cancer Gene Ther 1997;4(4):222–8.

[70] Parker JN, Gillespie GY, Love CE, et al. Engineered herpes simplex virus expressing IL-12 in the treatment of experimental murine brain tumors. Proc Natl Acad Sci U S A 2000;97(5): 2208–13.

[71] Andreansky S, He B, van Cott J, et al. Treatment of intracranial gliomas in immunocompetent mice using herpes simplex viruses that express murine interleukins. Gene Ther 1998;5(1): 121–30.

[72] Yoshikawa K, Kajiwara K, Ideguchi M, et al. Immune gene therapy of experimental mouse brain tumor with adenovirus-mediated gene transfer of murine interleukin-4. Cancer Immunol Immunother 2000;49(1):23–33.

[73] Liu Y, Ehtesham M, Samoto K, et al. In situ adenoviral interleukin-12 gene transfer confers potent and long-lasting cytotoxic immunity in glioma. Cancer Gene Ther 2002;9(1):9–15.

[74] Yamini B, Yu X, Gillespie GY, et al. Transcriptional targeting of adenovirally delivered tumor necrosis factor alpha by temozolomide in experimental glioblastoma. Cancer Res 2004;64(18):6381–4.

[75] Allen C, Vongpunsawad S, Nakamura T, et al. Retargeted oncolytic measles strains entering via the EGFRvIII receptor maintain significant antitumor activity against gliomas with increased tumor specificity. Cancer Res 2006;66(24):11840–50.

[76] Eguchi J, Hatano M, Nishimura F, et al. Identification of interleukin-13 receptor alpha2 peptide analogues capable of inducing improved antiglioma CTL responses. Cancer Res 2006;66(11):5883–91.

[77] Okano F, Storkus WJ, Chambers WH, et al. Identification of a novel HLA-A*0201-restricted, cytotoxic T lymphocyte epitope in a human glioma-associated antigen, interleukin 13 receptor alpha2 chain. Clin Cancer Res 2002;8(9):2851–5.

[78] Bobo RH, Laske DW, Akbasak A, et al. Convection-enhanced delivery of macromolecules in the brain. Proc Natl Acad Sci U S A 1994;91(6):2076–80.

[79] Chiocca EA, Broaddus WC, Gillies GT, et al. Neurosurgical delivery of chemotherapeutics, targeted toxins, genetic and viral therapies in neuro-oncology. J Neurooncol 2004;69(1–3): 101–17.

[80] Hall WA, Rustamzadeh E, Asher AL. Convection-enhanced delivery in clinical trials. Neurosurg Focus 2003;14(2):1–4.

[81] Rainov NG, Heidecke V. Long term survival in a patient with recurrent malignant glioma treated with intratumoral infusion of an IL4-targeted toxin (NBI-3001). J Neurooncol 2004;66(1–2):197–201.

[82] Weber F, Asher A, Bucholz R, et al. Safety, tolerability, and tumor response of IL4-pseudo-monas exotoxin (NBI-3001) in patients with recurrent malignant glioma. J Neurooncol 2003; 64(1–2):125–37.

[83] Rand RW, Kreitman RJ, Patronas N, et al. Intratumoral administration of recombinant circularly permuted interleukin-4-pseudomonas exotoxin in patients with high-grade glioma. Clin Cancer Res 2000;6(6):2157–65.

[84] Kunwar S. Convection enhanced delivery of IL13-PE38QQR for treatment of recurrent malignant glioma: presentation of interim findings from ongoing phase 1 studies. Acta Neurochir Suppl 2003;88:105–11.

[85] Joshi BH, Plautz GE, Puri RK. Interleukin-13 receptor alpha chain: a novel tumor-associated transmembrane protein in primary explants of human malignant gliomas. Cancer Res 2000;60(5):1168–72.

[86] Sampson JH, Reardon DA, Friedman AH, et al. Sustained radiographic and clinical response in patient with bifrontal recurrent glioblastoma multiforme with intracerebral infusion of the recombinant targeted toxin TP-38: case study. Neuro Oncol 2005;7(1):90–6.

[87] Weber FW, Floeth F, Asher A, et al. Local convection enhanced delivery of IL4-pseudomonas exotoxin (NBI-3001) for treatment of patients with recurrent malignant glioma. Acta Neurochir Suppl 2003;88:93–103.

ELSEVIER
SAUNDERS

Surg Oncol Clin N Am
16 (2007) 1005–1013

SURGICAL
ONCOLOGY CLINICS
OF NORTH AMERICA

Index

Note: Page numbers of article titles are in **boldface** type.

United States Postal Service

Statement of Ownership, Management, and Circulation
(All Periodicals Publications Except Requester Publications)

1. Publication Title	2. Publication Number	3. Filing Date
Surgical Oncology Clinics of North America	0	1	2	-	5	6	5	5	9/14/07

4. Issue Frequency	5. Number of Issues Published Annually	6. Annual Subscription Price
Jan, Apr, Jul, Oct	4	$187.00

7. Complete Mailing Address of Known Office of Publication (Not printer) (Street, city, county, state, and ZIP+4)

Elsevier Inc.
360 Park Avenue South
New York, NY 10010-1710

Contact Person: Stephen Bushing
Telephone (Include area code): 215-239-3688

8. Complete Mailing Address of Headquarters or General Business Office of Publisher (Not printer)

Elsevier Inc., 360 Park Avenue South, New York, NY 10010-1710

9. Full Names and Complete Mailing Addresses of Publisher, Editor, and Managing Editor (Do not leave blank)

Publisher (Name and complete mailing address)

John Schrefer, Elsevier, Inc., 1600 John F. Kennedy Blvd. Suite 1800, Philadelphia, PA 19103-2899

Editor (Name and complete mailing address)

Catherine Bewick, Elsevier, Inc., 1600 John F. Kennedy Blvd. Suite 1800, Philadelphia, PA 19103-2899

Managing Editor (Name and complete mailing address)

Catherine Bewick, Elsevier, Inc., 1600 John F. Kennedy Blvd. Suite 1800, Philadelphia, PA 19103-2899

10. Owner (Do not leave blank. If the publication is owned by a corporation, give the name and address of the corporation immediately followed by the names and addresses of all stockholders owning or holding 1 percent or more of the total amount of stock. If not owned by a corporation, give the names and addresses of the individual owners. If owned by a partnership or other unincorporated firm, give its name and address as well as those of each individual owner. If the publication is published by a nonprofit organization, give its name and address.)

Full Name	Complete Mailing Address
Wholly owned subsidiary of	4520 East-West Highway
Reed/Elsevier, US holdings	Bethesda, MD 20814

11. Known Bondholders, Mortgagees, and Other Security Holders Owning or Holding 1 Percent or More of Total Amount of Bonds, Mortgages, or Other Securities. If none, check box. ☐ None

Full Name	Complete Mailing Address
N/A	

12. Tax Status (For completion by nonprofit organizations authorized to mail at nonprofit rates) (Check one)
The purpose, function, and nonprofit status of this organization and the exempt status for federal income tax purposes:
☐ Has Not Changed During Preceding 12 Months
☐ Has Changed During Preceding 12 Months (Publisher must submit explanation of change with this statement)

PS Form 3526, September 2006 (Page 1 of 3 (Instructions Page 3)) PSN 7530-01-000-9931 PRIVACY NOTICE: See our Privacy policy in www.usps.com

13. Publication Title	14. Issue Date for Circulation Data Below
Surgical Oncology Clinics of North America	July 2007

15. Extent and Nature of Circulation			Average No. Copies Each Issue During Preceding 12 Months	No. Copies of Single Issue Published Nearest to Filing Date
a. Total Number of Copies (Net press run)			1250	1200
b. Paid Circulation (By Mail and Outside the Mail)	(1)	Mailed Outside-County Paid Subscriptions Stated on PS Form 3541. (Include paid distribution above nominal rate, advertiser's proof copies, and exchange copies)	433	418
	(2)	Mailed In-County Paid Subscriptions Stated on PS Form 3541 (Include paid distribution above nominal rate, advertiser's proof copies, and exchange copies)		
	(3)	Paid Distribution Outside the Mails Including Sales Through Dealers and Carriers, Street Vendors, Counter Sales, and Other Paid Distribution Outside USPS®	190	186
	(4)	Paid Distribution by Other Classes Mailed Through the USPS (e.g. First-Class Mail®)		
c. Total Paid Distribution (Sum of 15b (1), (2), (3), and (4))		►	623	604
d. Free or Nominal Rate Distribution (By Mail and Outside the Mail)	(1)	Free or Nominal Rate Outside-County Copies Included on PS Form 3541	94	78
	(2)	Free or Nominal Rate In-County Copies Included on PS Form 3541		
	(3)	Free or Nominal Rate Copies Mailed at Other Classes Mailed Through the USPS (e.g. First-Class Mail)		
	(4)	Free or Nominal Rate Distribution Outside the Mail (Carriers or other means)		
e. Total Free or Nominal Rate Distribution (Sum of 15d (1), (2), (3) and (4))		►	94	78
f. Total Distribution (Sum of 15c and 15e)		►	717	682
g. Copies not Distributed (See instructions to publishers #4 (page #3))			533	518
h. Total (Sum of 15f and g)		►	1250	1200
i. Percent Paid (15c divided by 15f times 100)			86.89%	88.56%

16. Publication of Statement of Ownership

If the publication is a general publication, publication of this statement is required. Will be printed in the October 2007 issue of this publication. ☐ Publication not required.

17. Signature and Title of Editor, Publisher, Business Manager, or Owner

[signature]

John Bassett – Executive Director of Subscription Services

Date: September 14, 2007

I certify that all information furnished on this form is true and complete. I understand that anyone who furnishes false or misleading information on this form or who omits material or information requested on the form may be subject to criminal sanctions (including fines and imprisonment) and/or civil sanctions (including civil penalties).

PS Form 3526, September 2006 (Page 2 of 3)